Clinical Speech and Voice Measurement

Laboratory Exercises

Robert F. Orlikoff, Ph.D.
Memphis State University
Memphis, Tennessee

R. J. Baken, Ph.D.
Columbia University
New York, New York

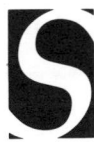

SINGULAR PUBLISHING GROUP, INC.
SAN DIEGO, CALIFORNIA

Singular Publishing Group, Inc.
401 West "A" Street, Suite 325
San Diego, California 92101-7904

19 Compton Terrace
London, N1 2UN, U.K.

e-mail: singpub@mail.cerfnet.com
Website: http://www.singpub.com

© 1993 by Singular Publishing Group, Inc.
Second Singular Printing May 1994
Third Singular Printing April 1998

All rights, including that of translation reserved. No part of this publication may be reproduced, stored in a retrieval system, or transmitted in any form or by any means, electronic, mechanical, recording, or otherwise, without the prior written permission of the publisher.

Typeset in 12/14 Palatino by CFW Graphics
Printed in the United States of America by McNaughton & Gunn

Library of Congress Cataloging-in-Publication Data

Orlikoff, Robert F.
    Clinical speech and voice measurement : laboratory exercises / Robert F. Orlikoff, R. J. Baken.
      p.   cm.
    Includes bibliographical references.
    ISBN 1-879105-91-8
    1. Speech disorders—Diagnosis—Problems, exercises, etc.
2. Speech disorders—Laboratory manuals.   3. Speech—Measurement—Problems, exercises, etc.   4. Voice—Measurement—Problems, exercises, etc. I. Baken, R. J. (Ronald J.), 1943–   . II. Title.
    [DNLM: 1. Speech Production Measurement—examination questions. WV 18 071c 1993]
RC428.O73 1993
616.85'5075—dc20
DNLM/DLC
for Library of Congress   94–14930
                                                                          CIP

Contents

Introduction   1

    UNIT 1   A Word or Two to Our Student Readers   3

    UNIT 2   A Few Technicalities   7

Background Skills and Information   17

    UNIT 3   Basic Skills: Physical Examination   19

    UNIT 4   Tutorial: Descriptive Statistics   39

    UNIT 5   Tutorial: Relative Measures and Logarithmic Scaling   51

    UNIT 6   Tutorial: Plotting Data   61

    UNIT 7   Tutorial: Semitones   71

    UNIT 8   Tutorial: Decibels   79

    UNIT 9   Basic Skills: The Oscilloscope   87

    UNIT 10   Basic Skills: Reading Oscillograms   103

    UNIT 11   Basic Skills: Calibration   119

Vocal Fundamental Frequency   127

    UNIT 12   Clinical Application: Vocal Fundamental Frequency   129

    UNIT 13   Clinical Application: Fundamental Frequency Perturbation (Vocal Jitter)   147

Vocal Intensity   163

    UNIT 14   Clinical Application: The Sound Level Meter, Vocal Intensity, and the Voice Range Profile   165

Vocal Intensity (continued)

| UNIT 15 | Clinical Application: Vocal Rise Time | **187** |
| UNIT 16 | Clinical Application: Amplitude Perturbation (Vocal Shimmer) | **197** |

Air Pressures for Speech and Voice — **211**

| UNIT 17 | Clinical Application: Intraoral Pressure During Consonant Production | **213** |
| UNIT 18 | Clinical Application: Estimating Subglottic Pressure | **227** |

Airflows for Speech and Voice — **239**

UNIT 19	Clinical Application: Mean Phonatory Airflow Using a Pneumotachograph	**241**
UNIT 20	Clinical Application: Airflow During Speech Production	**255**
UNIT 21	Clinical Application: Estimating Glottal Resistance	**267**
UNIT 22	Clinical Application: Determining Lung Volume Change and Mean Phonatory Airflow from Spirometric Records	**287**
UNIT 23	Clinical Application: Estimating Mean Speech Airflow from Spirometric Records	**299**

Nasalization — **313**

| UNIT 24 | Clinical Application: Nasalance | **315** |
| UNIT 25 | Clinical Application: Nasalization | **331** |

Electroglottography — **347**

| UNIT 26 | Basic Skills: Electroglottography | **349** |

Sound Spectrography 365

UNIT 27	Basic Skills: Sound Spectrography I — Getting Acquainted	367
UNIT 28	Basic Skills: Sound Spectrography II — Identifying "Source" and "Filter" Contributions to the Speech Signal	381
UNIT 29	Clinical Application: Spectrography — Vowel Formants	395
UNIT 30	Clinical Application: Spectrography — Sonorants	413
UNIT 31	Clinical Application: Spectrography — Fricatives	425
UNIT 32	Clinical Application: Spectrography — Plosives and Affricates	437

Appendixes 455

APPENDIX A	Sample Vocal Tract Examination Form	457
APPENDIX B	The Angle Classification System of Malocclusions	461
APPENDIX C	Common Logarithm Table	465
APPENDIX D	Standard Reading Passage: The Rainbow	469
APPENDIX E	Mathematical Definitions of Vocal Jitter Measures	471
APPENDIX F	Mathematical Definitions of Vocal Shimmer Measures	473
APPENDIX G	Predicted Normal Forced Vital Capacity (FVC)	475
APPENDIX H	Low-Flow Reading Passage: Marvin Williams	477
APPENDIX I	High-Flow Reading Passage: Harrison Cook	479

To our spice:

JENNIFER EIKENBERRY ORLIKOFF

and

JOAN WALD BAKEN

To my seasoning:

RUSSELL, EMILY, and ERIKA ORLIKOFF

And to:

JOSEPH PUJOL (1857–1945),

who, perhaps more than anyone, understood the relationship between physiology and acoustics.

INTRODUCTION

UNIT 1

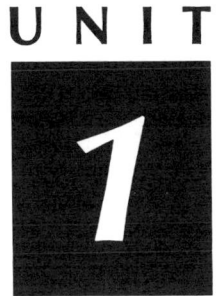

A Word or Two to Our Student Readers

By now, we suspect, you've leafed through this book to get some idea of what's in store for you.[1]

Our guess is that you're a student in a program in speech-language pathology. We also suspect that you've bought this book because it is required for some course.[2] And, having looked through this book, we hope that your reaction is "Wow! What a great course *this* is going to be! I'm really going to need this stuff when I get out there in the field."

But, we are realists, so we assume that there might be one or two of you who are muttering, "What's all this about? Another batch of useless academic rigmarole to plod through before I can get to the real clinical stuff!" If you're one of these, we'd like to have a word with you. The others are also encouraged to read on. But it is to those of you who are muttering that we really want to speak. We want to explain why all the stuff in this book is important for clinical practice.

Let's remind ourselves of something very elementary but generally ignored. And that is, *speech and voice are not tangible "things."* That is, they have no independent existence. They are, rather, a *product*, the result of physiologic processes. To say that a voice is "rough" or that consonants are "distorted" is to describe a symptom, not a disorder. The problem itself lies somewhere deeper — in an aberrant function of

---

[1] If, because of some strange lack of curiosity, you have NOT looked this book over, we urge you to do so now. Who knows what you might find?

[2] Okay, so it doesn't take a Perry Mason to figure that out. Even we, as enthusiastic about this stuff as we are, recognize that this book is not the sort of thing you're likely to curl up with in the hammock on a lazy summer afternoon.

the vocal tract or the nervous system that controls it. The purpose of therapy is to improve speech or voice. That means that — to put it as simply as possible — the therapist's goal is to eliminate the patient's symptoms. And that's fine as a broad objective. But the only way to achieve that goal is to change function. So therapy depends on knowing — as precisely as possible — how the system is functioning. Getting that information is what assessment is all about.

Now you might think you could pinpoint abnormal function by listening carefully to the patient's speech or by watching the patient's oral movements. And in some cases you can. But, in an awful lot of cases, you can't. You don't have to know very much about speech or voice to realize that most of the relevant action takes place well hidden in the recesses of the vocal tract. And a lot of the visible events happen far too fast to be accurately assessed by an observer's eyes.

You ears are not nearly as reliable as you might think, either. Perception is a very complicated affair and is influenced by all sorts of variables that may well be irrelevant to the specific function that needs to be assessed. Furthermore, a single perceptual characteristic can frequently be produced by totally different processes or vocal tract adjustments — and how can you know which one of the several possibilities is responsible in a given case? And, finally, the human auditory system is configured to make sense out of the totality of the speech signal. That contributes a great deal to our efficiency at decoding messages, but it also deprives us of a conscious awareness of the components of the speech signal. Unfortunately, it is those components — that the ear receives but we don't hear — that usually contain the important clues about what is going on. Auditory perception may tell us that there is something "funny" about the message we are receiving, and that's important because it tells us that there's a problem. But, all too often, auditory impressions leave us with no way of being certain about why the message is distorted. That's too bad, because it's the "why" that therapy needs to address. So, in addition to a subjective analysis of how a patient sounds, we need to outline as specifically as possible those physical elements that cause and perpetuate the speech symptoms that *are* the speech pathology. As indicated in the figure below, information may be assembled from an examination of the speech structure (anatomy), speech physiology (structural movement and the aerodynamic consequences of that movement) and the speech signal itself.

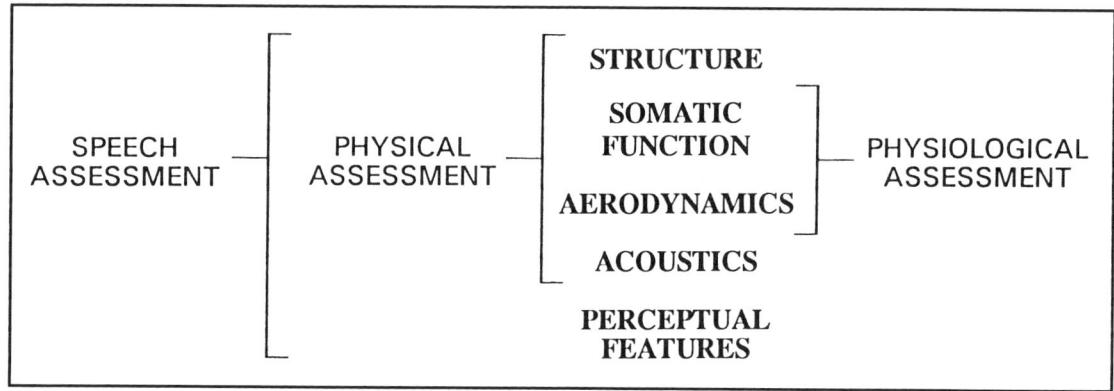

So, in spite of how it might look to the uninitiated,[3] this is not a laboratory manual for a course in the theories of speech and voice production.[4] It is a means of helping you develop hands-on clinical skills — manual *and* cerebral. This book is about ways of finding out what a patient's speech is actually like, rather than what it sounds like. And it's about determining why speech is the way it is. This book is about techniques of speech and voice measurement. Valid and appropriate measurement is central to accurate diagnosis, and accurate diagnosis is at the heart of competent therapy. *You can hardly find more clinical stuff than that.*

There are a few things you should understand about this book and about the coursework that you will be doing with it. The first is that neither we nor your instructor intend to teach you every possible "test" or technique for evaluating speech or voice. If you even thought that we might try to do this, you seriously misperceive what "testing" is all about. It is true that hundreds of specific tests and procedures have been devised and are documented in our professional literature. Many of these have proven to be useful in clinical practice, and it is important that you know about and understand them. A fair selection of these tools is included in the work you are probably going to do in your course. More critical to your ultimate clinical needs, however, will be the ability to observe and document speech characteristics or speech system behaviors in ways that are valid and reliable. This book and the course in which you will use it are intended to help you learn the principles for doing this kind of observation and documentation. The focus is not going to be so much on specific "tests," but on general methods that are applicable to a wide variety of circumstances.

But that omits the most critical aspect of the task of evaluating speech. The tests, measurements, examination, and analyses that you will perform — now as a student and later as a practitioner — will never give you answers to clinical problems. They will provide you only with data — that is, *information* — describing speech or its origins. YOU, a trained speech-language pathologist, will develop the answers on the basis of the data you obtain. Doing so will demand that you really *understand* speech production. The clinical conclusions you arrive at will be no better than the knowledge that informs them. (*That's* why you had to do all that coursework in phonetics, anatomy/physiology, perception, and the like!) But it is equally true that your conclusions can't be more valid that the data upon which they are based.

So, rather than teaching you the methods of specific tests, we have established two different goals for you. One objective is for you to understand how testing of various aspects of speech production needs to be conducted in order to get useful results. It would be impossible for you to master all the different instrumental

---

[3] We're talking mainly to the unenlightened, remember?

[4] Don't get us wrong! We think courses in theories of speech production are a good thing. Not only because we earn our living teaching them, but also because it seems self-evident to us that you can't fix something that's broken unless you know how it's supposed to work. Which, by the way, is a not-very-subtle way of warning you that the experiences we have planned for you will make you exercise your knowledge of speech science a lot!

methods available to us (we presume that you would actually like to *finish* your degree program some day!), so we have selected procedures that are likely to be most commonly used or that promise to be the most broadly educational.

Our other aim is for you to think about and ultimately understand the nature of the data that result from the various observational methods. To do this you will have to know where the data come from and how they need to be manipulated. Therefore, we minimize the use of computers in the exercises you will do. We are going to ask you to get information the "old fashioned" way — *by hand* — whenever it is possible. You'll sometimes find this tedious, but it has its virtues.[5] The most important is that with luck, some work, and a bit of thinking, you will end up really understanding what you are doing and what the data represent when you later use more automated, computerized, convenient equipment in the "real" clinical world. Don't underestimate the importance of that understanding. We have seen some very foolish things done, invalid interpretations made, and silly conclusions reached because a professional did not understand the nature of the information at issue.

What we and your instructor have in mind is to help make you competent speech-language pathologists, *clinical* speech-language pathologists, of the 21st century.

We even hope you have some fun!

---

[5] One is that you may come to have greater admiration and respect for the many great researchers who laid the foundations of much of our current understanding of speech and voice using data derived in just this way!

UNIT 2

A Few Technicalities

You're going to be looking at speech and voice in this course. You're going to use *instruments* to observe that which often can't be seen or heard, to measure and to quantify at a more fundamental level than you're likely to have worked at before. You're going to learn to use instrumentation — some of it quite sophisticated — to expand your clinical horizons. And this book, we hope, will help you to do it.

Now, you may find the whole idea of electronic instrumentation to be a little intimidating. That's both unwarranted and completely justified. After all, you've been using electronic devices for a long time — stereo systems, VCRs, microwave ovens, computers, and so on. Almost none of the instrumentation you will use in this course is more complicated than those, and most of it is much simpler. The problem, of course, is that most of the devices you've used are specially designed to work in a certain way. By and large they're built so that you can't screw things up too badly. Then, too, most of the "instruments" that you've used represented ends in themselves. But the instruments you'll use professionally are intended only to give you (or your patient) information on which to base conclusions. Finally, unless you have a very strange and kinky life-style, this is probably the first time you'll be using electronic instrumentation *on someone.* All of these differences make it seem prudent to take a few minutes to clarify some things before you get started.

BASIC ANATOMY OF AN INSTRUMENT

Let's begin by considering exactly what we mean by an *instrument.* Obviously it is a device or system used to visualize the details of some phenomenon or process in an objective and perhaps even quantifiable way. Usually (but not always) an instrument is "electronic," which is to say that its function depends on electrical circuits. No matter how complex, almost any instrument is built around three kinds of functional units.

The Input Stage

First, there must be some way for the instrumentation to make contact with the real world and, more particularly, for it to "hook into" whatever the instrument is supposed to observe or measure — an acoustic signal, air pressure, nasal airflow, and so on. This part of the instrument is known as the *input stage*. Connecting to the events or phenomena to be observed or measured is, like most things, easier said than done. There are two problems. The first is that the speech process that we want to watch often goes on in a very out-of-the-way place, or else it occurs amidst a pack of other events that we're not interested in. So the input system has to be designed to go where the action is and to remain unperturbed (and unaffected) by the irrelevant goings-on in its neighborhood. Sometimes the problem is easily solved. Simply putting a microphone near the mouth gives it the needed "front-row seat" for following the action of the speech signal, and choosing the right kind of microphone (a "unidirectional" one, of course!) and pointing it at the patient minimizes its response to the music class practicing tuba solos next door. But all too often, the difficulties are not so simply overcome. How, for instance, do you sample the pressure in the mouth without having your input system batted around by a tongue that is busy articulating? (There's an exercise further along that will show you one way of doing it.)

Restraining the tongue would prevent interference with the pressure-measuring system. But that would interfere with lingual articulation and, if you're going to do *that*, what's the point of doing speech measurement? After all, the objective is to find out what's happening during *speech*, right? So another thing that instrument input systems have to do is to stay out of the way. Their presence should not alter the speaker's usual pattern of speech production. That's a very lofty goal, and it's almost never actually met. Fortunately, with a little care and foresight we can usually come close enough to meeting it for routine clinical purposes. You can see, though, that in selecting an instrument, some serious thought needs to be given to the characteristics of its input section.

All of the care taken in getting the input system to where the action is and in ensuring that it remains simply an onlooker of — and not a player in — that action is only a way of optimizing the *real* task of the input stage: energy conversion.[1]

Except in the very simplest of apparatus, the form of energy of the input is unsuitable for processing by the rest of the system. Candles produce light, but the brain

---

[1] Following this line of reasoning, it is misleading to refer to the kind of instruments we will be discussing as "machines." Like a ruler, scale, or magnifying glass, clinical equipment is designed as an observation or measurement *tool*. For obvious reasons, the first and foremost rule of instrumentation is that a measurement tool must not alter the event being measured. The term "machine," however, implies that our equipment performs some sort of work — that, in fact, it creates, destroys, or changes something. You, the speech pathologist, are truly the only clinical "machine." (For a more detailed discussion, see *Principles of Applied Biomechanical Instrumentation*, 2nd ed., by L. A. Geddes and L. E. Baker, 1975. New York: John Wiley and Sons.)

processes electrical signals. Unless light energy can be converted to electrical energy, vision is impossible. Speech actions produce pressure changes (sound waves) in the atmosphere. But no matter how loudly you shout at a listener's skull the pressure waves can't be heard unless they've been converted into the appropriate electrical code. Any device that converts one form of energy to another is called a *transducer*. A microphone converts sound pressure to an electrical voltage. It is therefore a transducer. Eyes and ears convert light and acoustic energy into electrical pulses. They are transducers, too.

A transducer forms the real "business end" of almost any input system. Its job is to change the energy produced by or representing the process being measured into an electrical signal that is suitable for further processing by the instrument. How a transducer accomplishes this conversion depends in large measure on the kind of energy it is expected to convert. But, just as there are many ways to skin any given cat, so there are generally several ways to convert any given form of energy into an electrical signal. Therefore, there is almost always an assortment of different transducers available for a given job. Each kind has its virtues and its defects; each is best suited to a given set of circumstances. No measurement can be better than the transducer that provides the instrument with the information on which its analysis is based. The obvious moral is that transducer options need to be clearly understood, that the selection needs to be well informed, and that any transducer limitations or peculiarities be appropriately considered when interpreting results.

The Signal Conditioning Stage

The transducer only provides raw material for later processing. In general, that raw material is not quite good enough to provide the information that we are looking for. That is, it usually requires some degree of refinement. Any transducer, for example, is likely to produce a *very* small electrical signal that is too weak to be effectively worked on. It will need to be made stronger (that is, *amplified*). Many transducers will pick up a certain amount of noise along with the useful information to be converted. This unwanted material may have to be removed by *filtering*. In short, the second stage of the instrument is designed to improve the transducer's signal to make it suitable for the purposes at hand. This is called *signal conditioning*. Commonly, signal conditioning techniques include not only amplification and filtering, but also conversion of the transducer signal to a series of numbers (*analog-to-digital conversion*), averaging (*integration*), removal of signal peaks (*clipping*), and the like.

Sometimes quite simple signal conditioning is all that is needed to provide us with the information we require. But often more elaborate processing is called for. We might, for example, want to know which frequencies are present in a speech signal. (That is, we might want to derive the signal's *spectrum*.) Or we might be interested in knowing the *rate* at which the vocal folds are vibrating. (In other words, we want to know the *fundamental frequency* of the voice.) These and many other questions we might have clearly will require further — often quite complex — analysis. The second stage of the instrument, the signal conditioning section — irrespective of the simplicity or complexity of the processing involved — is really the very "heart" of the instrument.

The Output Stage

After signal conditioning and analysis we have the information that we want, but it exists in the form of electrons whizzing around electrical circuits, which does us no good whatever. Clearly, what we now need is another conversion, this time from electrical energy to some format that we can perceive. This is the job of the *output stage* of the instrument. It, too, consists of a transducer, which is intended to convert the information into a form that we find useful and, hopefully, convenient. One kind of output stage that we're all familiar with is the picture tube of a television set. The signal conditioning portions of a TV do, quite successfully, manage to extract an image from the electrical energy radiated by the local broadcaster. That image is purely electrical in form, which might be fine if you're a robot or a computer, but is not so good if you're endowed with the usual mammalian brain. The picture tube — the TV's output stage — converts that electrical image to patterns of light energy that we can (depending on the nature of the program being broadcast!) make sense of.

The output stage of an instrument might resemble a TV picture tube (a computer's output stage certainly does, an oscilloscope is little more than a TV set with a different signal processing stage). But the output might also take other forms. Pen writers, which produce traces on paper, are a popular output stage. Printers, which write numbers and letters on paper, are common as well. But flashing lights, moving pointers, buzzers, and loudspeakers are all to be found.

In summary, then, an instrumentation system has the following basic functional units:

Input Transduction	*Signal Conditioning*	*Output Transduction*
Sensing devices such as: microphones, strain gauges, pressure and flow transducers, force transducers.	Manipulation of the input signal for modification such as: amplification, filtering, computer digitization, data calculation.	Conversion of the conditioned signal and display on an output device such as: computer screen, pen recorder, voltmeter, printer, loudspeaker.

Block Diagrams

It is often important to describe the instrumentation system that was used to obtain the particular data on which clinical decisions have been based. This can be done in words, but it is usually more convenient to do a simple drawing that provides the necessary information. Called *block diagrams,* these sketches use simple geometric shapes connected by lines to represent the major elements of the instrumentation and their interconnections. Labeling adds any essential details. For instance, a block diagram of a simple public address system might look like this:

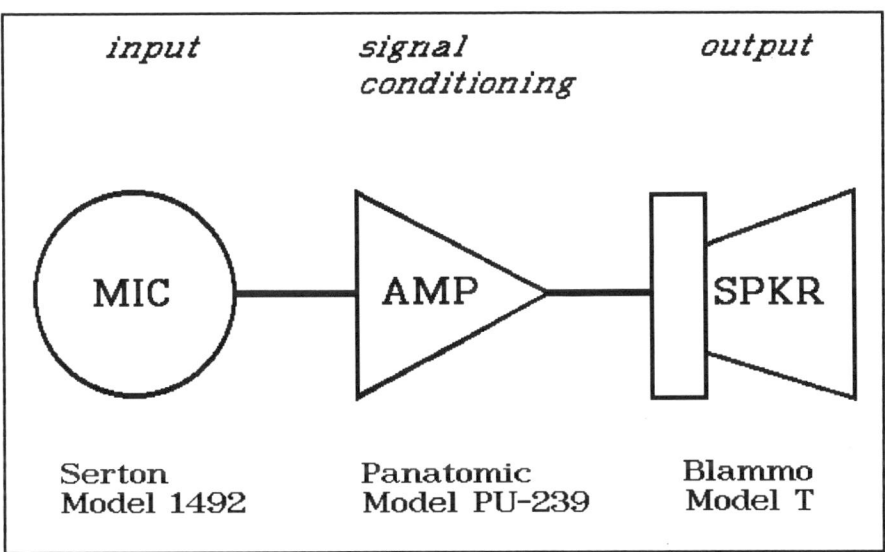

(The "input," "signal conditioning," and "output" labels have been added for your guidance. They do not usually appear on a block diagram.) Note that there are some conventional symbols; the ones for amplifier and speaker are used here. Details that might prove useful to the reader (such as the model number of the amplifier) are typed into the diagram. Note that the diagram does not resemble a picture of a public address system in any way, but it conveys all the critical information about setting one up. Of course, block diagrams can be more complex. The figure at the top of the following page shows one for a standard audio tape recorder.

This block diagram says:

> The input transducer for this system is a microphone whose signal is amplified and then filtered before being stored on tape by the "record head" during the recording process. For playback the signal is retrieved from the tape by a "playback head." The signal is then amplified, filtered, and transduced into acoustic energy by a loudspeaker.

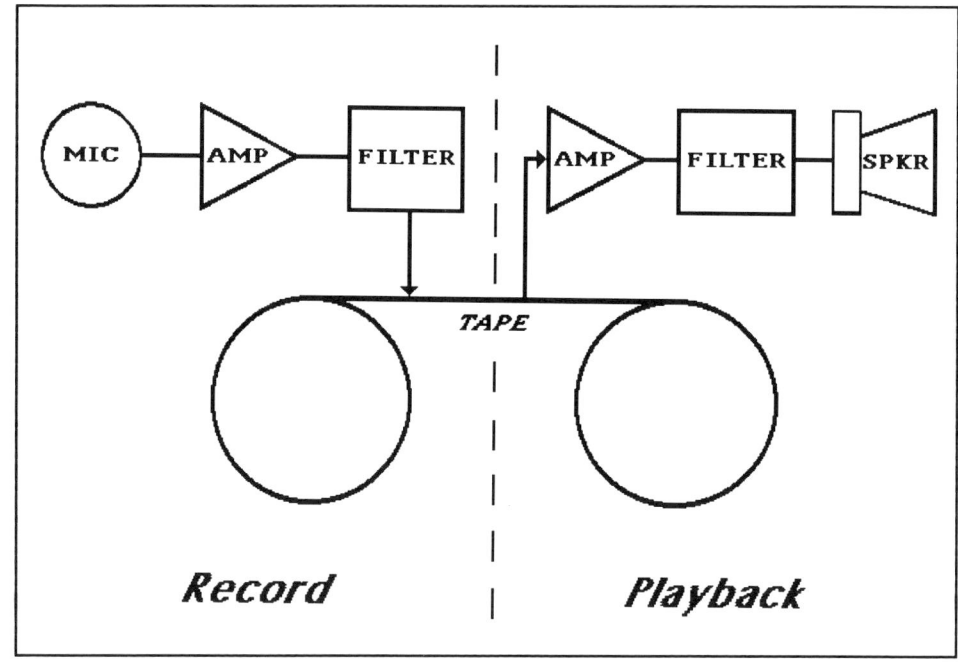

Finally, here is the block diagram for an instrumentation array that records physiologic data for determination of velopharyngeal orifice area.[2] See how well you can read it!

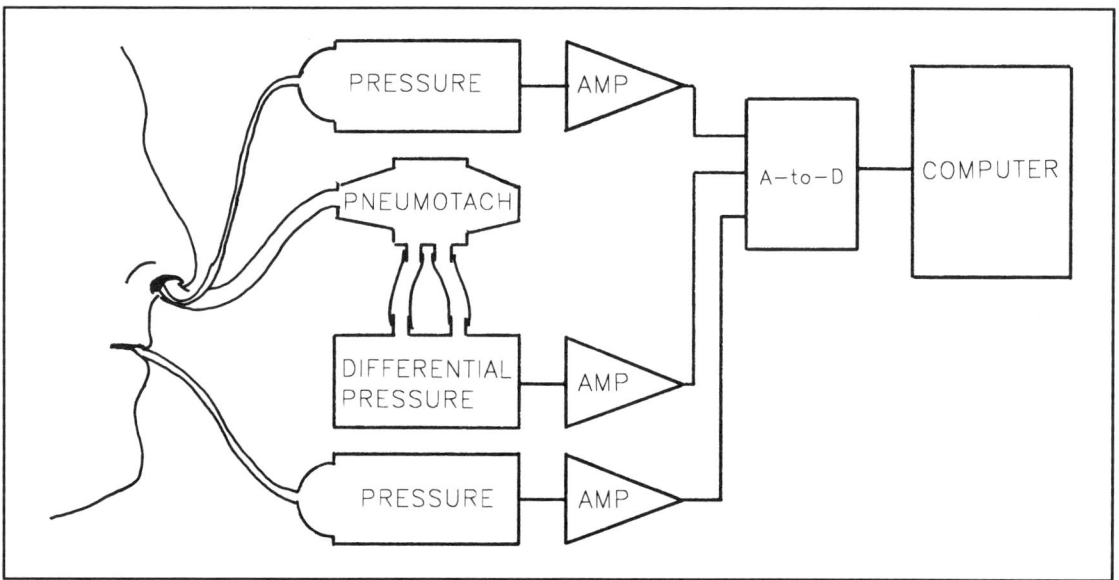

Based on Warren, D. W., Dalston, R. M., et al. (1989). The speech regulating system: Temporal and aerodynamic responses to velopharyngeal inadequacy. *Journal of Speech and Hearing Research, 32,* 566–575.

---

[2] According to the method described in "A Pressure-Flow Technique for Measuring Velopharyngeal Orifice Area During Continuous Speech," by D. W. Warren and A. B. DuBois, 1964, *Cleft Palate Journal, 1,* 52–71.

SAFETY

The fact that our instrumentation is used on people raises certain concerns and imposes certain obligations on us. Specifically, and preeminently, those concerns and obligations center on the moral and legal requirement that we not expose our patients to avoidable risk. The dangers that instrumentation poses are of two kinds: electrical and infectious.

Electrical Safety

The electricity that you use comes to you via a transmission system beginning at a generating plant and ending at the outlet into which you plug your instruments. The system is obviously complex, but one simple set of facts dominates all of our safety concerns.

Electric current always needs to travel a round trip to and from the place of production. If it is produced by a battery, there must be a wire routing the electrical current to the instrument being powered, and another wire that brings the "used" electricity back to the battery. A big electrical generator — like the one used by a local utility company — also has an "outgoing" electrical cable and a "return" electrical cable. Only there is a catch: the utility company uses the earth itself as the return cable! One of the two active contacts in every outlet is (at least indirectly) connected to the generator; it is called the "hot" side of the power line. The other contact is (again, indirectly) connected to "mother earth." This one is called the "cold" side of the power line. The voltage (that is, the *electrical pressure*) at the hot connector is high (about 115 V in the United States), while the voltage at the cold connector is (at least in theory), zero volts, which is the voltage of the earth itself. We get usable power out of this system by allowing the voltage (electrical pressure) to drop as the current (electrical flow) goes from the hot to the cold side. Anything which is (relatively directly) connected to the earth is said to be "grounded."

It's not only the electrical generator that is connected to *terra firma*: we often are, also. That is, we are often touching some electrical conductor that is grounded. Water pipes and faucets are good examples. So are the cover plates of electrical outlets.

All of this would be of little more than academic interest were it not that an electrical current tends to travel via the easiest possible path (technically, the path with the least resistance) from the hot side of the line to ground. The pathway through a circuit is a relatively unattractive path for the current, but it will follow this path if there is nothing easier available. But human tissue presents a relatively easy path for electrical current to follow. If, therefore, part of a person is in contact with the hot side of the power supply and, at the same time, another part of a person is grounded, the electricity will tend to flow from one part of the person to the other as it takes the easiest path to ground. At best, this flow is likely to be unpleasant. At worst, it can be fatal.

This still seems rather irrelevant until one realizes that things can go wrong in circuits. And Murphy's law states that if something can go wrong, it will. Imagine a not-unlikely scenario. The amplifier that you routinely use for picking up the speech signal is old and well used. Unknown to you, one of the power supply wires in it has cracked, and its bare end is resting on the inside of the amplifier's metal case. The result of this, given how the amplifier is wired, is that the metal case on the microphone that your patient is holding is now connected to a power supply wire. You have your patient hold the microphone and, ready to get a good audio recording, you turn on the amplifier. What happens? If you're lucky, your patient feels a mild tingle and you get an "interesting," unintended speech sample. But, if you're not so fortunate, your patient may be leaning on a radiator cover that is grounded, and a large jolt of the electric company's product goes surging through your soon-to-be former patient.

How do you protect yourself and your patient against this set of possibilities? The best way is to make sure that all of your equipment is grounded. That is, the case and any exposed conductive parts of your instruments should be more-or-less directly connected to earth. That precaution ensures that the easiest path to ground for the current is not through your patient, but rather through the ground connection that is attached to the instrument itself. How do you arrange this? By making certain that the outlet you use has a grounding connection — which is the third (round) contact on the outlet. Your instruments will have three-prong plugs. The one that connects to the grounding contact of the outlet handles grounding of the instrument's exposed conductors.

So, before you use any electrical instruments:

1. Be sure that the electrical outlets you use have a valid ground contact.
2. Never defeat the grounding function by using an adapter to plug a three-prong plug into a two-prong outlet.
3. Never use any equipment that has broken or frayed wires *anywhere*.
4. And, just to be on the safe side, never allow your patient to be in contact with anything other than your equipment that is grounded.

Infection Control

One would have to have been in a coma for the last several years to be unaware of the variety of serious infections prevalent around us: hepatitis, herpes, tuberculosis, AIDS, and many others. And few locations in the human body are as bacteriologically dirty as the mouth, the object of so much of our attention. Our obligation to protect our own health and that of our patients means that we need to take infection control measures very seriously. This is not to say that we need to maintain the aseptic conditions of a surgical operating room, but there are reasonable precautions that we can take and sensible procedures that we can institute to minimize the risk of spreading infection.

It is impossible to overstate the benefits of washing one's hands. Soap and water will not kill germs, but do wash them away, removing them from the skin before they can penetrate to cause an infection and before they can be passed on to someone else. *Handwashing is mandatory immediately before and immediately after any examination.* Your hands should go directly from the wash basin to your patient — stopping only at a clean towel in between. And hands should go from the patient to the wash basin along a similarly direct route. Anything going into a mouth should be handled only with freshly washed hands. Hands should be washed immediately after handling anything that has been in any part of a vocal tract.

Anything that has been in a mouth, nose, ear, or pharynx should be considered contaminated. Anything that the object has touched is similarly unclean. Avoid putting contaminated objects directly on countertops. Such objects should go into collection bins reserved for dirty items (and for dirty items alone). Tongue depressors are cheap — throw them away after one use. (If there is any possibility of children being around, break the tongue depressor against the inside of the trash container, making it less attractive to a child who is looking for something to play with.)

Surgical gloves protect your hands in infectious environments. Gloves are changed after every patient, thereby preventing spread of infection from one patient to another. Gloved hands touch nothing except the patient and the instruments used in the examination.

Finally, everything that might be contaminated must be washed and then (because soap does not kill germs) sterilized with a suitable disinfectant. It is wise to wash down countertops and other surfaces with a disinfectant as well.

Safety becomes a habit after a while. Start practicing now!

BACKGROUND SKILLS AND INFORMATION

UNIT 3

Basic Skills: Physical Examination

A physical examination is used by the speech pathologist to assess those structures and functions that are involved with and subserve speech aerodynamics and neuromotor control. The ability to discriminate between normal variability and abnormal status comes only with practice and experience allied to a logical and knowledge-based approach.

Purpose: In these exercises you will

- Learn to position your patient and ensure adequate illumination for a physical examination.
- Become familiar with the techiniques of clinical palpation of structures and with the correct use of several examination instruments.

Observational data may be recorded on the hand-in sheet or in a more comprehensive manner, using either a familiar vocal tract examination form or the one provided in Appendix A.

Recommended/suggested equipment and supplies: You will need an examination chair, diffused and color-balanced light source, head mirror, incandescent lamp, wooden tongue depressors, gauze, nasopharyngeal mirror, laryngeal mirror, alcohol lamp, otoscope, neurological (tendon) hammer, nasal speculum, and disposable gloves/finger cots.

General preparation: An examination chair allowing you to flexibly position and support the patient will facilitate the examination, as will a chair that can be elevated to bring the subject's face closer to your eye level.

1. Comfortably position your patient in the examination chair so that his head, arms, and legs are well supported and seated so that you have easy physical access to his face and mouth.
2. Position your light source to illuminate the patient's lower face and neck. Be sure to avoid shining the light directly into the patient's eyes.

> **CLINICAL NOTE:** For your patient's safety, do not undertake this exercise if you have fingernails that extend more than one-half cm (about 1/4") beyond your fingertips.

I. PALPATION

1. Instruct your patient to alternately clench and unclench his teeth while you place your hands on both sides of his head. Using the fleshy parts of your fingers and fingertips, palpate the parietal and frontal areas down to the level of the zygomatic arches ("cheek bones"). Determine the extent (origin) of the right and left temporalis muscles. Placing your fingers and palms against the patient's cheeks, determine the mass and symmetry of the right and left masseter muscles. Record your observations on the hand-in sheet.

2. Instruct your patient to swallow. (You may wish to supply a sip of water or a small morsel of food.) Again, placing your hands on the patient's cheeks, feel for masseter contraction. How did this differ from what was felt during clenching? Explain.

3. Instruct your patient to alternately depress and elevate his mandible. Placing a fingertip slightly below and in front of the external auditory meatus (see figure on facing page), feel for the action of the temporomandibular joint (TMJ). With an open jaw, have your patient alternately lateralize the mandible. Be sure to examine and compare the right and left TMJs. Describe what you feel. While continuing palpation, have the patient open and close his jaw repetitively.

4. Instruct your patient to turn his head to one side. Oppose this action by placing your open palm on the side of your patient's jaw (see figure on facing page). With the thumb and forefinger of your opposite hand, palpate (using a gentle pinch) the sternocleidomastoid muscle from the mastoid process to the sternum. (You may also use the fleshy parts of your fingers as shown.) Repeat to examine the opposite sternocleidomastoid muscle and compare what you feel.

5. Using your fingers and fingertips, gently palpate your patient's neck to locate the following structures and landmarks: (a) hyoid bone, (b) thyroid prominence and notch, (c) thyroid laminae, (d) cricothyroid space, (e) cricoid arch, (f) tracheal rings, and (g) sternal notch.

6. Placing your thumb or forefinger gently on the thyroid prominence, describe what you feel as your patient swallows.

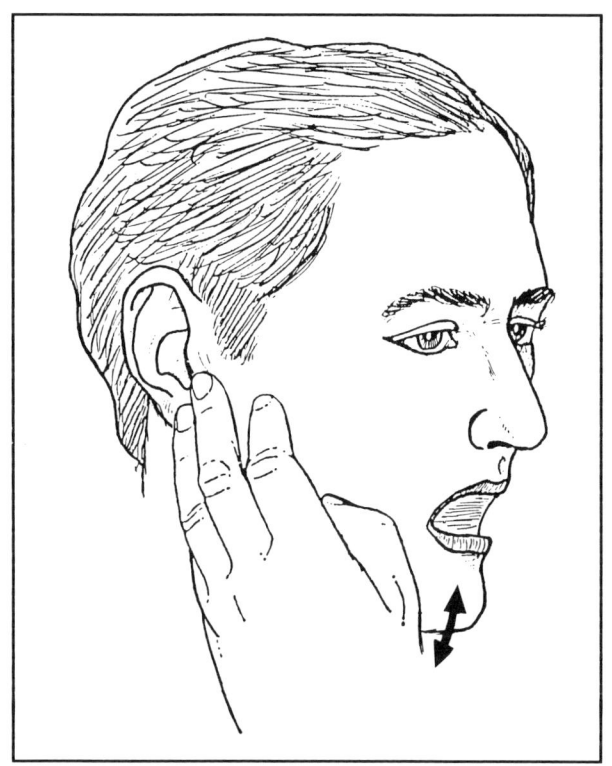

Palpation of the right temporomandibular joint.

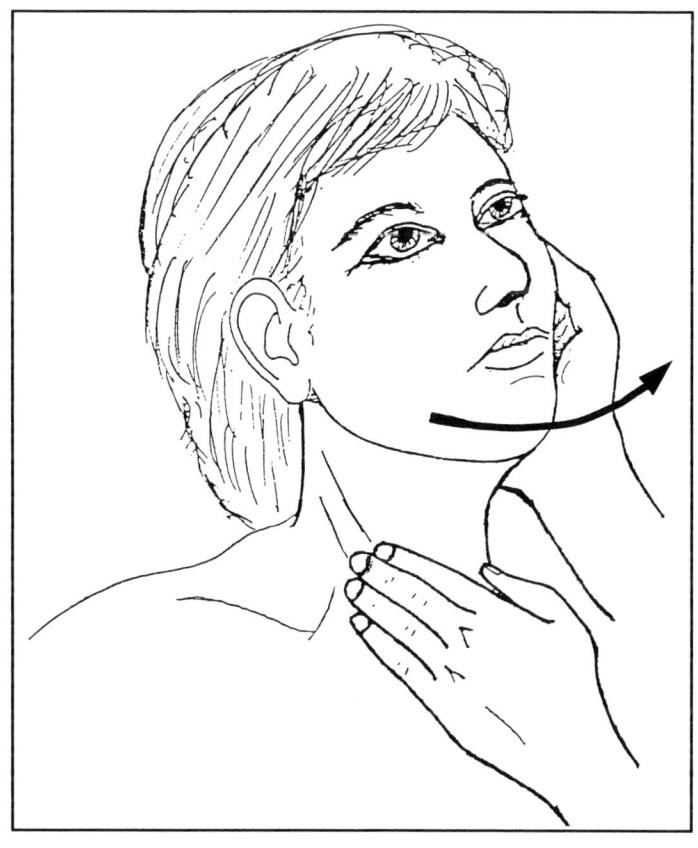

Palpation of the right sternocleidomastoideus.

7. Wearing a disposable glove or fingercot, slowly palpate your patient's hard palate, in particular the rugae and alveolar ridge. Describe the central/medial region of the palate in terms of its "vaulting" and smoothness. Determine if there are any palpable depressions or protrusions of the palate.

II. OBSERVATION OF STRUCTURE

1. Place an unobstructed incandescent light source slightly behind your patient, not far from her head.

2. Adjust the headband of your head mirror to fit snugly but comfortably. Position your head mirror over your preferred eye so you can see easily through the central hole. (The mirror should be positioned relatively close to your eye.)

3. Sitting or standing directly in front of your patient, observe her face, head, neck, and oral cavity. Avoid adjusting your position to aid illumination; the light directed on your patient should *follow* your gaze/head movements.

> **WARNING:** Basic considerations of infection control dictate that you never place a tongue depressor or other examination instrument on a table top or other surface. Disposable instruments are thrown away after use. When finished using nondisposable instruments, they are immediately placed in a sterilizing solution (see Unit 2, "A Few Technicalities").

4. Obtain a clean tongue depressor and hold it firmly with your thumb and forefinger in a clenched fist. Standing to one side of the patient, instruct her to open her mouth. Insert the end of the depressor in the corner of her mouth and, orienting the blade vertically, forcefully push the lips back in the direction of her ear. Have the patient close her jaws in a bite and, using the orientation of the upper and lower first molars as a guide, assess your patient's occlusion (see figure on opposite page). According to Angle's classification system (Appendix B), what class of occlusion (or malocclusion) does your patient have?

5. With a firm grip on the tongue depressor, press down on the posterior part of the tongue. Using the head mirror, illuminate and view the following structures: (a) posterior pharyngeal wall, (b) palatine tonsils, (c) palatoglossal arch (anterior faucial pillars), and (d) palatopharyngeal arch (posterior faucial pillars). When the tongue obstructs your view, carefully but forcefully push it downward and/or laterally with the depressor. Record your observations on the hand-in sheet.

6. Warm an angled nasopharyngeal mirror over an alcohol lamp to prevent fogging when inserted into your patient's mouth. Check the temperature of the mirror by pressing its unmirrored surface against the back of your hand.

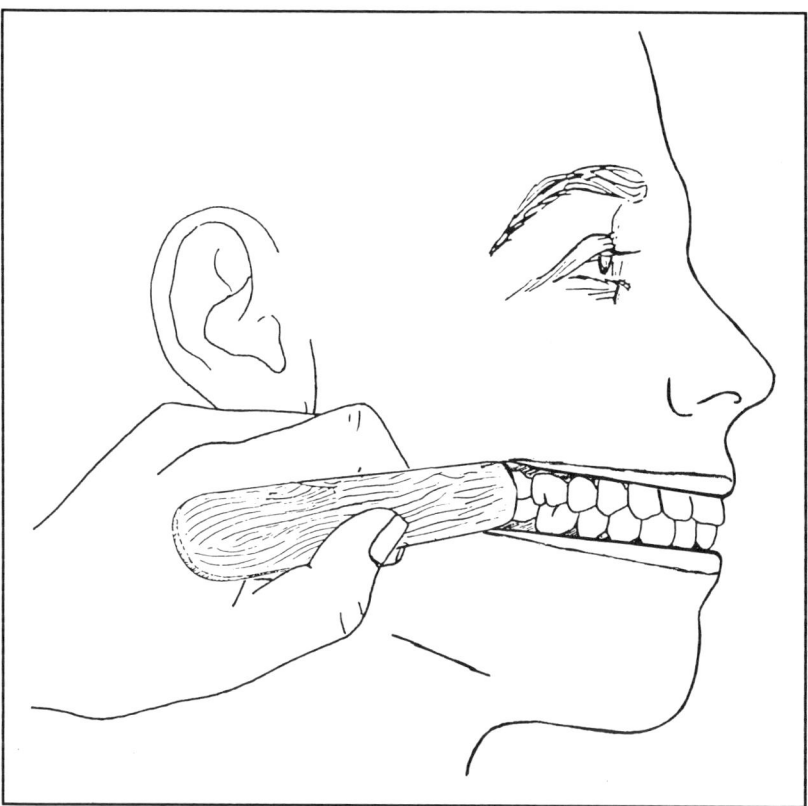

Examination of the first molars to determine the occlusal relationship of the upper and lower jaws.

7. Press down again on the posterior tongue with the depressor as you did for #5 above. Orient the warmed angled mirror upward and place it on top of the depressor. Slide this mirror along the depressor until the nasopharynx is visible (see figure on the following page). With your head mirror, direct light toward the angled mirror. Rotate the mirror to observe the entire nasopharyngeal region. Have your patient breathe through her nose and pant, if necessary, to inhibit gagging. Identify and describe the following structures: (a) adenoidal tissue, (b) the auditory tube orifices, and (c) the posterior portion of the vomer (nasal septum).

8. After removing the mirror and depressor, note the mobility of the velum and pharyngeal walls during yawning, sustained phonation, and slowly repeated short vowel productions. Record your observations on the hand-in sheet.

III. INDIRECT LARYNGOSCOPY

1. With your head mirror and incandescent lamp positioned as before, place your patient so he is sitting erect with his lower back against the examination chair. His chin should be slightly forward and elevated.

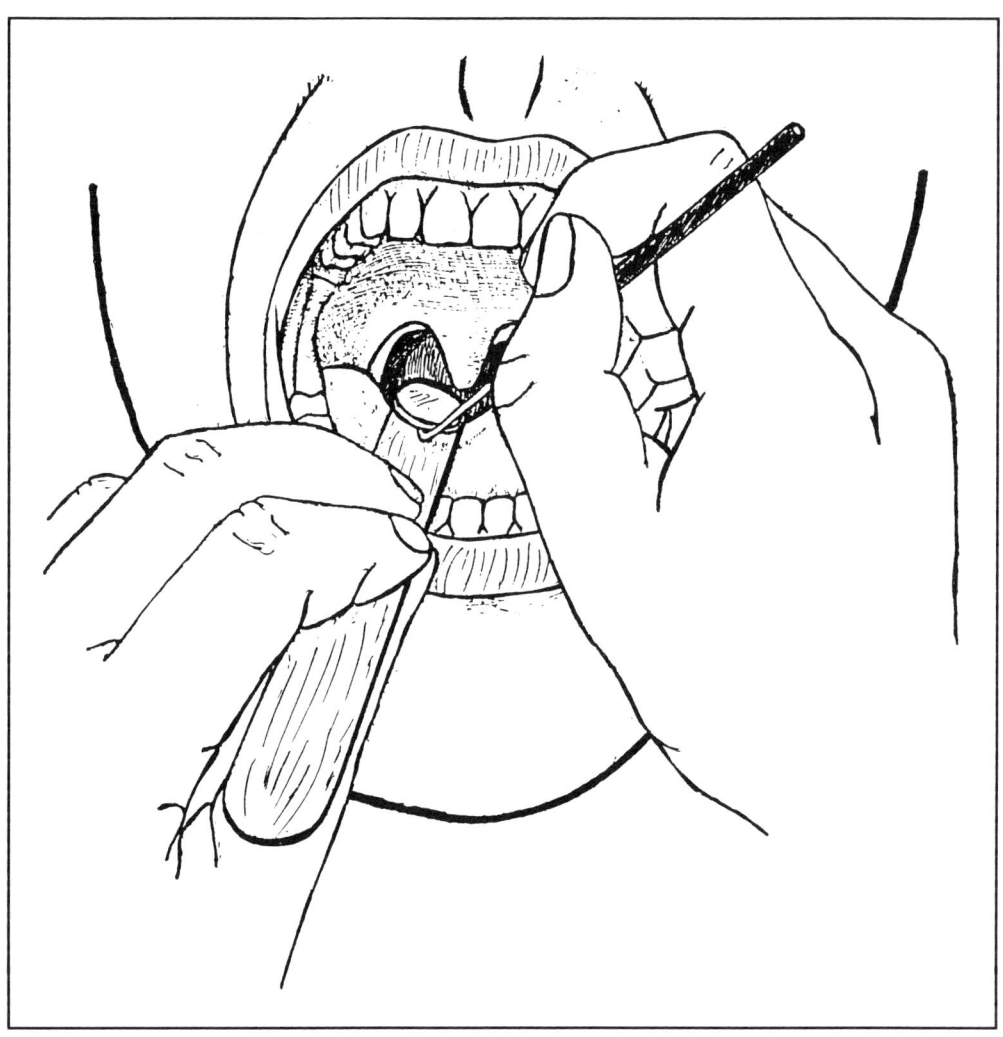

Indirect examination of the nasopharynx.

2. As in #6 above, warm an angled mirror over an alcohol lamp until it is warmer than your patient's exhaled breath. Again, check the mirror temperature by placing it against the back of your hand.

3. Instruct your patient to protrude his tongue. Using a piece of sterile gauze, carefully grasp the tongue between your thumb and forefinger and gently pull forward and downward. Insert the laryngeal mirror into the pharyx and, using the back of the mirror, press upward on the uvula and velum. With your head mirror, direct light toward the angled mirror. Adjust the placement of the mirror until the vocal folds and glottis are visible (see figure on facing page). Have your patient relax his shoulders and instruct him to breathe quietly (or to pant if he is prone to gagging). Identify and describe the following structures: (a) epiglottis, (b) vestibular (ventricular) folds, (c) vocal folds, and (d) tubercles.

4. Note the movement and position of the vocal folds during: (a) quiet breathing, (b) panting, (c) yawning, (d) coughing, and (e) sustained phonation.

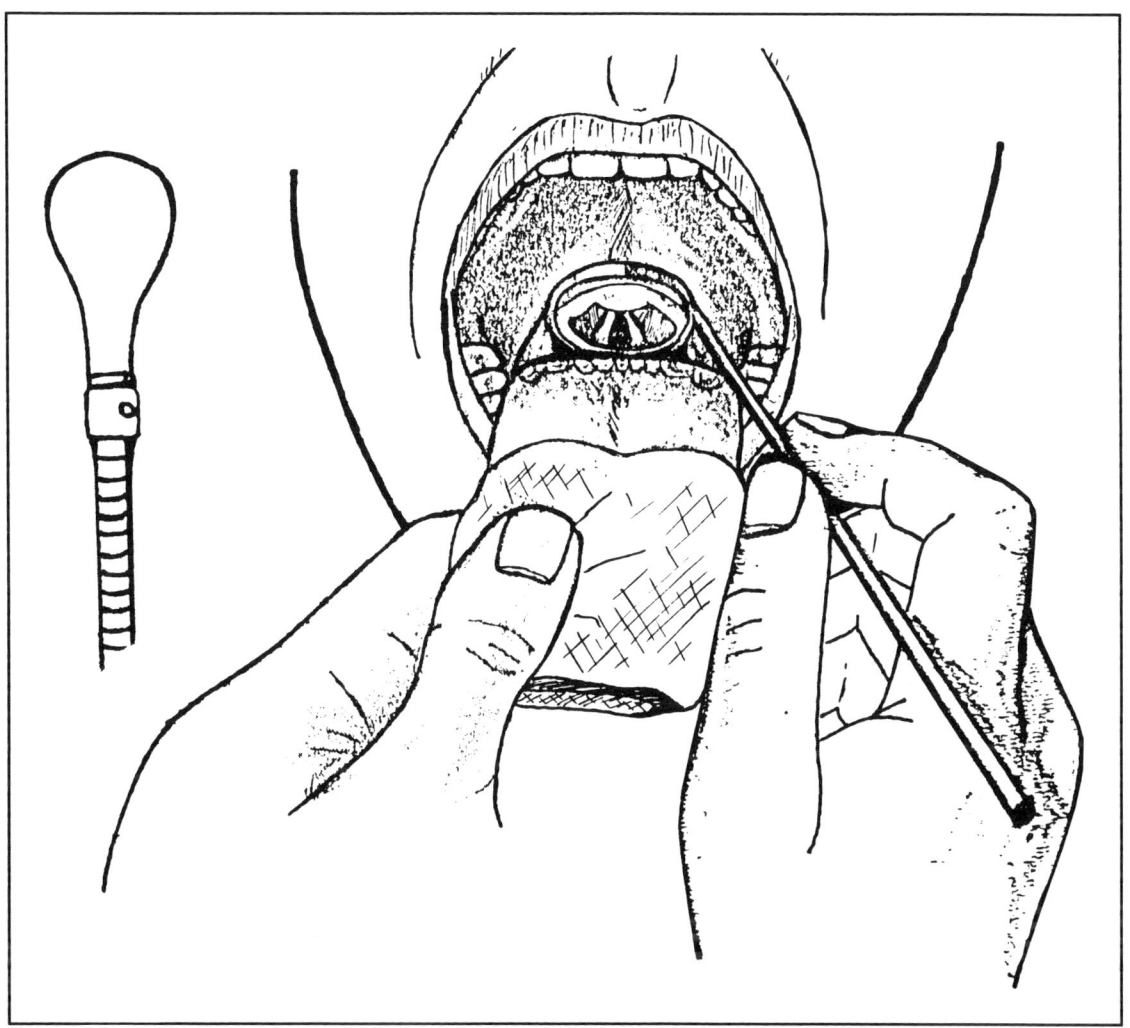

Indirect examination of the larynx and laryngopharynx.

5. On the hand-in sheet, modify the schematic illustration of a laryngoscopic view to reflect what you observe during quiet (eupneic tidal) breathing.

IV. USING THE OTOSCOPE

1. Gently retract the patient's auricle upwards and backwards with your thumb and forefinger, using the other hand to insert the aural speculum of the otoscope (see figure on next page). Adjust the otoscope so that the meatus is clearly illuminated.

2. Modify the drawings of the right and left tympanic membranes shown schematically on the hand-in sheet to reflect what you observe, including the cone of light, if seen.

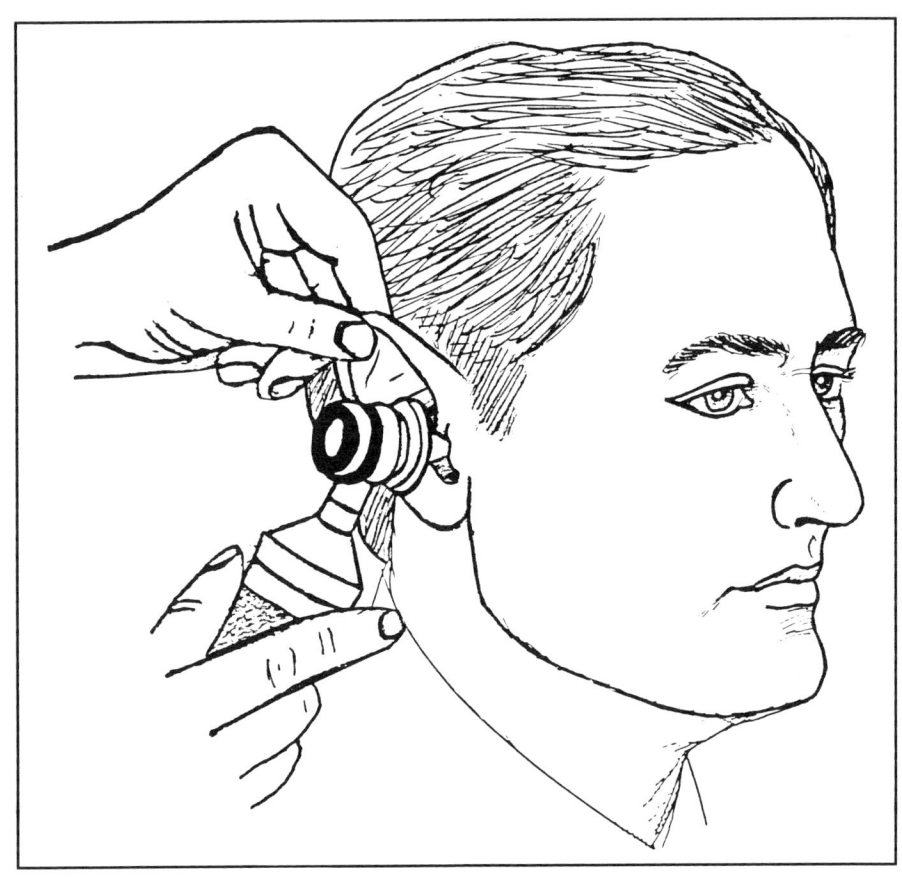

An otoscopic examination.

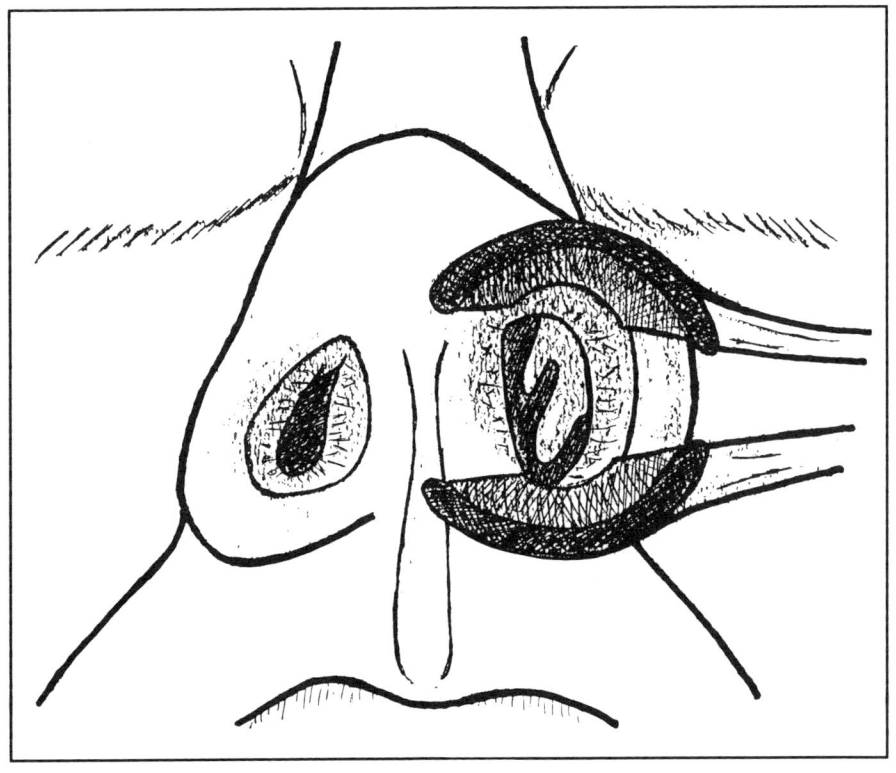

Examination of the nasal cavity.

V. USING THE NASAL SPECULUM

1. Instruct the patient to sit back in the examination chair and to look straight upward, placing her head against the chair headrest. Observe the size, shape, and symmetry of the nares. Record your observations on the hand-in sheet.

2. Place one hand on the patient's forehead, and with the other, insert a nasal speculum into the nasal vestibule. Orient the speculum in an up-and-down direction (see figure on facing page).

3. Using an otoscope, illuminate the nasal vestibule through the speculum. Gently and slowly manipulate the position of the head to afford the best view. On the hand-in sheet, modify the drawing of the nasal septum and turbinates to reflect what you see.

VI. USING THE NEUROLOGICAL HAMMER

1. Seat your patient so that his lower legs hang freely. Lightly but quickly tap the patellar tendon just below the kneecap using a neurological hammer. Observe the quadriceps muscle of the thigh for a quick, bulging contraction. Repeat this on the opposite leg and compare results.

2. Have your patient sit comfortably with his mouth open and relaxed. Place your thumb over the mentum (midline) of the patient's chin (see figure on the next page). Using the hammer, apply a quick tap to your thumb to stretch the masseter muscles. Observe the jaw for a rapid twitch or closure. Describe the strength of the response.

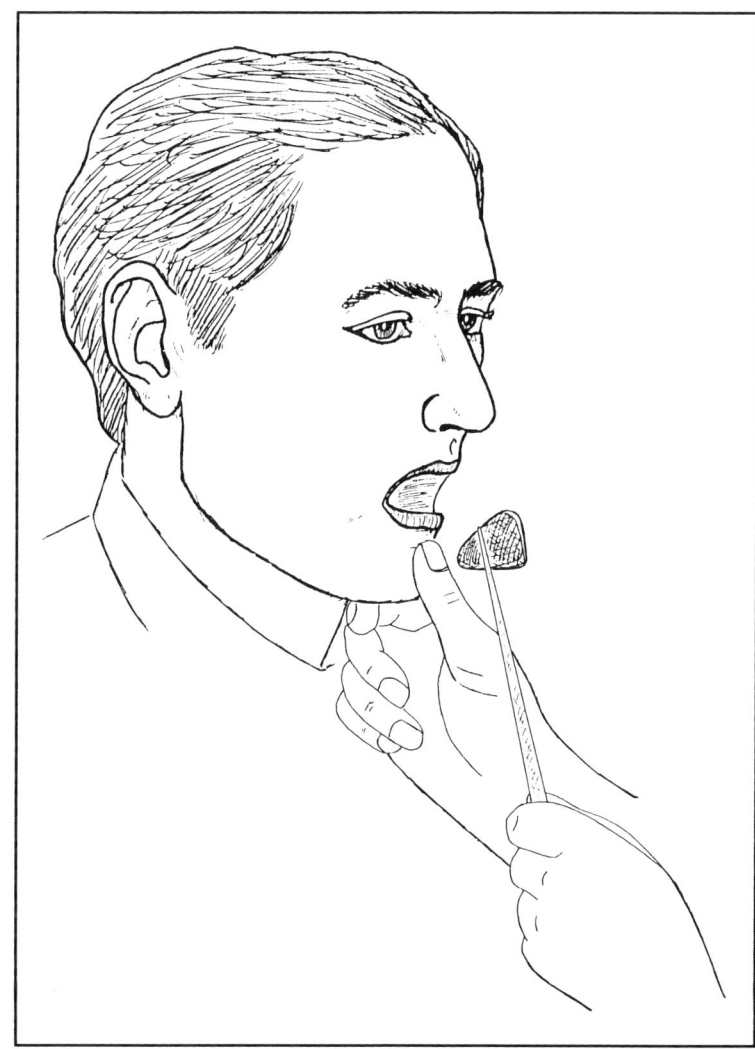

Eliciting a jaw-jerk (myotatic) response.

READ MORE ABOUT IT!

Barrett, R. H., & Hanson, M. L. (1974). *Orofacial myofunctional disorders.* St. Louis: Mosby.

Bates, B. (1991). *A guide to physical examination and history taking* (5th ed.). Philadelphia: J. B. Lippincott.

Collins, R. D. (1982). *Illustrated manual of neurologic diagnosis* (2nd ed.). Philadelphia: J. B. Lippincott.

Cummings, C. W., Fredrickson, J. M., Harker, L. A., Krause, C. J., & Schuller, D. E. (Eds.). (1986). *Otolaryngology-head and neck surgery* (4 vols.). St. Louis: Mosby.

DeWeese, D. D., & Saunders, W. H. (1987). *Textbook of otolaryngology* (7th ed.). St. Louis: Mosby.

Fricke, J. E. (Ed.). (1970). *Speech and the dentofacial complex: The state of the art (ASHA Reports No. 5).* Washington, DC: American Speech and Hearing Association.

Greenberger, N. J., & Hinthorn, D. R. (1993). *History taking and physical examination: Essentials and clinical correlates.* St. Louis: Mosby.

Hale, S. T., Kellum, G. D., Richardson, J. F., Messer, S. C., Gross, A. M., & Sisakun, S. (1992). Oral motor control, posturing, and myofunctional variables in 8-year-olds. *Journal of Speech and Hearing Research, 35,* 1203–1208.

Hearer, A. F. (1992). *De Jong's the neurological examination* (5th ed.). Philadelphia: J. B. Lippincott.

Hirano, M. (1981). *Clinical examination of voice.* New York: Springer-Verlag.

Jung, J. H. (1989). *Genetic syndromes in communication disorders.* San Diego: Singular Publishing Group.

Kahane, J. C. (1982). Anatomy and physiology of the organs of the peripheral speech mechanism. In N. J. Lass, L. V. McReynolds, J. L. Northern, & D. E. Yoder (Eds.), *Speech, language, and hearing* (Vol. 1, pp. 109–155). Philadelphia: W. B. Saunders.

Kahane, J. C. (1986). *Anatomy and physiology of the speech mechanism.* Austin, TX: PRO-ED.

Kahane, J. C., & Folkins, J. F. (1984). *Atlas of speech and hearing anatomy.* Columbus, OH: Charles E. Merrill.

MacLeod, J., & Munro, J. (Eds.). (1987). *Clinical examination* (7th ed.). Edinburgh: Churchill Livingstone.

Miller, R. M., & Groher, M. E. (1990). *Medical speech pathology* (pp. 190–221). Rockville, MD: Aspen.

Pannbacker, M. (1985). Common misconceptions about oral pharyngeal structure and function. *Language, Speech, and Hearing Services in Schools, 16,* 29–33.

Peterson-Falzone, S. J. (1982). Resonance disorders in structural defects. In N. J. Lass, L. V. McReynolds, J. L. Northern, & D. E. Yoder (Eds.), *Speech, language, and hearing* (Vol. 2, pp. 526–555). Philadelphia: W. B. Saunders.

Robbins, J., & Klee, T. (1987). Clinical assessment of oropharyngeal motor development in young children. *Journal of Speech and Hearing Disorders, 52,* 271–277.

Saunders, W. H. (1964). The larynx. *Clinical Symposia, 16,* 67–99.

Shelton, R. L., Morris, H. L., & McWilliams, B. J. (1973). Anatomical and physiological requirements for speech. *ASHA Reports, 9,* 2–18.

Spriestersbach, D. C. (1965). The effects of orofacial anomalies on the speech process. *ASHA Reports, 1,* 111–129.

Subtelny, J. D., Mestre, J. C., & Subtelny, J. (1964). Comparative study of normal and defective articulation of /s/ as related to malocclusion and deglutition. *Journal of Speech and Hearing Research, 29,* 269–285.

Travis, L. E. (Ed.) (1971). *Handbook of speech pathology* (2nd ed.). New York: Appleton-Century-Crofts.

Weinberg, B., Christensen, R., Logan, W., Bosma, J., & Wornell, A. (1969). Severe hypoplasia of the tongue. *Journal of Speech and Hearing Disorders, 34,* 157–168.

West, R. W., & Ansberry, M. (1968). *The rehabilitation of speech* (4th ed.). New York: Harper and Row.

Yanagisawa, E., Owens, T. W., Strothers, G., & Honda, K. (1983). Videolaryngoscopy: A comparison of fiberscopic and telescopic documentation. *Annals of Otology, Rhinology and Laryngology, 92,* 430–436.

Zemlin, W. R. (1988). *Speech and hearing science: Anatomy and physiology* (3rd ed.). Englewood Cliffs, NJ: Prentice-Hall.

Student _____   Date _____

PHYSICAL EXAMINATION

I. PALPATION

1. Palpation of temporalis and masseter muscles: _____

_____
_____
_____
_____
_____
_____
_____
_____

2. Masseter contraction during swallowing: _____

_____
_____
_____
_____
_____

3. Palpation of the TMJ: _____

_____
_____
_____
_____

Student _____   Date _____

_____

_____

4. Palpation of the sternocleidomastoideus: _____

_____

_____

_____

_____

_____

6. Laryngeal palpation during swallowing: _____

_____

_____

_____

_____

_____

_____

7. Palpation of the hard palate: _____

_____

_____

_____

_____

_____

_____

_____

Student _____ Date _____

II. OBSERVATION OF STRUCTURE

4. Angle classification: _____

5. Observation of oropharynx: _____

_____
_____
_____
_____
_____
_____
_____
_____
_____
_____

7. Observation of nasopharynx: _____

_____
_____
_____
_____
_____
_____
_____
_____
_____

Student _____   Date _____

8. Mobility of the velum and pharyngeal walls: _____

_____

_____

_____

_____

_____

III. INDIRECT LARYNGOSCOPY

3. Observation of the laryngopharynx: _____

_____

_____

_____

_____

_____

_____

_____

_____

_____

4. Movement and position of the vocal folds: _____

_____

Student _____ Date _____

_____
_____
_____
_____
_____
_____
_____
_____

5. Schematized laryngoscopic view.

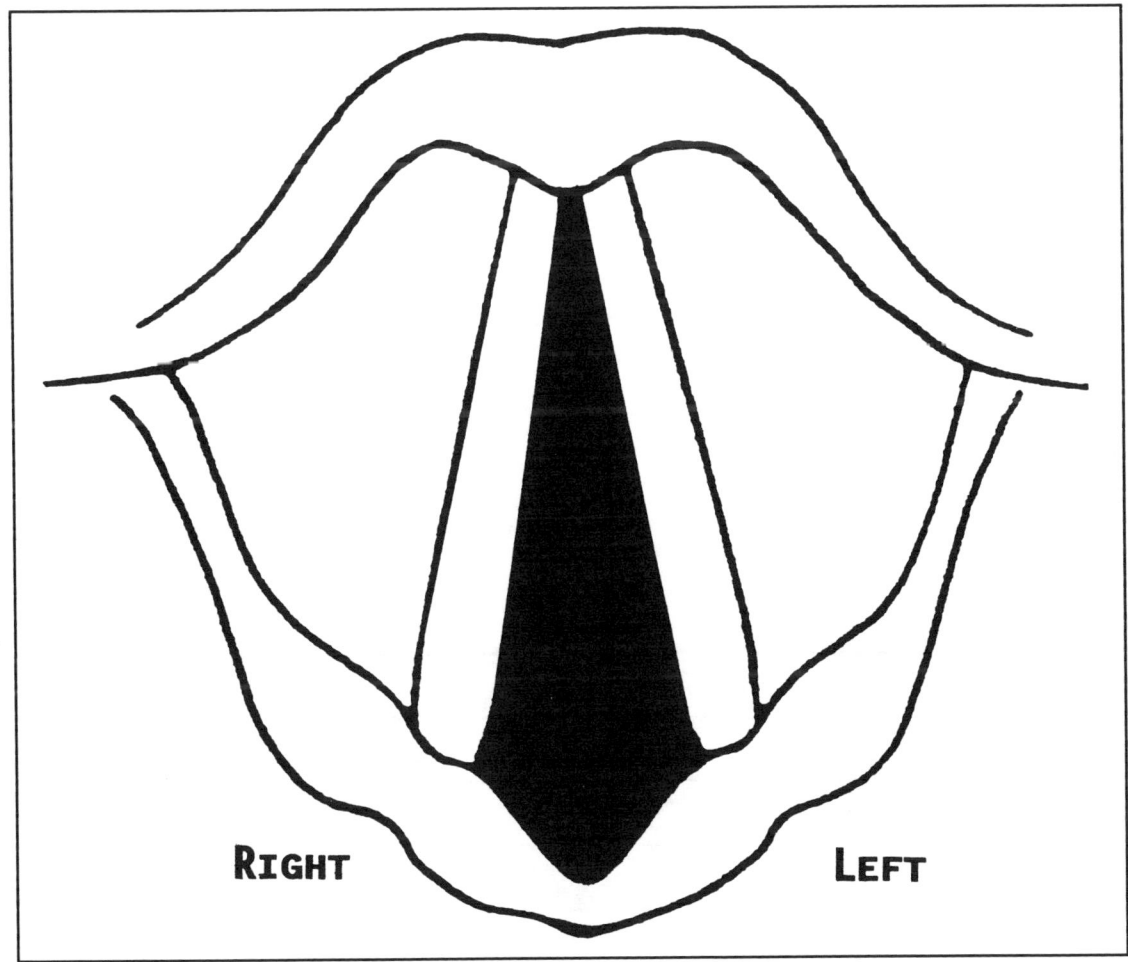

Student _____   Date _____

IV. USING THE OTOSCOPE

2. Schematic illustration of the tympanic membranes.

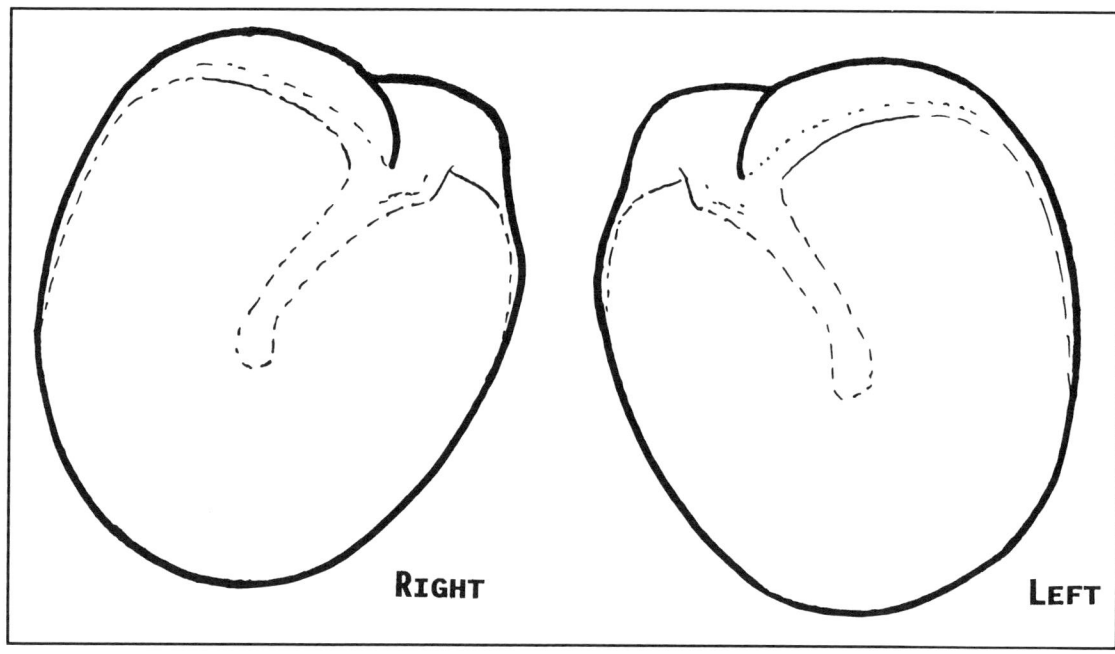

V. USING THE NASAL SPECULUM

1. Examination of the nares: _____

_____

_____

_____

_____

_____

_____

_____

Student   Date

3. Schematic illustration of the nasal septum and turbinates.

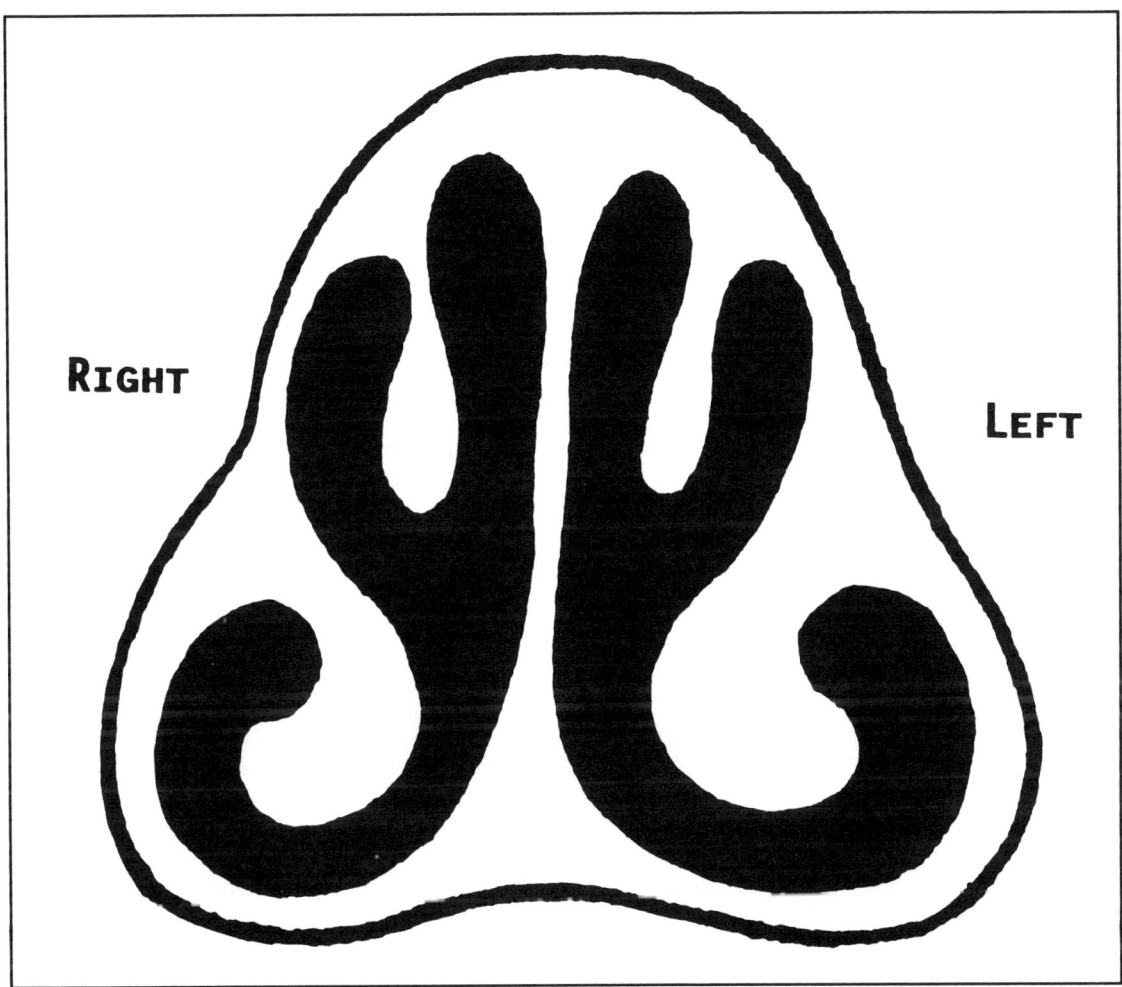

VI. USING THE NEUROLOGICAL HAMMER

1. Myotactic responses (patellar): _____

_____

_____

_____

_____

Student _____ Date _____

_____
_____
_____
_____

2. Myotactic response (mandibular): _____

_____
_____
_____
_____
_____
_____
_____
_____
_____

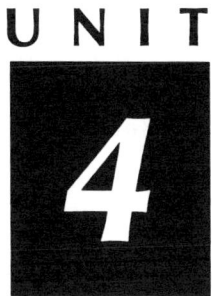

UNIT 4

Tutorial: Descriptive Statistics

I. SUMMARY STATISTICS

The use of appropriate summary statistics is essential to our ability to make clear sense of clinical data that are expressed in numerical, rather than in graphic, form. In general, such statistics attempt to answer two important questions about the data: (a) How much (or how little)? and (b) How variable (or how consistent)? The arithmetic mean, median, and mode are the most common measures of *central tendency*. Colloquially, these measures are associated with the average, most typical, and most common datum values, respectively. Calculation of the mean simply involves dividing the sum of all values by the number of values. To determine the median, list the data in rank order and, for an odd number of values, find the middle score in the list. For an even number of data, the median is the mean of the two middle scores. The mode is the datum that occurs most often.

Measures of *variability*, on the other hand, reflect the dispersion, or spread, of the data. The most common indices of variability include the range and standard deviation (usually designated by *SD* or by the lowercase Greek letter sigma, σ). The range reflects the extent (extremes) of data distribution, while the standard deviation describes the average amount by which the data deviate from the mean. The range is often expressed as the maximum value minus the minimum value. The definitional formula for the standard deviation is:

$$SD = \sqrt{\frac{\sum(\bar{X} - X)^2}{n}}.$$

Thus to calculate *SD*, you must: (a) find the mean value ($\bar{X} = \Sigma X/n$), (b) subtract each value from the mean ($\bar{X} - X$), (c) square these differences $(\bar{X} - X)^2$, (d) add the squared differences $\Sigma(\bar{X} - X)^2$, called the sum of squares), (e) find the mean square $\Sigma(\bar{X} - X)^2/n)$, and (f) extract the square root of the mean square. The greater the dispersion of data from the mean, the larger the *SD*.

Exercises

Provide your answers to the exercises on the hand-in sheet.

Table 1. Mean Maximal Syllable Repetition Rates (syllables/second) for /pʌ/ Produced by 18 Adult Dysarthric Speakers.

Speaker	Rate	Speaker	Rate	Speaker	Rate
1	3.1	7	6.3	13	2.4
2	5.0	8	5.3	14	2.8
3	4.5	9	2.8	15	4.4
4	3.9	10	6.6	16	3.3
5	6.7	11	4.2	17	4.9
6	3.6	12	2.8	18	4.8

Data from "Tongue Strength and Alternate Motion Rates in Normal and Dysarthric Subjects, by J. P. Dworkin and A. E. Aronson, *Journal of Communication Disorders*, 19, 115–132. Table 1, pp. 118–120. Used with permission.

1. Using the data in Table 1 determine:

   a. The number of repetitions per second of the syllable /pʌ/ that the *average* dysarthric subject produced;

   b. The repetition rate that was *most typical* of the dysarthric subjects;

   c. The *most common* repetition rate produced by the dysarthric subjects; and

   d. The *range* of repetition rates produced by the dysarthric subjects.

2. On the average, the repetition rates varied by how many syllables per second?

3. How do these patients compare with normal speakers?

4. Measure your own mean maximal repetition rate. How does your rate compare with available norms for /pʌ/?

II. CORRELATION

It is often necessary to examine whether two variables (call them X and Y) are related to each other. When two variables are related and the relationship can be approximated by a straight line, we say that these variables are *linearly correlated.* The most common equation used to compute a linear correlation yields what is called the Pearson product-moment correlation coefficient (Pearson *r*). A perfect positive correlation is indicated by an *r* of +1, a perfect negative (inverse) correlation is associated with an *r* of −1, and a complete absence of correlation is associated with an *r* of 0. A perfect positive correlation means that if you know the value of X, the relative value of Y can be determined with certainty: As one gets larger, so does the other. In the case of a perfect negative correlation ($r = -1$), the value of X is also a precise indicator of the value Y, only in this case as X gets larger, Y gets smaller. However, as the value of *r* approaches zero, the ability to predict one variable on the basis of the other becomes less and less precise. Most commonly the Pearson *r* is determined as follows:

$$r_{X,Y} = \frac{n\Sigma XY - (\Sigma X)(\Sigma Y)}{\sqrt{[n\Sigma X^2 - (\Sigma X)^2][n\Sigma Y^2 - (\Sigma Y)^2]}}.$$

The figure below shows the frequency and intensity contours produced by a normal adult woman during the utterance "Hello," based on data provided by Horii.[1]

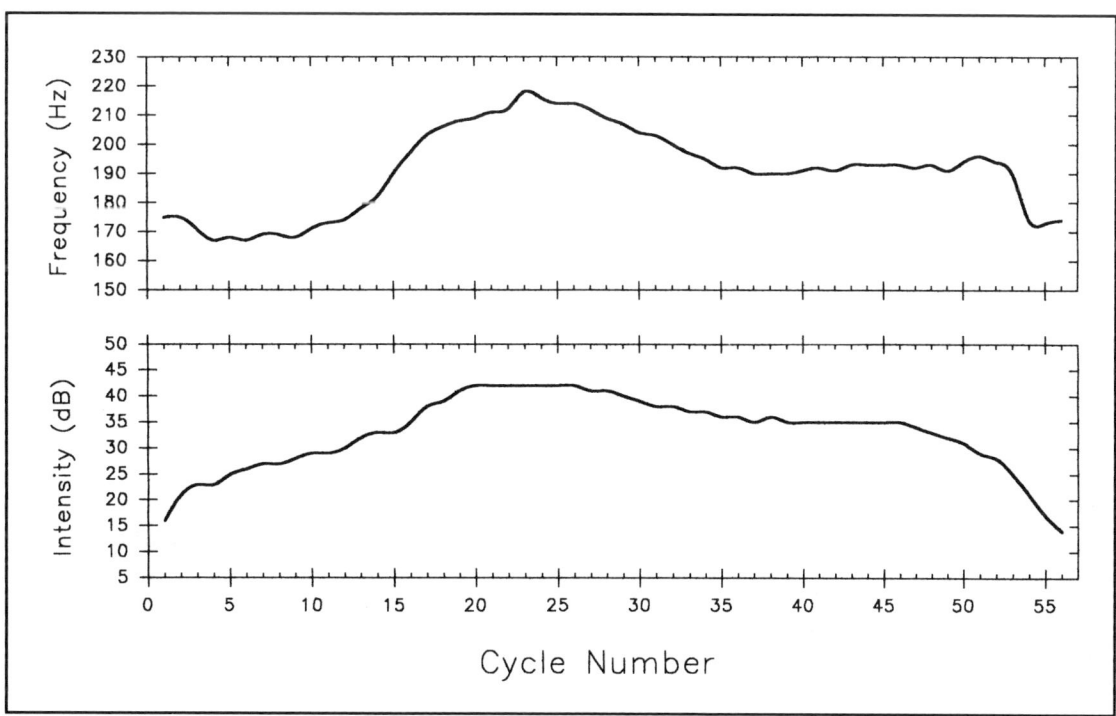

---

[1] Horii, Y. (1983). Automatic analysis of voice fundamental frequency and intensity using a Visi-Pitch. *Journal of Speech and Hearing Research, 26,* 467–471.

These data are shown numerically (in boldface) in Table 2 (opposite), along with other derived values that will be necessary for our calculation of correlation. For this example, the X variable will be fundamental frequency and the Y variable will be vocal intensity. The large sums and somewhat cumbersome calculations result from the relatively large number of data pairs ($n = 56$) used for the analysis.

Using the values in Table 2, we can calculate the Pearson product-moment correlation for the data:

$$r_{F_0 I} = \frac{n\Sigma(F_0 \times I) - (\Sigma F_0)(\Sigma I)}{\sqrt{[n\Sigma F_0^2 - (\Sigma F_0)^2][n\Sigma I^2 - (\Sigma I)^2]}}$$

$$= \frac{56(358,017) - (10,703)(1,847)}{\sqrt{[56(2,057,675) - (10,703)^2][56(63,729) - (1,847)^2]}}$$

$$= \frac{20,048,952 - 19,768,441}{\sqrt{[675,591][157,415]}}$$

$$= \frac{(280,511)}{\sqrt{106,348,157,300}}$$

$$= \frac{280,511}{326,110.6}$$

$$r = .86$$

This correlation coefficient indicates that F_0 and intensity are fairly closely related; one increases somewhat predictably with the other.

We may wish to estimate the proportion of variance in Y (i.e., intensity) that is predictable from X (i.e., F_0). The *coefficient of determination* provides this estimate, and is obtained simply by squaring the Pearson *r*. In this case $r^2 = .86 \times .86 = .74$. Thus 74% of the variance in intensity is predictable from the coincident frequency in this sample.

Table 2. Sequential Frequency (F_0, in Hz) and Intensity (I, in dB) Data.

Cycle [Pair]	F_0 [X]	I [Y]	$F_0 \times I$ [XY]	F_0^2 [X^2]	I^2 [Y^2]
1	175	16	2,800	30,625	256
2	175	21	3,675	30,625	441
3	171	23	3,933	29,241	529
4	167	23	3,841	27,889	529
5	168	25	4,200	28,224	625
6	167	26	4,342	27,889	676
7	169	27	4,563	28,561	729
8	169	27	4,563	28,561	729
9	168	28	4,704	28,224	784
10	171	29	4,959	29,241	841
11	173	29	5,017	29,929	841
12	174	30	5,220	30,276	900
13	178	32	5,696	31,684	1,024
14	182	33	6,006	33,124	1,089
15	190	33	6,270	36,100	1,089
16	197	35	6,895	38,809	1,225
17	203	38	7,714	41,209	1,444
18	206	39	8,034	42,436	1,521
19	208	41	8,528	43,264	1,681
20	209	42	8,778	43,681	1,764
21	211	42	8,862	44,521	1,764
22	212	42	8,904	44,944	1,764
23	218	42	9,156	47,524	1,764
24	216	42	9,072	46,656	1,764
25	214	42	8,988	45,796	1,764
26	214	42	8,988	45,796	1,764
27	212	41	8,692	44,944	1,681
28	209	41	8,569	43,681	1,681
29	207	40	8,280	42,849	1,600
30	204	39	7,956	41,616	1,521
31	203	38	7,714	41,209	1,444
32	200	38	7,600	40,000	1,444
33	197	37	7,289	38,809	1,369
34	195	37	7,215	38,025	1,369
35	192	36	6,912	36,864	1,296
36	192	36	6,912	36,864	1,296
37	190	35	6,650	36,100	1,225
38	190	36	6,840	36,100	1,296
39	190	35	6,650	36,100	1,225
40	191	35	6,685	36,481	1,225
41	192	35	6,720	36,864	1,225

(continued)

Table 2. *(continued)*

Cycle [Pair]	F_0 [X]	I [Y]	$F_0 \times I$ [XY]	F_0^2 [X^2]	I^2 [Y^2]
42	191	35	6,685	36,481	1,225
43	193	35	6,755	37,249	1,225
44	193	35	6,755	37,249	1,225
45	193	35	6,755	37,249	1,225
46	193	35	6,755	37,249	1,225
47	192	34	6,528	36,864	1,156
48	193	33	6,369	37,249	1,089
49	191	32	6,112	36,481	1,024
50	194	31	6,014	37,636	961
51	196	29	5,684	38,416	841
52	194	28	5,432	37,636	784
53	190	25	4,750	36,100	625
54	174	21	3,654	30,276	441
55	173	17	2,941	29,929	289
56	174	14	2,436	30,276	196
Sum (Σ) =	10,703	1,847	358,017	2,057,675	63,729

Frequency and intensity data from: "Automatic Analysis of Fundamental Frequency and Intensity Using a Visi-Pitch," by Y. Horii, 1983, *Journal of Speech and Hearing Research, 26,* 467–471. Fig. 5, p. 470. Copyright © American Speech-Language-Hearing Association, Rockville, MD. Used with permission.

Exercises

1. Using the limited data shown below, examine the relationship between this dysarthric speaker's speech rate (let's call this variable X) and his intelligibility scores (let's call this variable Y).

Test Session	Speech Rate (syllables/s)	Intelligibility (percent)	XY	X^2	Y^2
1	1.2	52	62.4	1.4	2,704
2	3.0	34	102.0	9.0	1,156
3	2.7	36	97.2	7.3	1,296
4	2.7	49	132.3	7.3	2,401
5	2.3	48	110.4	5.3	2,304
Sum (Σ) =	11.9	219	504.3	30.3	9,861

   a. What is the sample correlation coefficient?

   b. What percent of the variance in speech intelligibility scores is predictable by the dysarthric's speech rate?

c. Describe the relationship between this patient's speech rate and intelligibility ratings.

2. Using the limited data in the table below, examine the relationship between this stutterer's mean speaking sound pressure level (variable X) and percentage of dysfluent syllables (variable Y).

Sample Number	Mean Sound Pressure Level (dB)	Dysfluent Syllables (percent)	XY	X^2	Y^2
1	53	0.3	15.9	2,809	0.09
2	75	1.4	105.0	5,625	1.96
3	81	0.8	64.8	6,561	0.64
4	66	2.2	145.2	4,356	4.84
5	48	1.5	72.0	2,304	2.25
Sum (Σ) =	323	6.2	402.9	21,655	9.78

a. What is the sample correlation coefficient?

b. What percent of the variance in relative dysfluency is predictable by the stutterer's mean sound pressure level?

c. Describe the relationship between this patient's sound pressure level and the percentage of stuttered syllables.

III. LINEAR REGRESSION

While the correlation coefficient tells us about how strongly two variables are related to each other, the *regression equation* states what the relationship is. The figure on the next page is a *scatterplot* of Horii's frequency and intensity data. For every cycle in the phonatory sample a point is plotted showing its F_0 (on the horizontal, or X-axis) and its intensity (on the vertical, or Y-axis).

The line that runs through the data points is called the *regression line*. It represents the best relationship we can determine for the association of the X and Y (frequency and intensity, respectively) variables. The regression line is drawn so that the average distance between it and any data point is minimized. The regression equation is the equation of this line. You will remember from elementary algebra that the equation of a straight line is:

$$Y = mX + b.[2]$$

---

[2] This is the form used in most algebra texts. Statisticians, however, often state the equation as $Y = bX + a$.

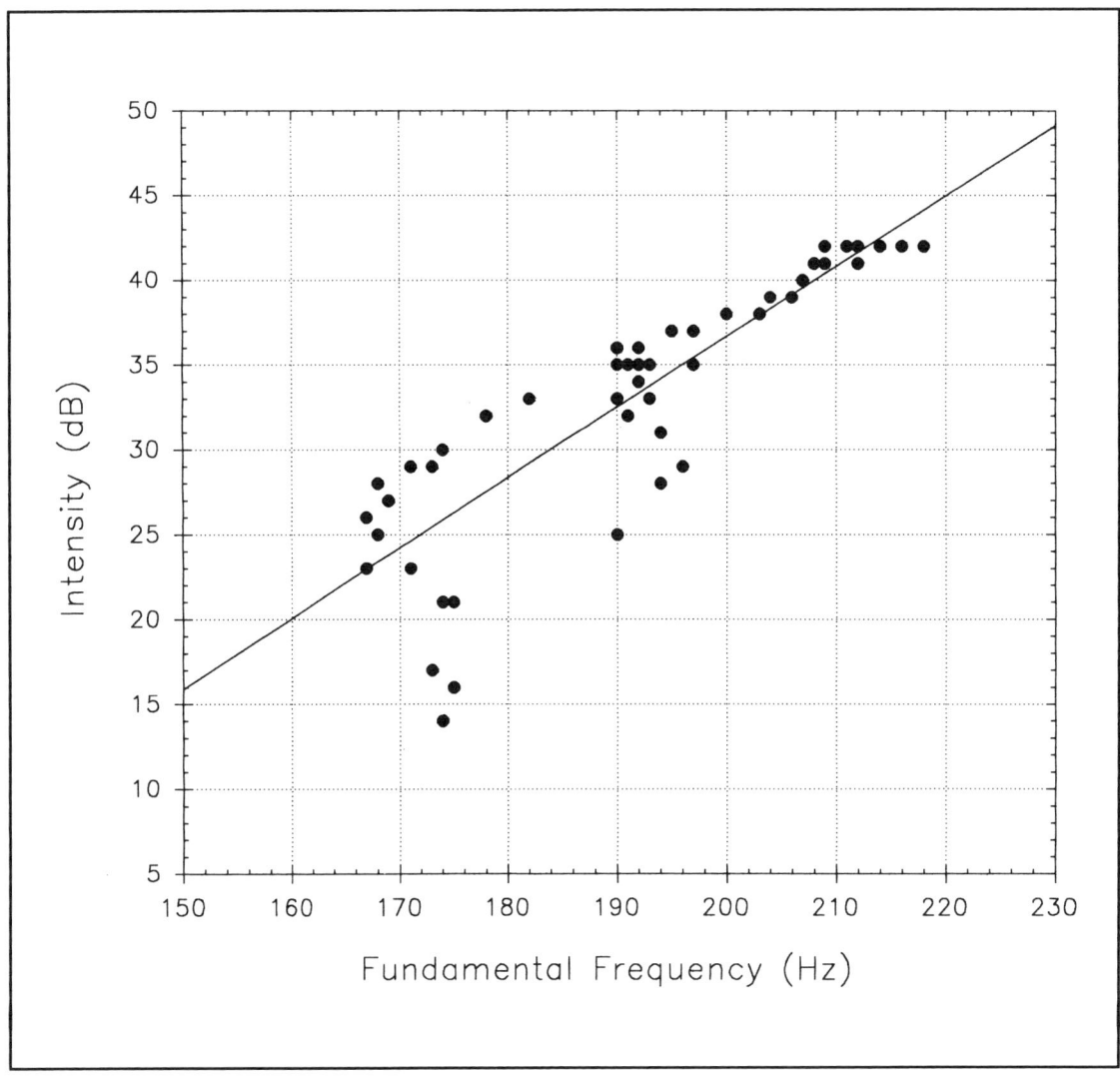

The term "m" is called the *slope* of the line, and describes the line's steepness. This tells us how rapidly Y changes as X changes. The "b" is the *Y-intercept*. It specifies how high on the graph the regression line is.

The slope and Y-intercept may be computed from the data as follows:

$$m_{Y,X} = \frac{n\Sigma XY - (\Sigma X)(\Sigma Y)}{n\Sigma X^2 - (\Sigma X)^2}, \text{ and}$$

$$b_{Y,X} = \bar{Y} - m_{Y,X}\bar{X},$$

where $\bar{Y}$ and $\bar{X}$ represent the respective means, that is, $\Sigma Y/n$ and $\Sigma X/n$, respectively.

Thus, for our frequency and intensity data:

$$m_{I,F_0} = \frac{56(358{,}017) - (10{,}703)(1{,}847)}{56(2{,}057{,}675) - (10{,}703)^2}$$

$$= \frac{280{,}511}{675{,}591}$$

$$= 0.415, \text{ and}$$

$$b_{I,F_0} = 33.0 - 0.415(191.1)$$

$$= -46.34$$

to yield the regression equation:

$$\text{Predicted Intensity} = 0.415(F_0) - 46.34.$$

Based on the data, then, a cycle with a frequency of 160 Hz, for example, would be predicted to have a concurrent intensity of $0.415(160) - 46.34$, or 20.06 dB. Mark this point on the scatterplot above with an "x."

Exercises

1. Clearly, using the same table, you should be able to predict vocal frequencies based on intensity data. Designating intensity as the X variable and F_0 as the Y variable in the slope and intercept equations, provide the appropriate regression equation.

2. Based on your regression line, what F_0 value would you predict is associated with an intensity of 40 dB?

3. Based on your regression line, what F_0 value would you predict is associated with an intensity of 5 dB?

READ MORE ABOUT IT!

Atkinson, J. E. (1978). Correlation analysis of the physiological factors controlling fundamental voice frequency. *Journal of the Acoustical Society of America, 63,* 211–222. **[A good example of the use of correlation analysis]**

Bland, M. (1987). *An introduction to medical statistics.* Oxford: Oxford University Press.

Bloom, M., & Fischer, J. (1982). *Evaluating practice: Guidelines for the accountable professional.* Englewood Cliffs, NJ: Prentice-Hall.

Duncan, R. C., Knapp, R. G., & Miller, M. C. III. (1983). *Introductory biostatistics for the health sciences* (2nd ed.). New York: Wiley.

Kilpatrick, S. J., Jr. (1977). *Statistical principles in health care information* (2nd ed.). Baltimore: University Park Press.

O'Dell, J. W. (1984). *BASIC statistics — An introduction to problem solving with your personal computer.* Blue Ridge Summit, PA: Tab.

Shelton, R. L., Jr., Knox, A. W., Arndt, W. B., Jr., & Elbert, M. (1967). The relationship between nasality score values and oral and nasal sound pressure level. *Journal of Speech and Hearing Research, 10,* 549–557. **[Another example using correlation techniques]**

Silverman, F. H. (1993). *Research design and evaluation in speech language pathology and audiology* (3rd ed.). Englewood Cliffs, NJ: Prentice-Hall.

Ventry, I. M., & Schiavetti, N. (1986). *Evaluating Research in speech pathology and audiology* (2nd ed.). New York: Macmillan.

Wall, F. J. (1986). *Statistical data analysis handbook.* New York: McGraw-Hill.

Weisberg, H. F. (1992). *Central tendency and variability.* Newbury Park, CA: Sage Publications.

Yanagihara, N., Koike, Y., & von Leden, H. (1966). Phonation and respiration. *Folia Phoniatrica, 18,* 323–340. **[A good example of the use of regression analysis]**

Student _____   Date _____

DESCRIPTIVE STATISTICS

I. SUMMARY STATISTICS

1. **a.** Average repetitions per second (show arithmetic):

   _____

   b. Most typical repetition rate (show arithmetic):

   _____

   _____

   c. Most common repetition rate (describe how common):

   _____

   _____

   d. Range of repetition rates: _____

2. Average variation of the repetition rate (show arithmetic):

   _____

   _____

3. Comparison of dysarthrics to normal speakers: _____

   _____

   _____

   _____

   Source: _____

4. My maximal repetition rate for /p/: _____ rep/s.

   Comparison to normative data: _____

   _____

   _____

   Source: _____

Student _____ Date _____

II. CORRELATION

1. a. Sample correlation coefficient: _____

   b. Relationship of speech rate and intelligibility: _____

   _____

   _____

   _____

2. a. Sample correlation coefficient: _____

   b. Relationship of SPL and dysfluencies: _____

   _____

   _____

   _____

III. LINEAR REGRESSION

1. Regression equation: _____

2. If intensity = 40 dB, F_0 should be (show arithmetic): _____

   _____

3. If intensity = 5 dB, F_0 should be (show arithmetic): _____

   _____

UNIT 5

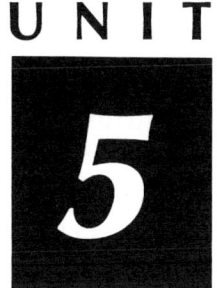

Tutorial: Relative Measures and Logarithmic Scaling

I. PERCENTAGES

The most basic statement of relationship is the proportion. To find a proportion, divide the data (or datum) of interest by the total of all the data. For instance, if within a group of 30 dysarthric speakers 6 are classified ataxic, the proportion of ataxic dysarthrics is 6/30 or 0.20. To then translate a proportion into a percentage, simply multiply the proportion by 100. Therefore 0.20 × 100 or 20% of the dysarthric speakers are ataxic. Another example of a proportion is the ventilatory I-fraction. The I-fraction is the inspiratory time relative to (that is, divided by) the duration of the entire breath cycle:

$$\frac{\text{inspiration}}{\text{inspiration} + \text{expiration}}.$$

The I-fraction, the proportion of the breath cycle devoted to inspiration, is a *relative* index of ventilatory behavior, whereas the inspiratory and expiratory times are *absolute measures.* In division, the time unit "cancels out" so that regardless of how ventilatory events may have been timed (for example, in seconds, in milliseconds, or even by the regular dripping of a leaky faucet), the inspiratory *proportion* will not change. The proportion is said to be *dimensionless.*

II. RATIOS

When we derive a proportion such as the I-fraction we are really making a comparison of a part to the whole. *Ratios* (sometimes called quotients) are proportions used to compare two quantities, neither of which may represent the whole. In our population of 30 dysarthrics, for instance, we may wish to compare the number of spastic speakers to hyperkinetic speakers. If there are 6 spastic and 12 hyperkinetic dysarthrics, the ratio of spastic to hyperkinetic dysarthrics is 6/12 or 0.5 (that is, there are half as many spastic as hyperkinetic speakers), while the ratio of hyperkinetic to spastic dysarthrics is 12/6 or 2.0 (there are twice as many hyperkinetic speakers as spastic speakers). The ratio is a relative number; it tells us the magnitude of the numerator relative to that of the denominator. The denominator thus serves as the *reference*.

III. LOGARITHMS AND LOGARITHMIC SCALING

In the expression 10^4, the number 10 is called the *base* and the number 4 is the called the *exponent*. The exponent tells you how many times to multiply the base by itself. In this case, 10^4 equals $10 \times 10 \times 10 \times 10$, or 10,000. Similarly, 10^5 would be $10 \times 10 \times 10 \times 10 \times 10$, or 100,000. Another name for an exponent is *logarithm* (or simply, *log*).[1] We can, therefore, say that the log of 10,000 equals 4, written log 10,000 = 4. Notice that the log is equal to the number of zeros following the "1": Log 10, therefore, would equal 1 since there is only one zero ($10^1 = 10$) and log 1 = 0 since there are no zeros ($10^0 = 1$). Logs of numbers less than 1 are negative: Log 0.1 = −1 ($10^{-1} = 0.1$). Compare the fact that log 10 = 1 and log 1/10 = −1. Thus, if log 100 = 2, log 1/100 (that is, log 0.01) must equal −2.

But how would you determine the log of a number like 2? Because 2 is not an even multiple of 10, its *log* is not an integer, but a decimal. Given that log 1 = 0 and log 10 = 1, log 2 must fall between those values, and is probably closer to 0 than to 1. Such nonobvious logs are typically derived by referring to a logarithm table such as the one provided in Appendix C.[2] In this case, you will find log 2 = 0.3. (This means, of course, that $10^{0.3} = 2$.)

On a logarithmic scale, two pairs of points will be the same distance apart if their ratios are equal, rather than the difference between the pairs. Consider, for instance, that although the absolute difference between the numbers 10 and 100 is *90* and the difference between 10,000 and 100,000 is *90,000*, their ratios both equal *0.1* (10/100 and 10,000/100,000, respectively).[3] This is to say that while the distance between 1 and 10, 10 and 100, 100 and 1,000 are equally spaced on a log scale, the linear distance between these points increases *exponentially*.

---

[1] Although one can apply exponents to other bases — 2, for instance, is popular — we will limit ourselves to a discussion of base 10.

[2] To look up a logarithm using Appendix C, follow this example: Let's say we want to find log 3.45. Find the row marked "3.4" and follow the columns of log values over to the one marked ".05". The log value that intersects this row and column (3.4 + .05) is 0.538. Thus log 3.45 = 0.538. See tutorial for determining logs of numbers lower than 0.01 and greater than 9.99. Be aware that many handheld calculators and all computer programming languages provide log functions.

[3] This fact explains why doubling a sound pressure always results in an increase of 6 dB, no matter what the original sound pressure might have been.

READ MORE ABOUT IT!

Speaks, C. E. (1992). *Introduction to sound: Acoustics for the hearing and speech sciences* (pp. 91–116). San Diego: Singular Publishing Group.

Stevens, S. S. (1951). Mathematics, measurement, and psychophysics. In S. S. Stevens (Ed.), *Handbook of experimental psychology* (pp. 1–49). New York: John Wiley.

Student _____   Date _____

RELATIVE MEASURES AND LOGARITHMIC SCALING

Complete the following exercises and hand them in to your instructor:

I. PERCENTAGES

1. Using the ventilatory data below, calculate the mean I-fraction for each breath cycle to complete the table.

Mean Inspiratory and Expiratory Times for a Normal Female Speaker During Spontaneous Utterances.

Breath Cycle	Inspiration (seconds)	Expiration (seconds)	I-fraction
1	0.333	2.511	_____
2	0.539	3.840	_____
3	0.768	6.481	_____
4	0.325	2.287	_____
5	0.487	4.010	_____

2. What unit of measurement is used to describe the I-fraction? _____

3. Do the mean inspiratory *or* expiratory times alone predict the subject's mean I-fraction? How well does the I-fraction predict the mean inspiratory or expiratory times? Explain.

_____

_____

_____

_____

4. If we know that the speech I-fraction will always approximate 0.12, can we then estimate expiratory duration based on the inspiration time? Explain.

_____

Student _____ Date _____

_____
_____
_____
_____
_____

II. RATIOS

1. Using the ventilatory data in the above table,

    a. Determine the mean ratio of expiratory time to inspiratory time (show arithmetic).

    _____

    b. How do you interpret this number? (Describe what this ratio means.)

    _____
    _____

    c. Based on this ratio, if a speech inspiration took 0.9 seconds, how long would you expect the ensuing expiration to last?

    _____
    _____

2. A stutterer produces a speech sample containing 60 syllables. Of these, 12 are spoken dysfluently.

    a. What is the percentage of dysfluent syllables in this sample?

    _____

    b. What is the ratio of dysfluent to fluent syllables?

    _____

    c. What is the ratio of fluent to dysfluent syllables?

    _____

Student _____   Date _____

III. LOGARITHMS AND LOGARITHMIC SCALING

NOTE: You may need to refer to the log table in Appendix C to answer some of the questions that follow.

1. Find the log of:

   a. 4/5: _____ , and

   b. 5/4: _____ .

   c. From these answers, what rule can you deduce concerning the logs of reciprocal numbers?

   _____

   _____

2. What is the log value of the *ratios* between the following pairs of numbers (the first log ratio is done for you):

0.1 & 0.3	log 0.33	= −0.481
1.0 & 3.0	log _____	= _____
100 & 300	log _____	= _____
1,100 & 1,300	log _____	= _____
5,100 & 5,300	log _____	= _____

3. Using Appendix C we find that log 7.38 = 0.868. Then, using a hand calculator with a log function we find that log 73.8 = 1.868. Based on these answers, can you predict log 738 and log 7,380 without the use of a log table or calculator? Explain:

   _____

   _____

   _____

   _____

Student   Date

4. a. A new test yields scores that may range anywhere between 0 and 100. The performance of 12 patients is shown below. Plot each of these scores by their log values on the graph provided on the next page.

Patient	Raw Score	Log Score
1	50.1	_____
2	20.0	_____
3	90.2	_____
4	10.0	_____
5	2.5	_____
6	99.0	_____
7	79.5	_____
8	5.1	_____
9	1.0	_____
10	40.0	_____
11	0.5	_____
12	64.6	_____

Student _____ Date _____

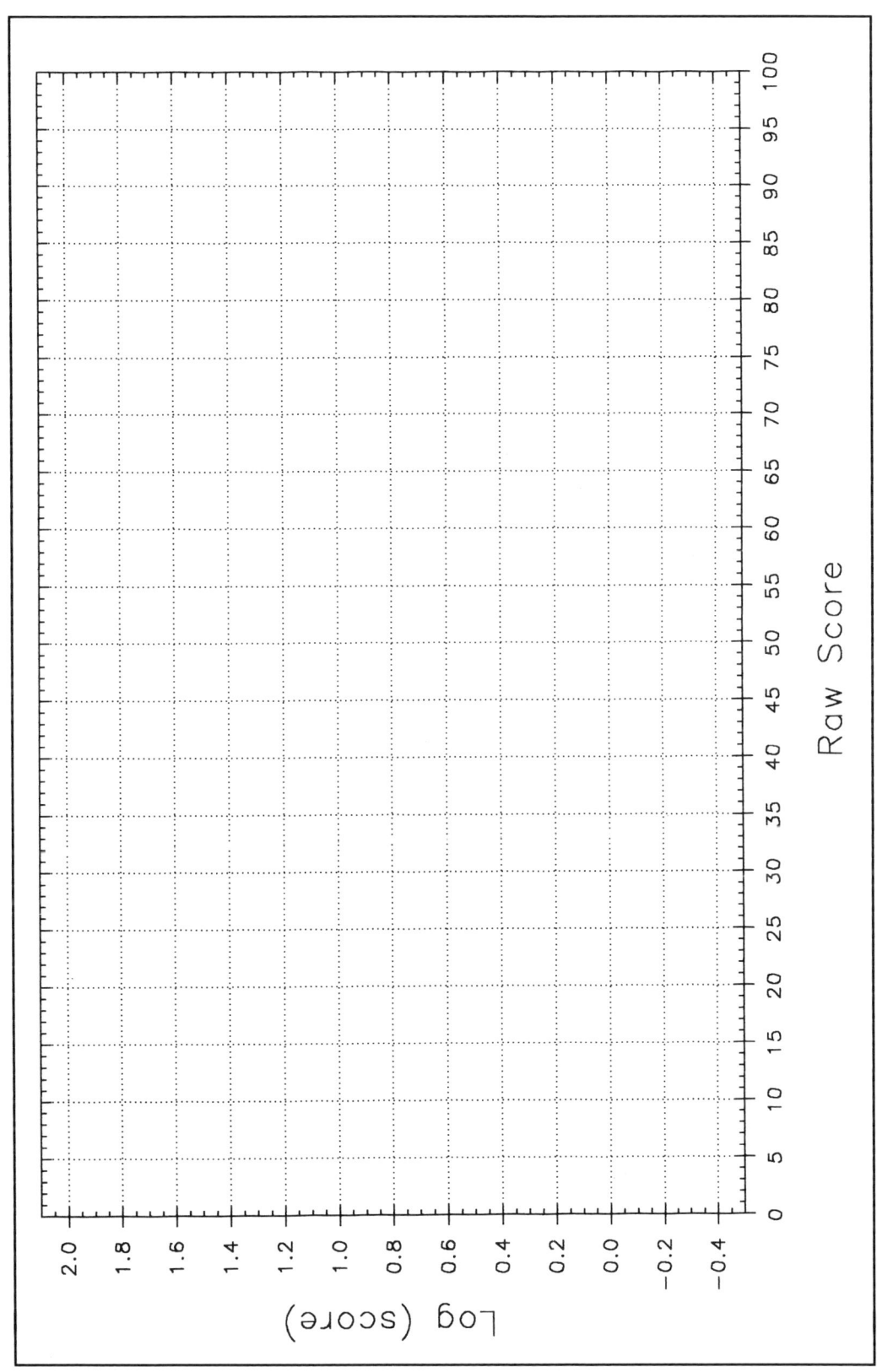

RELATIVE MEASURES AND LOGARITHMIC SCALING

Student   Date

    b. Suppose a 13th patient takes this test and obtains a score of 25.0. Examining the log values above, can you determine patient #13's log score? Explain.

    _____

    _____

    _____

    Indicate this score on your plot with an "x."

5. Use Appendix C to determine:

    a. log 4.95   = _____

    b. log 49,500 = _____

UNIT 6

Tutorial: Plotting Data

Much of the information available in our literature — and a significant amount of the data that we obtain from our patients — is in graph form. Not surprisingly, being able to read graphs and to plot data is a critical clinical skill. Although there are many, many ways to represent data graphically, almost all of the graphical information with which we need to deal is in the form of *Cartesian graphs,* the type of graph with which you are no doubt already familiar.

Purpose: These exercises will show you how to derive information from a graphic display and will provide you with a chance to hone your data-plotting skills.

General preparation: Review basic algebra, especially the principles of logarithms (see Unit 5 "Relative Measures and Logarithmic Scaling").

I. LINEAR GRAPHS

On all graphs, distances represent numbers. On a *linear* graph, the distance between two points is proportional to the size of the *difference* between two numbers; That is, the space between 10 and 20, for instance, is the same as the space between 1,010 and 1,020. Overall, linear graphs are probably the most common form of graphic display.

The vertical axis of the graph is generally referred to as the "Y axis" and the horizontal axis is the "X axis."[1] It is also common to name each axis for the variable displayed along it. (If "time" is one of the variables, it is almost always plotted on the X axis.) So, for instance, if one were to plot intraoral pressure as a function of time during an utterance, the vertical, or Y, axis might be called the "intraoral pressure axis"

---

[1] The X axis is sometimes referred to as the *axis of abscissas,* while the Y axis may be called the *axis of ordinates.*

and the horizontal, or X, axis, the "time axis." Any tick mark and/or label placed along an axis is called an *index*.

Exercises

1. Use the linear axes on the hand-in sheet to plot the following data points, and connect the points with straight lines:

   Mean Fundamental Frequency (F_0) of Non-Distress Vocalizations by Normal Infants.

Age (months)	Mean F_0 (Hz)
12	400
15	378
18	363
21	328
24	314

   Data adapted from "Developmental Trends in Vocal Fundamental Frequency of Young Children" by M. P. Robb and J. H. Saxman, 1985, *Journal of Speech and Hearing Research, 28*, 421–427. Table 4, p. 425. [Used with permission]

2. Write "Y =" in front of the label of the Y axis and write "X =" in front of the label of the X axis.

There are obviously many data points that aren't plotted. (That's because we don't have any information for them!) For instance, it is certainly true that children produce non-distress vocalizations at age 14 months, but their F_0 has not been studied by these researchers. Still, it is possible to "read between the data points" to get an estimate of what the F_0 at 14 months is likely to be. Such "reading between the data points" is called *interpolation*. It can be done simply with a little algebra. But if a highly precise answer is not needed, an interpolated value can be read directly from the graph.

Note carefully, however, that such interpolation is based on the assumption that the F_0 changes in a consistent way with age. That is, we don't expect any big surprises between 12 and 15 months! If that assumption is not likely to be valid, then you can't estimate in this way.

3. Do the following to find the expected F_0 of infant non-distress vocalizations at age 14 months:

   a. Draw a vertical line from age 14 months on the time index at the bottom of the graph, extending it straight up until it intersects the data line.[2]

---

[2] The distance traversed by this vertical line (extending from the X axis to the data point) is called the *ordinate* of that point.

b. From the point at which your line intersects the data line, extend a straight line to the left, until it intersects the "mean F_0" index.[3] **[The point at which this line intersects the index is the best estimate of the mean F_0 at age 14 months.]**

c. Add the F_0 that you have interpolated to the mean F_0 index.

4. Determine what mean F_0 should be at the age of 19 months. Add your 19-month estimate at the proper place on the mean F_0 index.

II. LOGARITHMIC GRAPHS

On a logarithmic graph, the location of numbers along the axis is proportional to the logarithm of the number. As a result, the distance between points is proportional to the *ratio* of the numbers plotted. Thus the distance separating 500 and 1,000 is the same as the distance that separates 5,000 and 10,000. Logarithmic graphs are convenient when a very large range of numbers must be plotted or when there is an inherently logarithmic relationship among the data points. Since the logarithm of 0 is an undefined quantity, there is no "zero point" on a logarithmic axis.

Exercises

1. Use the semi-logarithmic axes on the hand-in sheet to plot the following data. Your graph should have two data lines: one for the first-formant data, and another for the second-formant data.

Mean Formant Frequencies of /i/ at Different Ages.

Speaker Age (years)		Formant 1 (Hz)	Formant 2 (Hz)
3		484	3318
4		444	3050
5		408	3235
6		397	3108
7		411	3204
8		397	3104
9		403	3106
10		403	3028
11	(boys only)	397	2778
12	"	359	2877
13	"	355	2727

Data from "Development of speech sounds in children" by S. Eguchi and I. Hirsh, 1969, *Acta Otolaryngologica*, suppl. 257, 5–48. Table 1, pp. 9–13. [Used with permission]

---

[3] The distance traversed by this horizontal line (extending from the Y axis to the data point) is called the *abscissa* of that point. Together the ordinate and abscissa are called the *coordinates* of the data point.

2. Explain why a semi-logarithmic format was selected for this plot.

3. Use the full logarithmic axes on the hand-in sheet to prepare a "scatterplot" of the following data. For each vowel, plot formant 1 (X axis) against formant 2 (Y axis). (The data point for the vowel /i/ has already been plotted to give you an example.)

Mean Formant Frequencies of Women.

Vowel	Formant 1 (Hz)	Formant 2 (Hz)
/i/	310	2790
/ɪ/	430	2480
/ɛ/	610	2330
/æ/	860	2050
/ɑ/	850	1220
/ɔ/	590	920
/ʊ/	470	1160
/u/	370	950
/ʌ/	760	1400
/ɝ/	500	1640

Data from "Control methods used in a study of the vowels" by G. E. Peterson and H. L. Barney, 1952, *Journal of the Acoustical Society of America, 24,* 175–184. Table II, p. 183. [Used with permission]

The data plot on the opposite page shows the results of a study that investigated how speech intelligibility improved as sound pressure was increased. The questions that follow refer to this graph.

4. By interpolation, estimate the sound pressure level required to achieve 20% intelligibility?

5. Approximately how much intelligibility would be associated with a sound pressure level of 0.02 dynes?

6. How much must sound pressure be increased to change intelligibility from 15% to 30%?

7. Is intelligibility directly proportional to sound pressure?

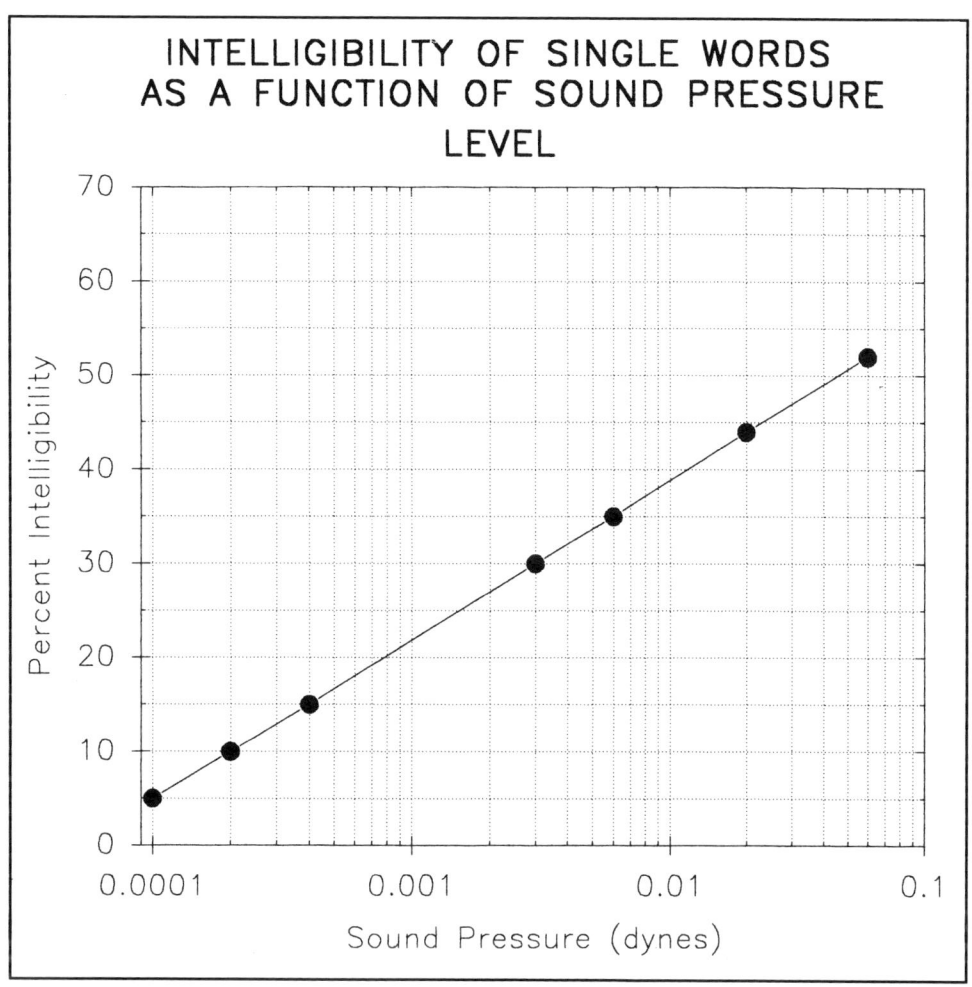

READ MORE ABOUT IT!

Bloom, M., & Fischer, J. (1982). *Evaluating practice: Guidelines for the accountable professional.* Englewood Cliffs, NJ: Prentice-Hall.

Silverman, F. H. (1993). *Research design and evaluation in speech language pathology and audiology* (3rd ed.). Englewood Cliffs, NJ: Prentice-Hall.

Tufte, E. R. (1983). *The visual display of quantitative information.* Cheshire, CT: Graphics Press.

Tufte, E. R. (1990). *Envisioning information.* Cheshire, CT: Graphics Press.

Ventry, I. M., & Schiavetti, N. (1986). *Evaluating research in speech pathology and audiology* (2nd ed.). New York: Macmillan.

Student _____ Date _____

PLOTTING DATA

I. LINEAR GRAPHS

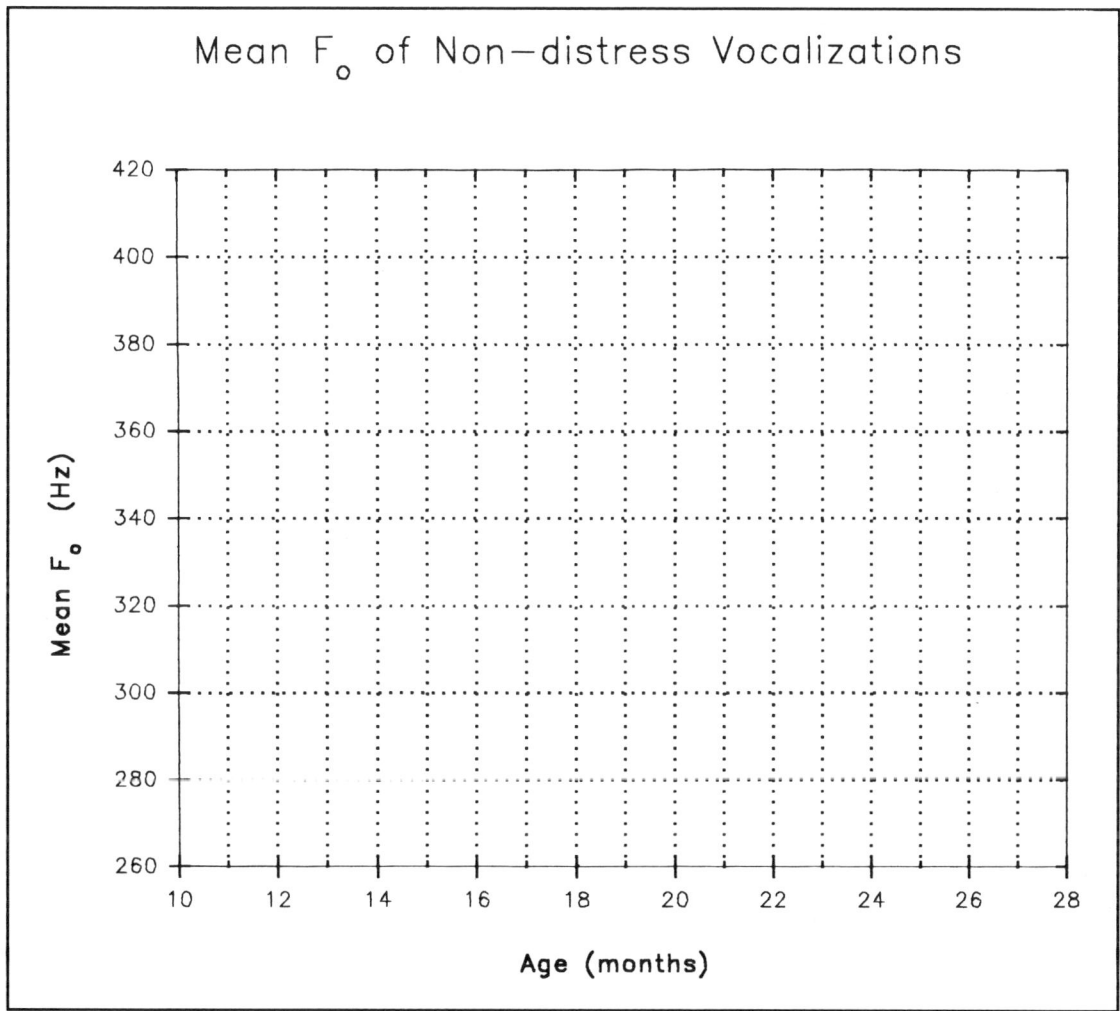

Student _____ Date _____

II. LOGARITHMIC GRAPHS

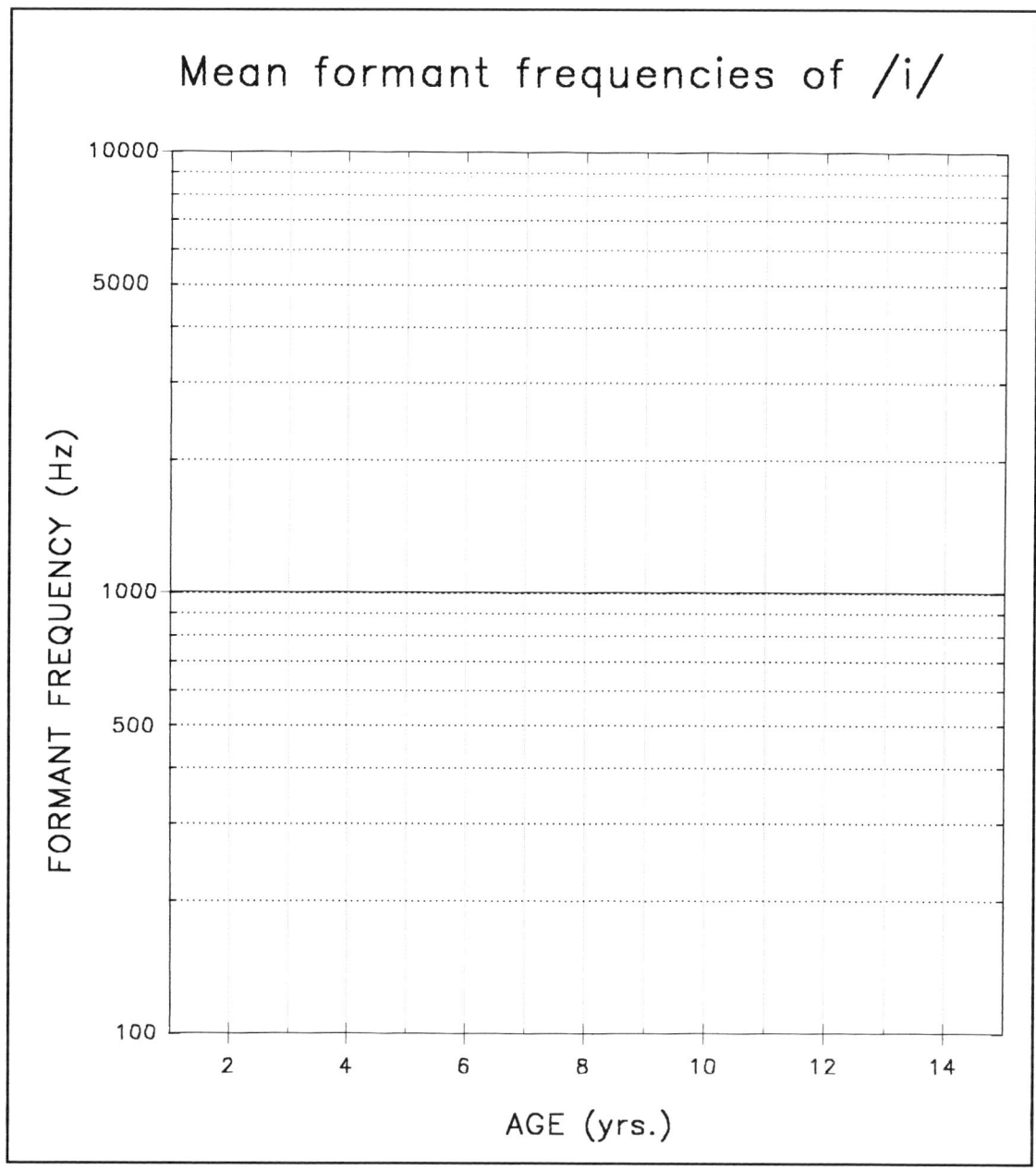

2. Reason for semi-logarithmic format: _____

_____

_____

Student _____ Date _____

_____
_____
_____
_____

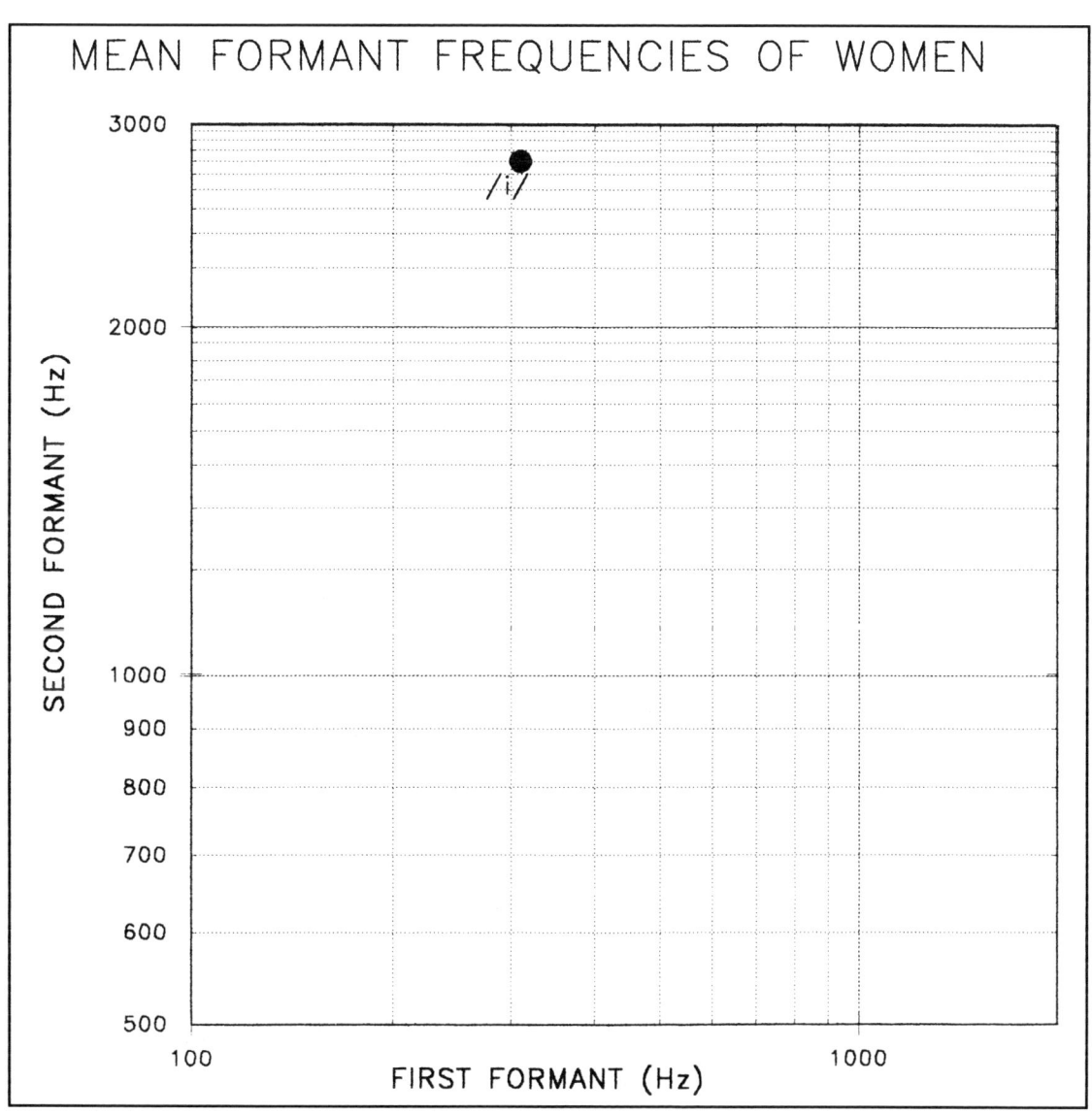

Student _____ Date _____

4. Sound pressure to achieve 20% intelligibility: _____

5. Intelligibility at 0.02 dynes: _____

6. Necessary sound pressure increase: _____
_____

7. Intelligibility and sound pressure: _____
_____
_____
_____

UNIT 7

Tutorial: Semitones

Just as we often compare two numbers in relative terms (for instance by expressing one as a percentage or proportion of the other as in the I-fraction), so it is often convenient to compare two frequencies in relative terms. For a number of reasons, the comparison of frequencies is a bit more complex. The *semitone* (ST) scale has been generally accepted as the best means of comparing frequencies. In the simplest sense, the semitone scale tells us how many notes of the musical scale (sharps and flats included) separate two frequencies.

The frequency, f_2, that is n semitones above or below another frequency, f_1, is

$$f_2 = 1.0595^n \times f_1$$

The number of semitones, n, that separates two frequencies, f_1 and f_2, is

$$n = 39.86 \times \log\left(\frac{f_2}{f_1}\right)$$

Purpose: In these exercises you will gain skill in calculating semitone values and will become familiar with the general principles of semitone scaling.

Equipment: Hand calculator with exponent and common logarithm functions.

General preparation: Review the bases of logarithmic scaling in general (see Unit 5 "Relative Measures and Logarithmic Scaling") and of ST scaling in particular (Baken, 1987, pp. 125–128).

EXAMPLES

1. You have an elderly male patient who can sustain a phonation as low as 85 Hz and as high as 150 Hz. The normative data in the literature (e.g., Ptacek, Sander, Maloney, & Jackson, 1966) indicate that an older male should have a range of about 25 ST. How does your patient compare to normal?

    The patient's frequency range in hertz is from:

    $$f_1 = 85 \text{ Hz, to}$$
    $$f_2 = 150 \text{ Hz.}$$

    The number of semitones between these limits is

    $$\begin{aligned} n &= 39.86 \times \log(f_2/f_1) \\ &= 39.86 \times \log(150/85) \\ &= 39.86 \times \log 1.765 \\ &= 39.86 \times 0.247 \\ &= 9.83 \text{ ST} \end{aligned}$$

    This patient has a much smaller frequency range than normal.

2. Actually, 85 Hz is not an unreasonable lower limit for a male's frequency range (e.g., Hollien, Dew, & Philips, 1971; Ptacek et al., 1966). The patient's problem seems to be in his inability to produce high frequencies. The norms indicate that he should be able to produce a frequency 25 ST above his lowest frequency. According to these norms, what is the highest frequency that your patient should be able to produce?

    We expect a frequency, f_2, that is ($n =$) 25 ST above an f_1 of 85 Hz. That frequency is

    $$\begin{aligned} f_2 &= 1.0595^n \times f_1 \\ &= 1.0595^{25} \times 85 \\ &= 4.242 \times 85 \\ &= 360.5 \text{ Hz} \end{aligned}$$

    According to the norms, this patient should be able to produce a frequency as high as 360.5 Hz.

    It is necessary occasionally to relate a frequency to a "standard." In this case the standard reference frequency is 16.35 Hz. That is, we agree that 16.35 Hz = 0 ST. Using this reference, then, any single frequency value may be converted to a semitone equivalent.

For example, a frequency of 500 Hz would equal:

$$n = 39.86 \times \log(f/16.35)$$
$$= 39.86 \times \log(500/16.35)$$
$$= 39.86 \times \log 30.581$$
$$= 39.86 \times 1.485$$
$$= 59.19 \text{ ST}$$

Thus, 500 Hz equals 59.19 ST re: 16.35 Hz.

Exercises

Provide your answers on the hand-in sheet.

1. What is the semitone equivalent of a mean speaking fundamental frequency of 133.68 Hz?

2. The A above middle C on a piano has a frequency of 440 Hz. The A that is one octave higher has a frequency of 880 Hz. How many semitones are in that octave?

3. The musical note high C has a frequency of 1046.5 Hz, and a C note one octave higher has a frequency of 2093.0 Hz. How many semitones are there in this octave?

4. From questions 2 and 3 above, deduce two rules concerning semitones: (a) How many semitones are in an octave? and (b) Moving up one octave on the musical scale represents how much frequency change?

5. Typically, people use a range of about 2.5 ST around their average F_0 when speaking. Therefore,

    a. If a male speaker uses an average F_0 of 120 Hz, about how high and how low would we expect his F_0 to range during normal speech?

    b. If a female's average speaking F_0 is 210 Hz, and her expected speaking range is $\pm$ 2.5 ST, what is the highest and lowest F_0 we would expect in her normal speech?

6. At the start of therapy, a young male patient uses a mean F_0 of 165 Hz while speaking. A goal of therapy is to lower his mean speaking F_0 to a more typical 120 Hz. By how many ST does the mean F_0 have to change?

7. A patient's maximal phonational frequency range (MPFR) extends from 140 Hz to 895 Hz. What is the patient's frequency range in ST?

8. Identify your own lowest modal register frequency and your highest falsetto register frequency. What is your MPFR as expressed in ST? How does it compare to ranges reported in the literature for normal speakers of your age and sex?

9. The note C below middle C has a frequency of 130.8 Hz. Use this information to complete the table on the hand-in sheet. Plot your results on the graph provided.

READ MORE ABOUT IT!

Baken, R. J. (1987). *Clinical measurement of speech and voice* (pp. 126–127). Boston: Little, Brown.

Fletcher, H. (1934). Loudness, pitch, and the timbre of musical tones and their relation to the intensity, the frequency, and the overtone structure. *Journal of the Acoustical Society of America, 6,* 59–69.

Hollien, H., Dew, D., & Philips, P. (1971). Phonational frequency ranges of adults. *Journal of Speech and Hearing Research, 14,* 755–760.

Jeans, J. (1937). *Science and music.* Cambridge: Cambridge University Press (reprinted by Dover, 1968).

Moravcsik, M. J. (1987). *Musical sound.* New York: Paragon.

Ptacek, P. H., Sander, E. K., Maloney, W. H., & Jackson, C. C. R. (1966). Phonatory and related changes with advanced age. *Journal of Speech and Hearing Research, 9,* 353–360.

Stevens, S. S., & Davis, H. (1938). *Hearing: Its psychology and physiology.* New York: John Wiley (reprinted by the Acoustical Society of America, 1983).

Young, R. W. (1939). Terminology for logarithmic frequency units. *Journal of the Acoustical Society of America, 11,* 134–139.

Student _____ Date _____

SEMITONES

Be sure to show your arithmetic along with your answer(s).

1. _____

2. _____

3. _____

4. _____
   _____
   _____

5. a. _____

   b. _____

6. _____

7. _____

8. _____
   _____
   _____
   _____
   _____
   _____

Student   Date

9. Determine the frequency of each of the notes in the following figure. Enter these values in the table on page 77 and plot them on the graph provided on page 78.

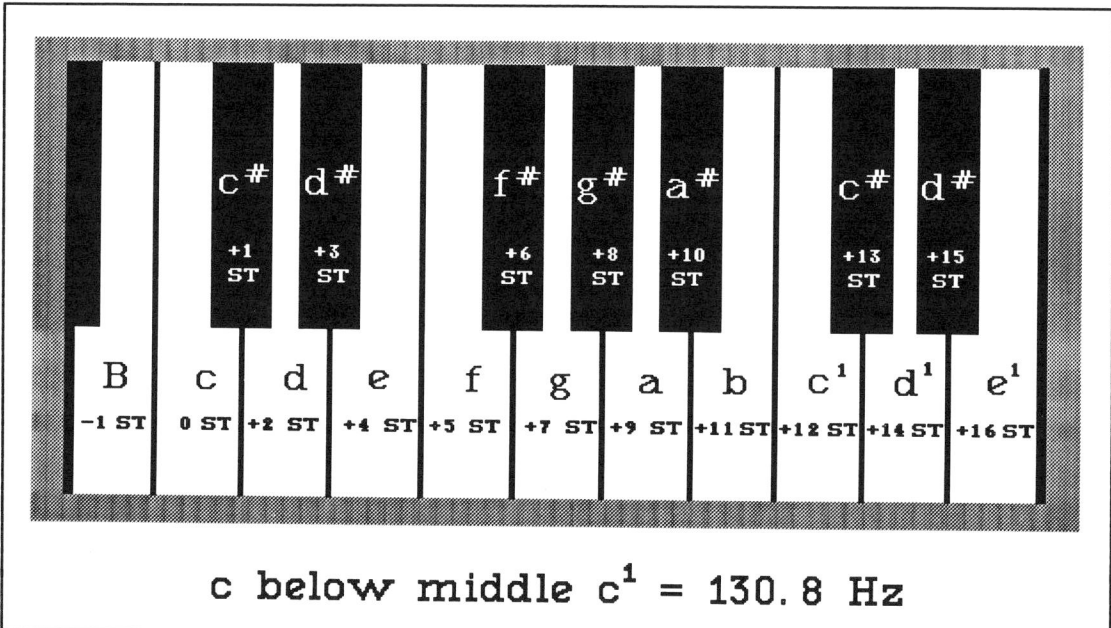

Student _____   Date _____

Note	Semitones re: c	Frequency in hertz
B	−1	_____
c	0	130.8
c#	+1	_____
d	+2	_____
d#	+3	_____
e	+4	_____
f	+5	_____
f#	+6	_____
g	+7	_____
g#	+8	_____
a	+9	_____
a#	+10	_____
b	+11	_____
c^1	+12	_____
$c\#^1$	+13	_____
d^1	+14	_____
$d\#^1$	+15	_____
e^1	+16	_____

Student					Date

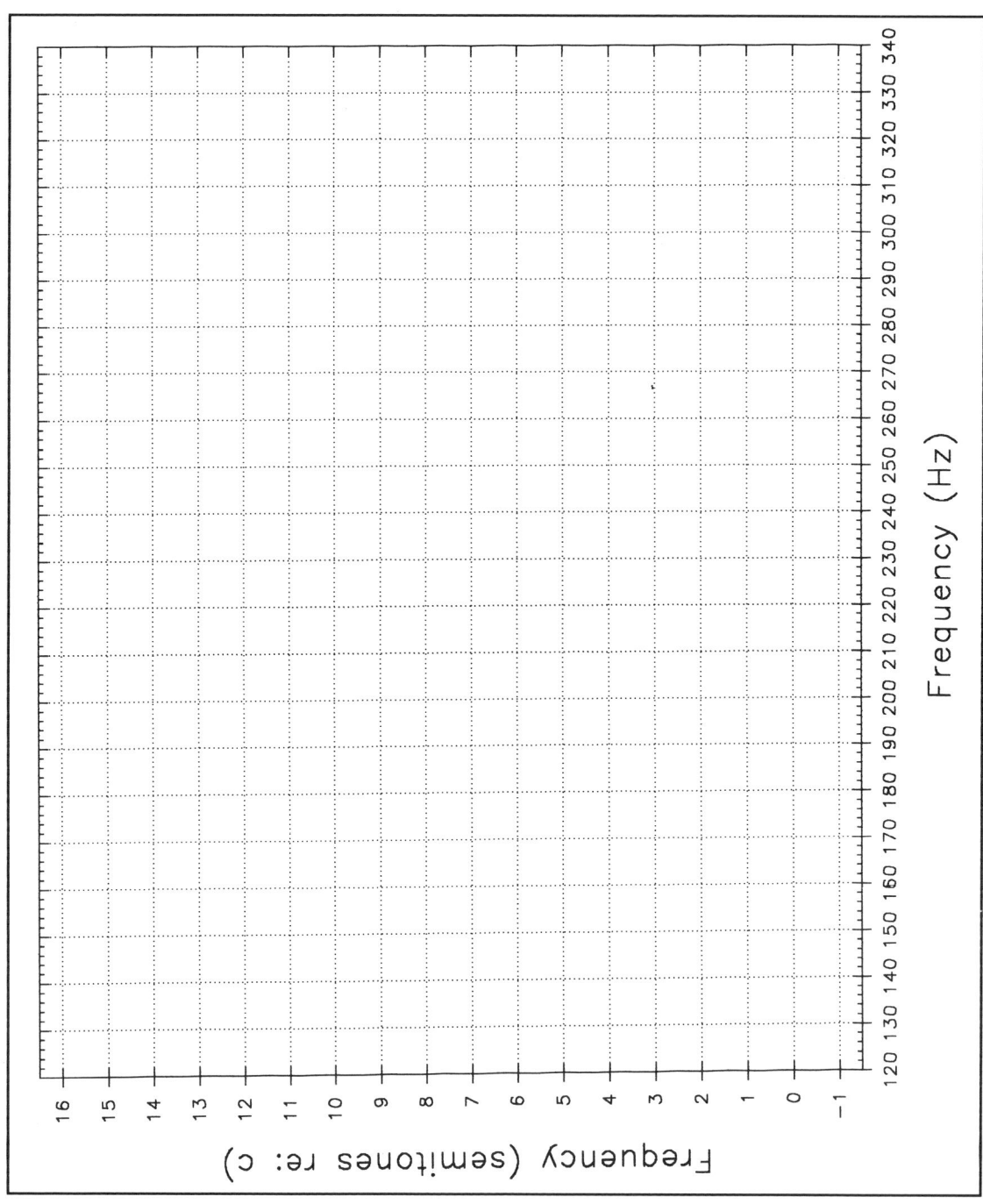

UNIT 8

Tutorial: Decibels

The most common form of relative scaling used in speech-language pathology is undoubtedly the decibel (dB)[1] scale. Unlike most of the relative measures we use, however, it is based not on a ratio, but on the *logarithm* of a ratio. It is therefore a *nonlinear* scale. In principle, almost any quantity (including, for example, air pressures or flows) can be scaled in terms of dB, but in practice the decibel scale is generally only used for sound pressure or sound power. There are several very good reasons why this seemingly complex system is used. The most important center on two facts. First, the human auditory system is sensitive to an enormous range of acoustic powers: from a just barely audible and amazingly small 10^{-16} watts (that is .0000000000000001 W) to a painfully loud 10^{-3} (.001 W). Dealing with so vast a range is cumbersome at best. The dB scale has the virtue of compressing the numerical range considerably. Second, auditory perception is not linear: the logarithmic nature of the dB transform more closely approximates the way in which perceived loudness grows as a function of sound power.

Purpose: In these exercises you will gain skill in calculating decibel values and will gain insight into general principles of decibel scaling.

General preparation: Review the bases of logarithmic scaling in general (see Unit 5 "Relative Measures and Logarithmic Scaling") and of dB scaling in particular (Baken, 1987; Speaks, 1992).

A value having the unit "dB" is *always* a comparison, either of one sound pressure to another or one sound power to another. This is clear in the statement, "As a result of therapy, vocal intensity increased by 11 dB." One readily understands that the statement indicates a comparison of pre-therapy and post-therapy vocal intensity. But very often the comparison involved is unstated and not obvious without a moment's thought. "Auditory threshold at 1000 Hz was 25 dB" is nonetheless a

---

[1] Note that "dB" is not an abbreviation but a *symbol* and thus is not written with a period.

comparative statement, even though the comparison is not stated. What it really says is "The smallest acoustic power of a signal of 1000 Hz to which the patient responds is 25 dB *greater than the power to which an average person responds.*" The comparison is there in the original statement, it's just not explicitly stated. Decibel values are *always, without exception, comparative.*

To say that a number represents a comparison implies that it is a ratio. Thus, a dB value is the expression of the ratio of sound powers (or sound pressures). If we let "I" denote sound power, then, in the case of the vocal therapy example, the ratio is $I_{\text{post-therapy}}/I_{\text{pre-therapy}}$. For the hearing threshold, the ratio is $I_{\text{patient's minimum}}/I_{\text{average minimum}}$. The power (or sound pressure) to which we are comparing (the denominator in the ratio) is called the *reference*.

The *Bel* is the logarithm (to the base 10) of this ratio:

$$\text{Bel} = \log (I_{\text{observed}}/I_{\text{reference}}).$$

But the Bel is a bit too coarse for everyday use. The entire range of normal hearing — the comparison of maximum audible sound power to minimum audible sound power — extends across only 13 Bels. Therefore we express the ratio in tenths of a Bel, or (using a standard metric-system prefix) *deci*bels. Thus, we define a decibel as

$$\text{dB} = 10 \times \log (I_{\text{observed}}/I_{\text{reference}}).$$

In words: dB is equal to *ten times the logarithm of the ratio of two powers.*

Exercises

Provide your answers on the hand-in sheet.

1. The "gain" of a system is the factor by which it increases the magnitude of an input. You are providing enhanced auditory feedback to your patient. The speech signal from the microphone has an average power of 3μW. The sound power reaching the patient's ears from the earphones is 182 μW. How much gain (in dB) have you provided?

2. As part of a research study you have determined that the average acoustic power for a subject's vowels is 442 μW. The same subject produces /s/ with an average power of 50 μW. What is the intensity (in dB) of the vowels compared to /s/?

It is also possible — and indeed quite common — to compare pressures rather than powers. (Note that electrical voltage is the equivalent of pressure.) Power, it turns out, is proportional to the square of pressure. Because of this, using the method we have employed so far, the dB relationship for two pressures (P) would be

$$dB = 10 \times \log (P_{observed}/P_{reference})^2.$$

Since the logarithm of the square of a number is equal to 2 times the log of the number, we can rewrite the dB pressure relationship as

$$dB = 10 \times 2 \times \log (P_{observed}/P_{reference}),$$

which is more conventionally written as

$$dB = 20 \times \log (P_{observed}/P_{reference}).$$

In words: dB is equal to *20 times the logarithm of the ratio of two pressures.*

3. A patient with a significant chest wall paralysis manages to produce an intraoral pressure (P_{io}) of only 2.5 cm H_2O during /t/. After therapeutic intervention, P_{io} for /t/ rises to 5.8 cm H_2O. Quantify the success of therapy in dB.

4. According to its manual, an amplifier used with a pressure transducer has a gain of 75 dB. If the transducer produces a maximum output voltage (electrical pressure) of 0.1 mV that serves as the input to the amplifier, what voltage would you expect the amplifier's output to be?

5. A patient with laryngeal paralysis can produce phonation with a sound pressure of 50 dB. After laryngeal surgery, her phonatory sound pressure doubled. By how many dB did her phonatory capability increase? (Hint: "Doubled" means the ratio of pre- and post-surgery phonatory sound pressure is 2).

6. Fill in the dB values in the table on the hand-in sheet.

7. Examine the values in the table. Can you deduce any rule about doubling and halving powers and pressures?

8. See if you can deduce a rule about multiplying a pressure or power by a factor of 10 and about dividing a pressure or power by 10.

9. Calculate the dB value of the pressure (all in µPa) on the table on the hand-in sheet. The reference pressure is 20 µPa. (The first one is done for you.) Plot your results on the graph provided. On the sheet with your plot, write any observations you may have about how dB increases with increasing pressure.

READ MORE ABOUT IT!

Baken, R. J. (1987). *Clinical measurement of speech and voice* (pp. 95–98). Boston: Little, Brown.

Borden, G. J., & Harris, K. S. (1984). *Speech science primer* (2nd ed., pp. 37–39). Baltimore: Williams & Wilkins.

Denes, P. B., & Pinson, E. N. (1993). *The speech chain: The physics and biology of spoken language* (2nd ed., pp. 37–43). New York: W. H. Freeman.

Deutsch, L. J., & Richards, A. M. (1979). *Elementary hearing science* (pp. 25–34). Baltimore: University Park Press.

Durrant, J. D., & Lovrinic, J. H. (1984). *Bases of hearing science* (2nd ed., pp. 52–62). Baltimore: Williams & Wilkins.

Fletcher, H. (1934). Loudness, pitch, and the timbre of musical tones and their relation to the intensity, the frequency, and the overtone structure. *Journal of the Acoustical Society of America, 6,* 59–69.

McPherson, D. L., & Thatcher, J. W. (1977). *Instrumentation in the hearing sciences* (pp. 73–78). New York: Grune & Stratton.

Speaks, C. E. (1992). *Introduction to sound: Acoustics for the hearing and speech sciences* (pp. 117–162). San Diego: Singular Publishing Group.

Zemlin, W. R. (1988). *Speech and hearing science* (3rd ed., pp. 430–431). Englewood Cliffs, NJ: Prentice-Hall.

Student _____   Date _____

DECIBELS

Be sure to show your arithmetic along with your answer(s).

1. Amplifier gain: _____

_____

_____

_____

2. /s/-vowel comparison: _____

_____

_____

_____

3. Intraoral pressure increase: _____

_____

_____

_____

4. Amplifier output: _____

_____

_____

_____

_____

5. Increase in phonatory capability: _____

_____

_____

_____

Student _____   Date _____

6. Fill in the dB values:

Input	Output	Ratio of Output to Input	dB
1. 10 mW (power)	20 mW	_____	_____
2. 47 μW "	94 μW	_____	_____
3. 10 mW "	5 mW	_____	_____
4. 2.5 W "	1.25 W	_____	_____
5. 3.4 V (pressure)	6.8 V	_____	_____
6. 8.7 cm H_2O "	17.4 cm H_2O	_____	_____
7. 13.2 cm H_2O "	6.6 cm H_2O	_____	_____
8. 14.6 mV "	7.3 mV	_____	_____

7. Doubling and halving: _____

_____

_____

_____

_____

8. Multiplication or division by 10: _____

_____

_____

_____

_____

Student _____ Date _____

9. Fill in the dB values. The reference pressure is 20 μPa.

Observed Pressure (μPa)	dB
5	−12.0
10	_____
15	_____
20	_____
40	_____
120	_____
200	_____
240	_____
320	_____
400	_____
500	_____
600	_____

Student _____ Date _____

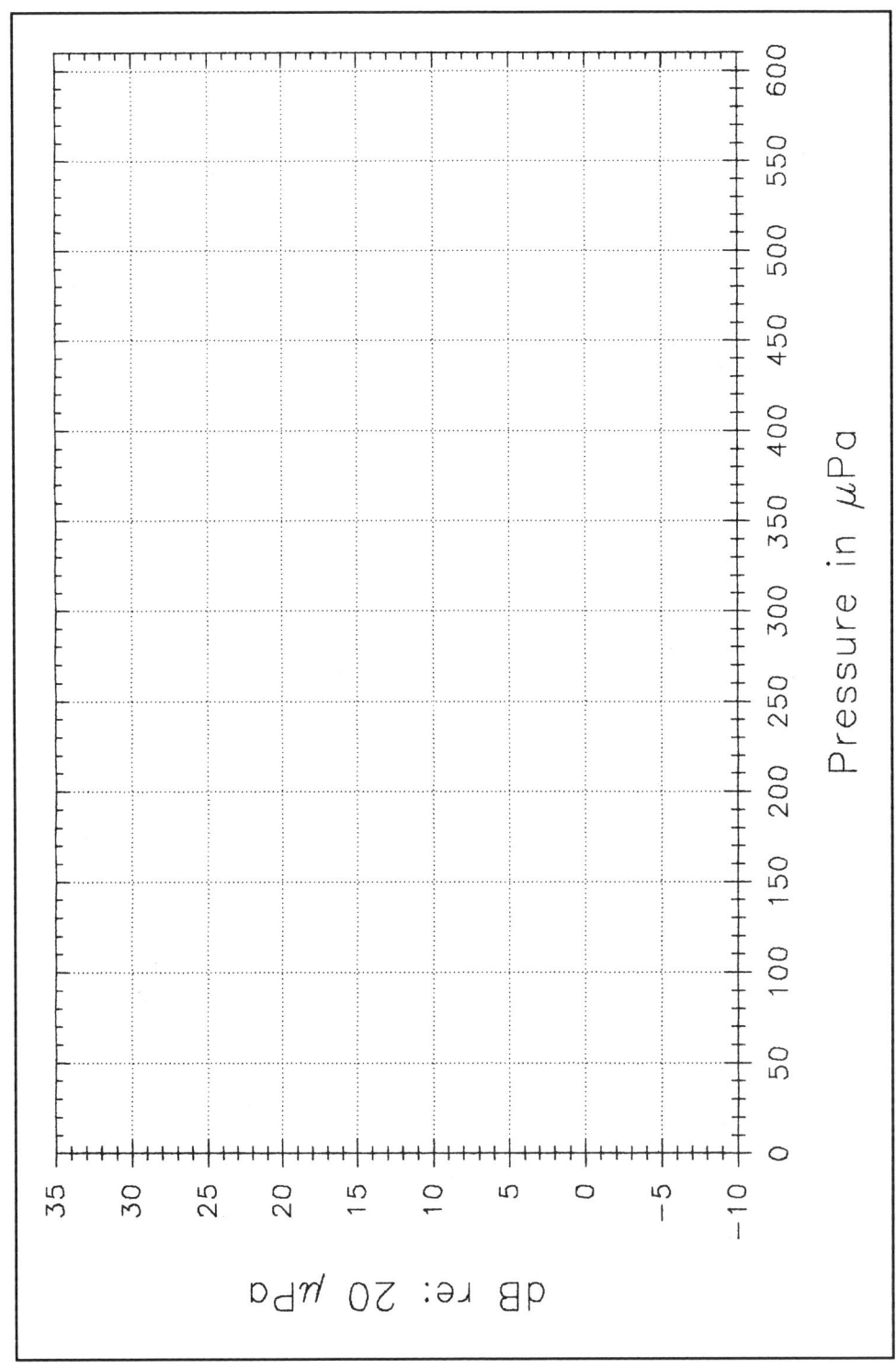

UNIT 9

Basic Skills: The Oscilloscope

The cathode-ray oscilloscope (commonly called a "scope") displays signals in visual form. Such signals might represent the changes in sound pressure transduced by a microphone or perhaps the nasal airflow sensed by a pneumotachograph system. Actually, any physical phenomenon that has been translated into an electrical voltage may be displayed as an *oscillogram*, which is a depiction of the signal as a two-dimensional (amplitude over time) waveform. An *oscillograph* functions like a scope, but instead provides a print (or "hard copy") of the oscillogram. While neither the oscilloscope nor the oscillograph analyzes signals, each facilitates subsequent measurement and analyses by providing a visualization of the waveforms.

The major components of any scope include two amplifiers and the cathode-ray tube (CRT), on which the waveform is actually shown. One of the amplifiers, called the horizontal or "time base" amplifier, controls the time scale of the display, and the other, referred to as the vertical amplifier, regulates the sensitivity of the vertical scale. A grid, or *graticule*, is typically placed in front of (or etched onto) the CRT screen to provide horizontal and vertical "divisions." The most useful scopes for clinicians are portable, allow for simultaneous display of at least two input signals (by employing two vertical amplifiers), and store waveforms on the CRT screen.

Purpose: In these exercises you will learn about the major components of the oscilloscope and you will practice obtaining and storing a clear display on the CRT screen.

Equipment: An oscilloscope (preferably a storage type), waveform (function) generator, tape recorder, microphone, and amplifier. An oscilloscope camera is optional, but recommended.

General preparation:

1. Read the instruction manual for your oscilloscope. Locate each of the following and briefly describe its function. Indicate the location of the controls on the outline of an oscilloscope provided on the hand-in sheet.

    a. Power switch
    b. Intensity control
    c. Focus
    d. Time base control (seconds/division)
    e. Vertical amplifier control (volts/division)
    f. Vertical trace position control
    g. Horizontal position control
    h. Automatic trigger control
    i. Trigger level control
    j. AC/DC/GROUND input switch
    k. Vertical input connector(s)
    l. CRT display graticule

    If you are using a *storage* oscilloscope, also locate and describe the following:

    m. Single sweep trigger control
    n. Storage control (for both upper and lower screen)
    o. Erase control
    p. Trigger reset

    If you are using a *dual-channel* oscilloscope (one with two vertical amplifiers), locate and describe:

    q. Alternate/chop selector

2. Turn on the oscilloscope and allow it to "warm up" for a few minutes. Set the time base (horizontal amplifier control) to 0.1 seconds per division (s/div) and be sure that the automatic trigger is activated. Adjust the beam intensity control so that the beam is clearly visible but is not surrounded by a "halo." Adjust the focus until the line is as sharply defined as possible.

I. FUNCTION OF THE VERTICAL AND HORIZONTAL AMPLIFIERS

1. To begin, disconnect all external inputs from the oscilloscope. Examine the controls for the scope's time base (horizontal) amplifier. There should be a setting marked "external." Set the control to the "external" setting. (The screen should show a single dot.) Now set the vertical amplifier's input control to GROUND.

2. You can now use the vertical and horizontal trace position controls to move the dot around the screen, as you would with an "Etch-A-Sketch" toy. Practice moving the dot around, but set it to the center of the screen when you are finished.

3. Now change the time base control to 1 s/div (or as close to that setting as your oscilloscope allows). The dot on the screen will move from left to right and then (invisibly) return to the left of the screen and move to the right once more, repeatedly. How long does it take the dot to move through one screen division? How long to traverse the entire screen?

   Because the dot is moving at a constant speed, each point on the horizontal axis of the CRT display represents a point in time during a single sweep of the dot. The horizontal axis of the screen has now become a *time* axis.

4. Change the time base setting to make the dot move faster. Keep increasing the dot's speed as you observe the screen. How does the appearance of the dot change? At what speed does the dot become a line? How do you explain this phenomenon?

5. Reset the time base control to a speed of about 0.5 s/div. Use the vertical amplifier control to move the dot up and down while the trace is moving across the screen.

   You are really creating a graph of the movement of the vertical-position control knob over time.

6. Now set the time base to about 5 milliseconds per division (5 ms/div) and again move the vertical position control. Are you still generating a graph of control-knob position over time? Explain.

II. AC/DC COUPLING

1. Set the time base amplifier for about 0.2 s/div. Leave the vertical input switch set to GROUND and use the vertical position control to locate the trace at the center of the CRT screen.

2. Set the vertical amplifier to its least sensitive setting (greatest number of volts/division). Connect the output of a waveform (function) generator to the input of the vertical amplifier. Turn on the waveform generator and set it to produce a *1-Hz square wave* of moderate amplitude (perhaps 1 volt).

3. Now change the vertical amplifier's input switch to obtain DC coupling. Adjust the vertical amplifier's sensitivity until the square wave takes up about 3/4 of the height of the screen. (If necessary, you may also adjust the amplitude control on the waveform generator.)

4. Draw the trace as it appears on the screen in the space provided on the hand-in sheet. (Alternatively, you may paste a photograph of the scope screen on the sheet.) Label your sketch (or photograph) to show the sensitivity of the vertical amplifier and the setting of the time base.

5. Now change the vertical amplifier's input switch to obtain AC coupling. Draw the wave as it now appears on the screen (or paste a photograph onto the hand-in sheet).

6. What has caused the change in waveshape that you have observed?

7. How might the choice of coupling (AC or DC) affect the display of slowly changing phenomena (such as nasal airflow) and rapidly changing signals (such as the acoustic wave of a vowel)?

III. ADJUSTING THE TIME BASE AND VERTICAL GAIN

1. Connect a microphone to an amplifier, and then connect the amplifier output to the vertical amplifier of the oscilloscope using AC coupling.

2. Sustain a vowel at a comfortable pitch and loudness while you observe the oscilloscope display. Adjust the time base so that approximately five cycles of your vowel waveform appear on the CRT screen. (If the display is not stable, try adjusting the trigger control.) Set the sensitivity of the vertical amplifier so that your signal covers between 2/3 and 3/4 of the height of the screen. What is the time base setting? If you have a camera, attach a photograph of the vowel waveform to the hand-in sheet.

3. Because you know the time base setting, you can calculate the mean fundamental frequency (F_0) of the vowel waveform that you have photographed. Indicate the F_0 on the hand-in sheet.

4. Now produce a different vowel at a higher pitch. Change the sensitivity of the vertical amplifier so that the waveform occupies between 2/3 and 3/4 of the screen height. Adjust the time base again, so that about 5 cycles appear on the screen. What is the new time base setting? Photograph this waveform, and attach it to the hand-in sheet.

5. Calculate the mean F_0 of this higher-pitched vowel production.

6. Using a tape recorder (or recording system), record the utterance "one-two-four-three" at a normal pitch and loudness and at a moderate rate. Disconnect the microphone and amplifier from the scope input, and instead connect the output of the tape deck (or recorder). Play back the recording and adjust the scope for a display of appropriate height. Use a fairly slow time base setting, so

that all of the syllables occupy a single screen. (You will probably have to play back your recording several times to adjust your scope properly.) What time base setting did you find most appropriate?

7. Examine the display carefully, trying to match features of the speech sounds to the acoustic record on the screen. Photograph the screen and attach it to the hand-in sheet. Also, using IPA symbols, show the location of various phones in the oscillogram. Add a word or two to your labels to indicate which features let you identify each speech sound.

READ MORE ABOUT IT!

Baken, R. J. (1987). *Clinical measurement of speech and voice* (pp. 78–89). Boston: Little, Brown.

Cooper, W. D. (1978). *Electronic instrumentation and measurement techniques* (2nd ed., pp. 200–268). Englewood Cliffs, NJ: Prentice-Hall.

Curtis, J. F., & Schultz, M. C. (1986). *Basic laboratory instrumentation for speech and hearing* (pp. 135–146). Boston: Little, Brown.

Decker, T. N. (1990). *Instrumentation: An introduction for students in the speech and hearing sciences* (pp. 59–64). New York: Longman.

Middleton, R. G. (1980). *Know your oscilloscope* (4th ed.). Indianapolis: Howard W. Sams.

Pronovost, W. (1947). Visual aids to speech improvement. *Journal of Speech Disorders, 12,* 387–391.

Schwartz, M. F. (1969). Use of a storage oscilloscope in speech therapy. *Journal of Speech and Hearing Disorders, 34,* 111–112.

Sessions, K. W., & Fischer, W. A. (1978). *Understanding oscilloscopes and display waveforms.* New York: Wiley.

Student   Date

THE OSCILLOSCOPE

GENERAL PREPARATION

1. Use the schematic illustration below to show the location of the controls on your oscilloscope.

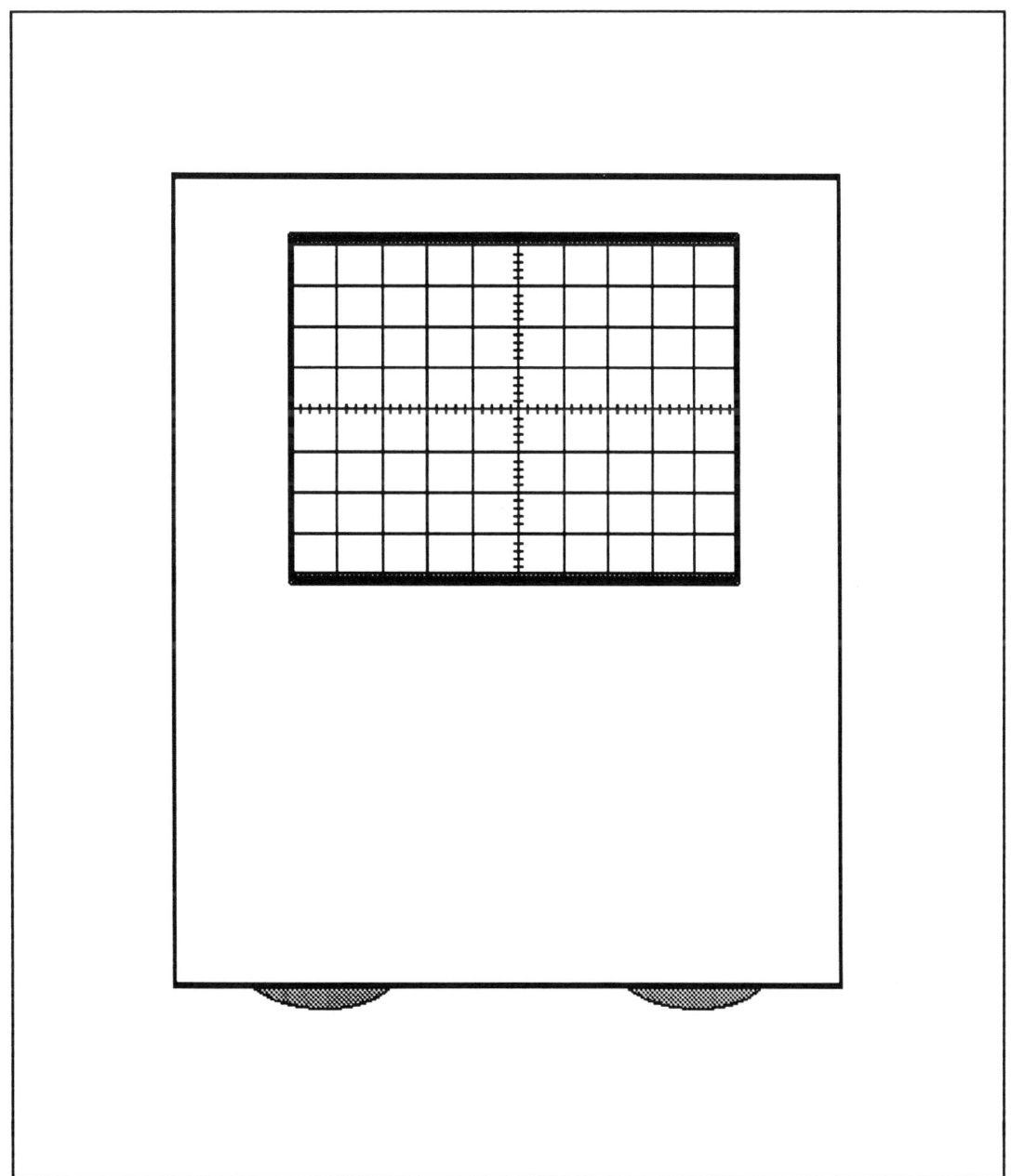

THE OSCILLOSCOPE **93**

Student _____ Date _____

Briefly describe the function of the oscilloscope's major controls:

a. Power switch: _____

_____

b. Intensity control: _____

_____

c. Focus: _____

_____

d. Time base: _____

_____

e. Vertical amplifier: _____

_____

f. Vertical trace position: _____

_____

g. Horizontal position: _____

_____

h. Automatic trigger: _____

_____

i. Trigger level: _____

_____

j. AC/DC/GROUND: _____

_____

k. Vertical input: _____

_____

Student _____   Date _____

l. CRT display graticule: _____

_____

m. Single sweep trigger: _____

_____

n. Storage control: _____

_____

o. Erase control: _____

_____

p. Trigger reset: _____

_____

q. Alternate/chop selector: _____

_____

I. FUNCTION OF THE VERTICAL AND HORIZONTAL AMPLIFIERS

3. Time to traverse one division: _____

Time to traverse entire screen: _____

4. Time base setting when dot becomes line: _____

Explain: _____

_____

_____

6. Graph of knob position over time? _____

_____

_____

_____

THE OSCILLOSCOPE

Student _____ Date _____

II. AC/DC COUPLING

4 and **5.** Draw your square waves below or attach your photographs.

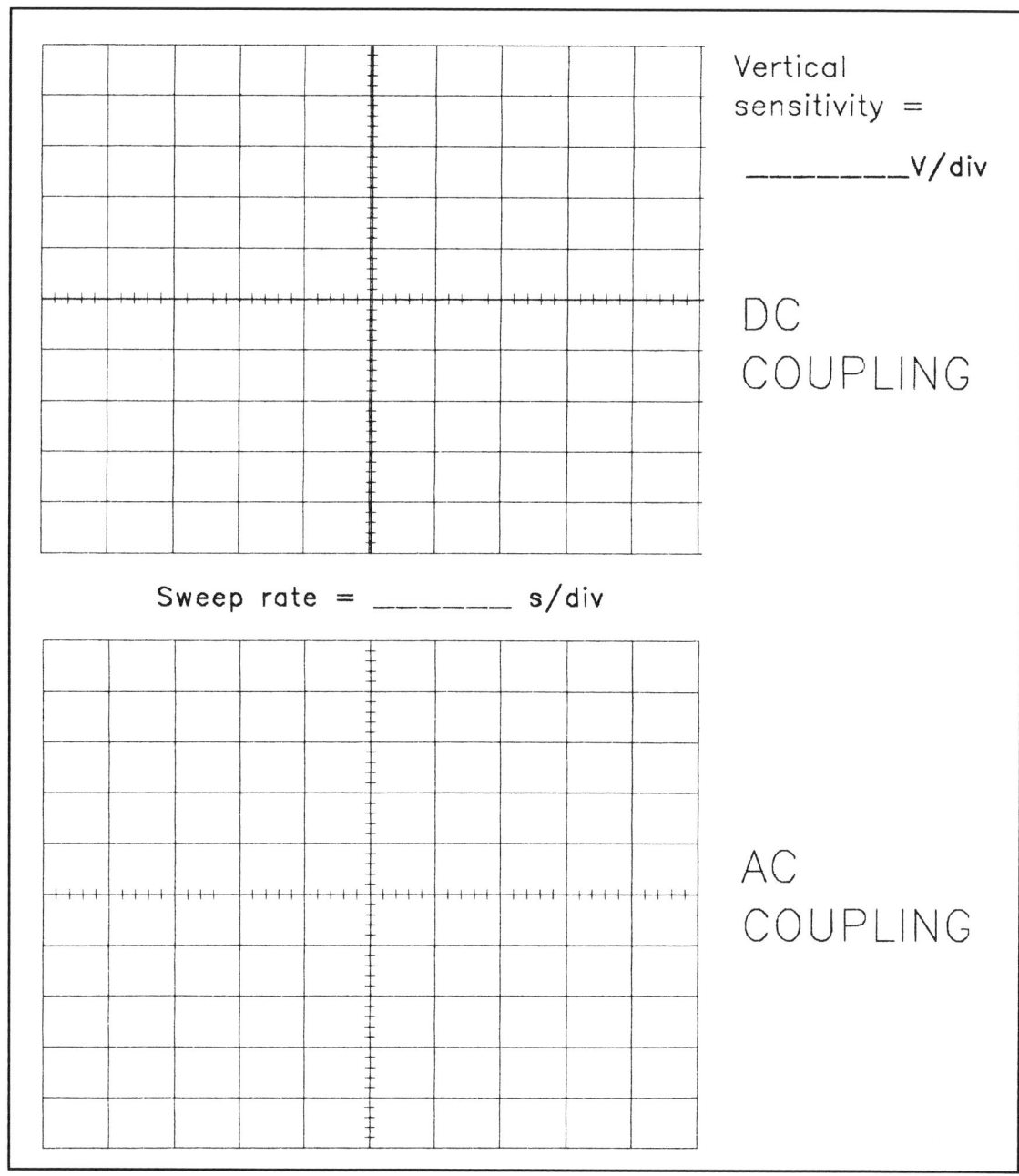

Student   Date

(You may use these oscillograms of square waves instead of producing your own):

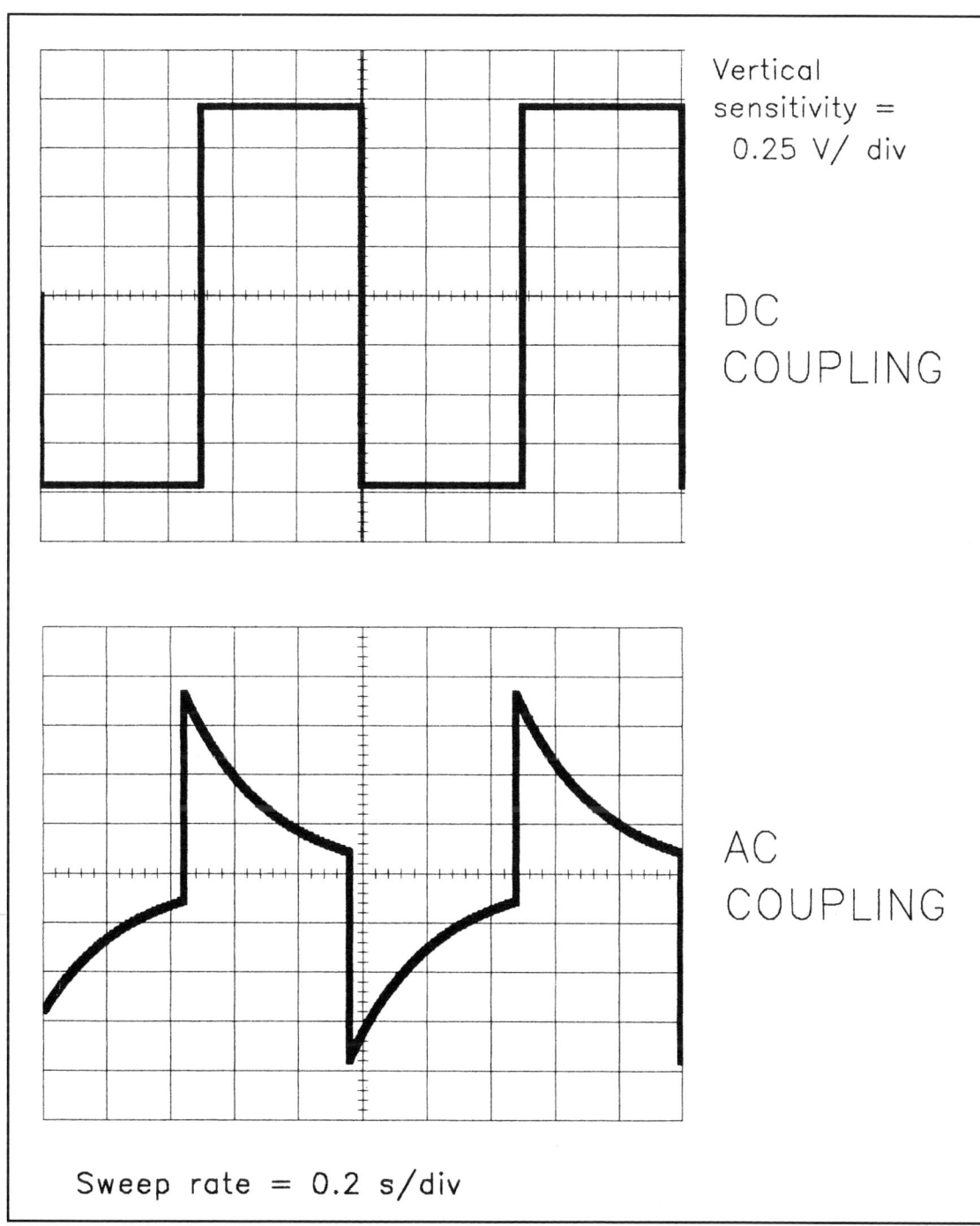

Student   Date

6. Why has changing DC to AC coupling changed the appearance of the square wave?

7. How might the choice of coupling affect the display of slowly changing phenomena?

Student _____ Date _____

III. ADJUSTING THE TIME BASE AND VERTICAL GAIN

2. Your sweep rate (time base setting): _____

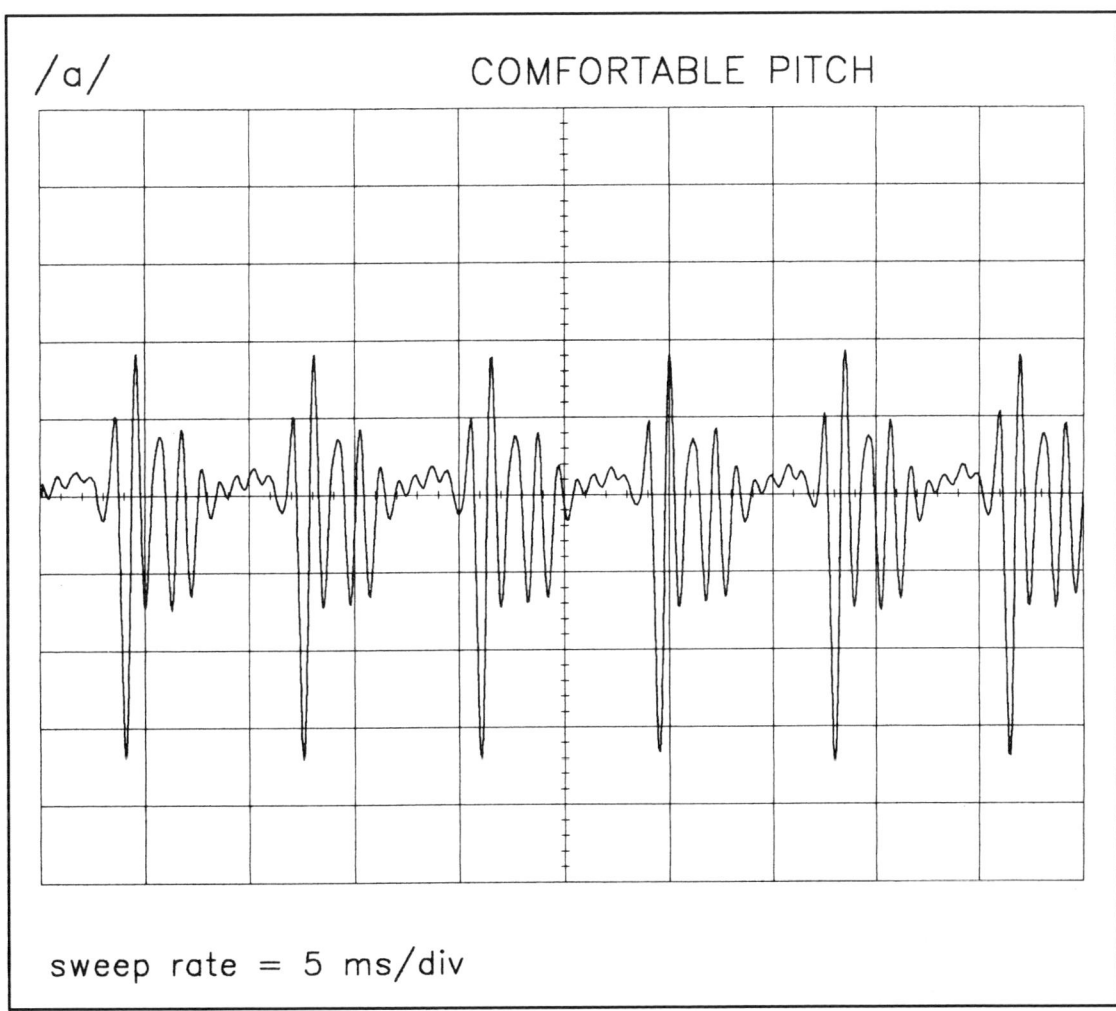

3. There are about _____ cycles in the _____-ms record above.

Therefore, mean fundamental frequency (F_0) is about _____.

Student   Date

4. Your sweep rate (time base setting): _____

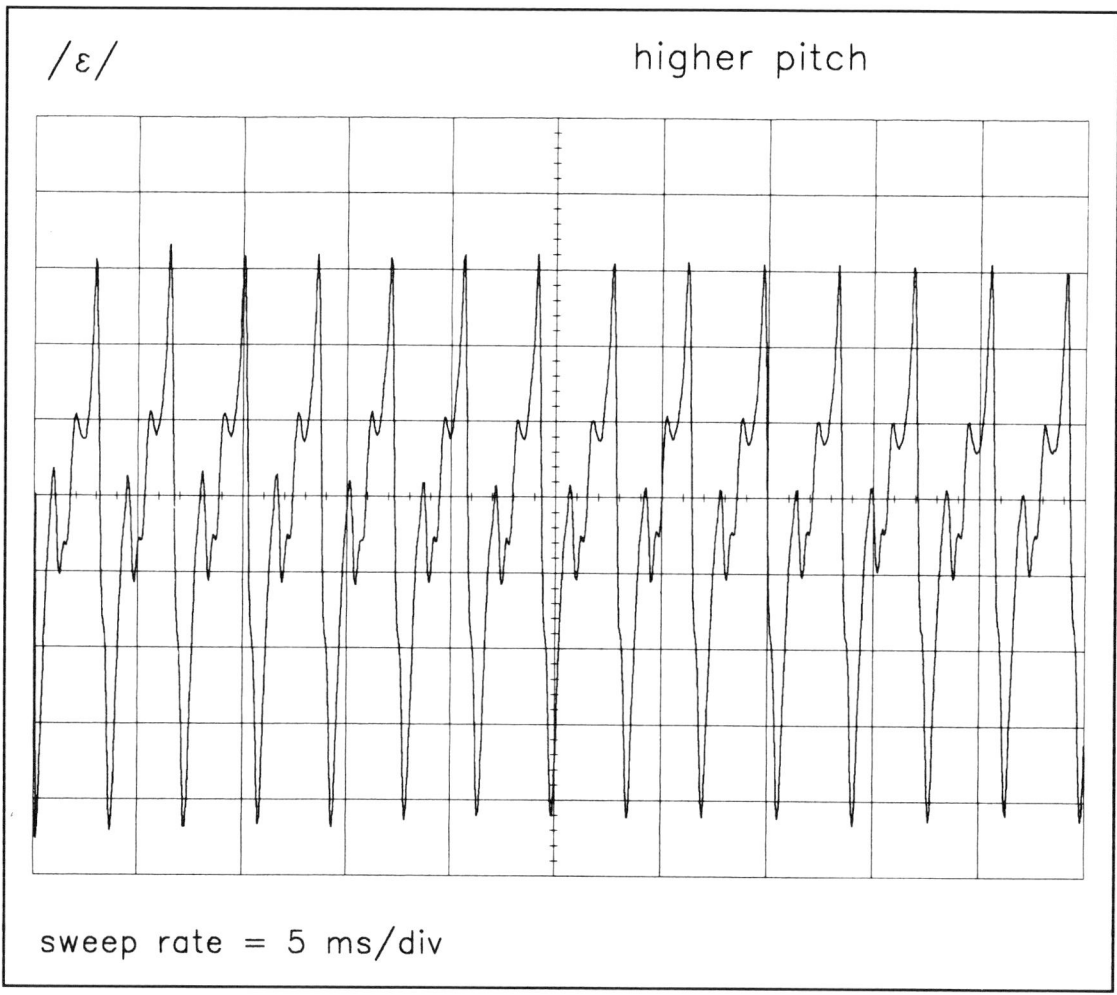

5. There are about _____ cycles in the _____-ms record above.

Therefore, mean fundamental frequency (F_0) is about _____ .

Student   Date

6 and 7. You may use the oscillogram of a tape recording provided below, or paste your own oscillogram over it.

Your sweep rate (time base setting): _____

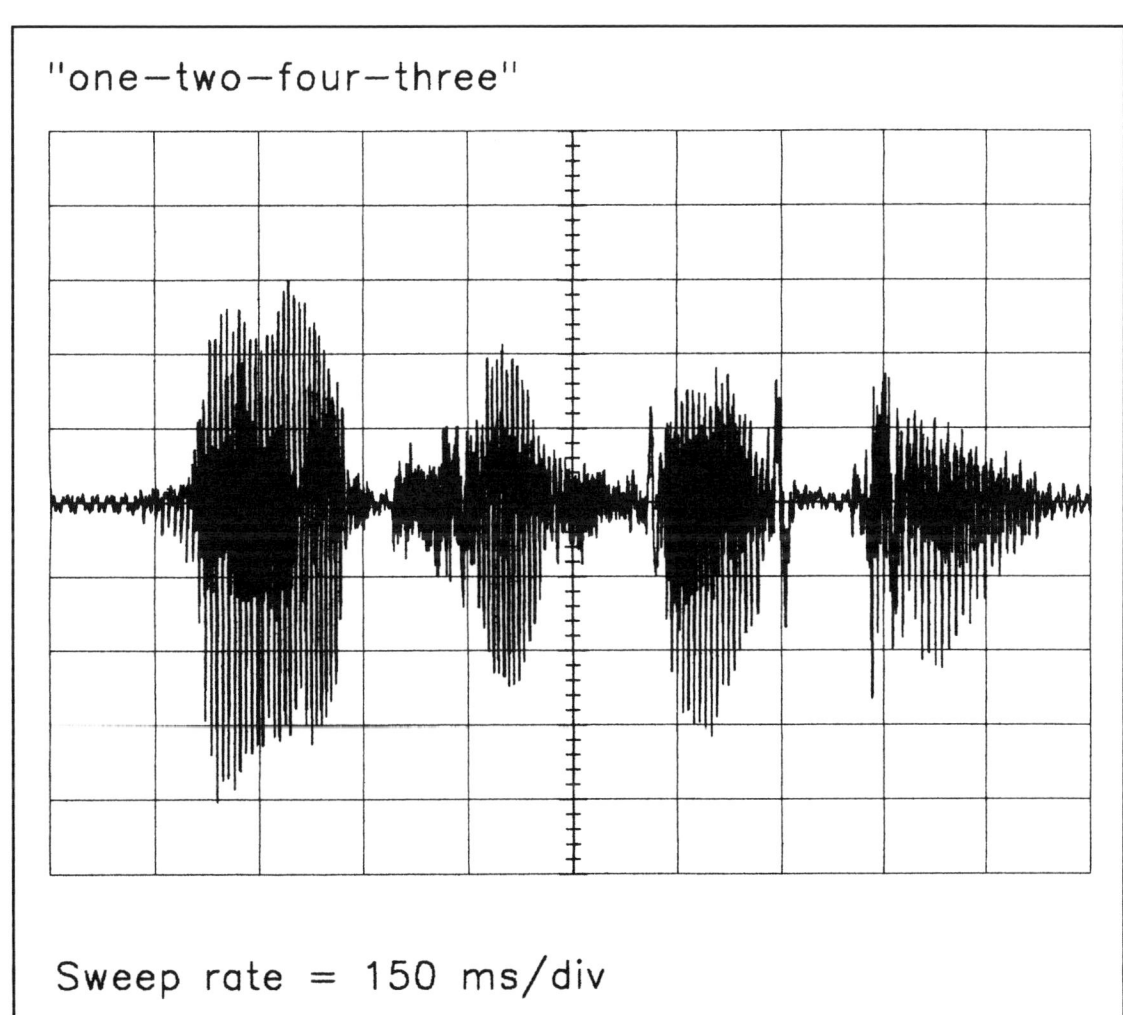

Basic Skills: Reading Oscillograms

Purpose: In these exercises you will use oscillograms of the acoustic signal to derive amplitude- and time-based data. In particular, you will determine the mean vocal period, fundamental frequency, and peak-to-peak amplitude of several sustained vowels. You will also practice segmenting speech utterances into their constituent phones based on the salient acoustic features.

Equipment: A microphone and a means of generating a printed oscillogram (for example, an oscilloscope and camera, visicorder/oscillograph, or computerized system).

I. SUSTAINED PHONATIONS

1. On the hand-in sheet are several oscillograms of short segments extracted from phonations sustained by five different speakers:

   A. Normal 33-year-old male
   B. Normal 31-year-old female
   C. Normal 16-month-old female
   D. Incomplete vocal mutation, 17-year-old male
   E. Vocal fold polyp, 6-year-old male

   a. Mark each of these oscillograms to delineate every vocal period and amplitude in the sample.

   b. Determine the mean vocal period (t, in seconds), fundamental frequency (F_0, in hertz), and peak-to-peak amplitude (in volts) of each sample and enter these data in the table on the hand-in sheet.

c. Obtain a sample of your own /ɑ/ sustained at a comfortable pitch and loudness (see Unit 9 "The Oscilloscope"). Measure the mean t, F_0, and amplitude characteristics of your production. Enter these values in the table for speaker "F," indicating your age and sex.

   d. Obtain a sample of /ɑ/ sustained by a dysphonic speaker at the patient's comfortable pitch and loudness. Enter these data in the table for speaker "G" along with some short descriptive information.

2. Which of the oscillograms above (A–G) proved most difficult when you attempted to determine the mean frequency and amplitude? Explain.

3. Compare speaker D's mean F_0 to those reported in the literature for young adult males sustaining a "comfortable" vowel or speaking (for example, Brown, Murry, & Hughes, 1976; Fitch & Holbrook, 1970; Hollien & Jackson, 1973; Murry & Doherty, 1980). Would you consider this speaker's mean F_0 "within normal limits"? What are some of the problems you face when trying to relate the present data to so-called "norms"?

4. Compare your patient's (speaker G's) data to those measured from your own sample. Describe possible reasons for any similarities or differences.

II. SPEECH

1. An oscillogram of a simple utterance as might be displayed on the commercially available Computerized Speech Lab (CSL™) system[1] is shown on the hand-in sheet. (The short vertical lines at the bottom of the display are "voicing marks" provided by the analysis software.) Mark this oscillogram to show:

   a. Any portion that is a vowel or vowel-like (V) sound;

   b. Any portion that is a fricative (F);

   c. Any portion that is a plosive (P);

   d. Any portion that is an affricate (A).

   e. If this utterance is likely to be a "yes/no" question, place a large question mark at its end.

   f. Explain the reasons for your choices in the space provided.

2. A similar acoustic record of the word "apples" is also shown on the hand-in sheet, along with a phonetic transcription. Using this display:

---

[1] CSL, model 4300, Kay Elemetrics Corporation, Pine Brook, NJ (software version 3.11).

a. Mark the "boundaries" between each of the indicated phones with vertical lines.

b. Why is it difficult to determine the exact location of isolated speech sounds within a spoken utterance?

c. Which syllable was stressed? Explain your answer.

3. Obtain an oscillogram of the phrase "Say apples again." Mark your oscillogram to identify the general location of each phone within the word "apples." Compare this production to that provided for #2 (page 116).

READ MORE ABOUT IT!

Baken, R. J. (1987). *Clinical measurement of speech and voice*. Boston: Little, Brown.

Brown, W. S., Jr., Murry, T., & Hughes, D. (1976). Comfortable effort level: An experimental variable. *Journal of the Acoustical Society of America, 60*, 696–699.

Fitch, J. L., & Holbrook, A. (1970). Modal vocal fundamental frequency of young adults. *Archives of Otolaryngology, 92*, 379–382.

Hollien, H., & Jackson, B. (1973). Normative data on the speaking fundamental frequency characteristics of young adult males. *Journal of Phonetics, 1*, 117–120.

Kent, R. D., & Read, C. (1992). *The acoustic analysis of speech*. San Diego: Singular Publishing Group.

Minifie, F. D. (1973). Speech acoustics. In F. D. Minifie, T. J. Hixon, & F. Williams (Eds.), *Normal aspects of speech, hearing, and language* (pp. 235–284). Englewood Cliffs, NJ: Prentice-Hall.

Murry, T., & Doherty, E. T. (1980). Selected acoustic characteristics of pathologic and normal speakers. *Journal of Speech and Hearing Research, 23*, 361–369.

Painter, C. (1979). *An introduction to instrumental phonetics* (pp. 25–33). Baltimore: University Park Press.

Pickett, J. M. (1980). *The sounds of speech communication*. Austin, TX: Pro-Ed.

Robb, M. P., & Saxman, J. H. (1985). Developmental trends in vocal fundamental frequency of young children. *Journal of Speech and Hearing Research, 28*, 421–427.

Schwartz, M. F. (1969). Use of a storage oscilloscope in speech therapy. *Journal of Speech and Hearing Disorders, 34*, 111–112.

Shoup, J. E., & Pfeifer, L. L. (1976). Acoustic characteristics of speech sounds. In N. J. Lass (Ed.), *Contemporary issues in experimental phonetics* (pp. 171–224). New York: Academic Press.

Weismer, G. (1984). Acoustic descriptions of dysarthric speech: Perceptual correlates and physiological inferences. *Seminars in Speech and Language, 5*, 293–314.

Student _____ Date _____

READING OSCILLOGRAMS

I. SUSTAINED PHONATIONS

1. Determine the mean period (t), fundamental frequency (F_0), and peak-to-peak amplitude of each of the speakers' oscillograms to complete the following table.

Speaker	Mean t (in s)	Mean F_0 (in Hz)	Mean Amplitude (in volts)
A. Male, 33 years	_____	_____	_____
B. Female, 31 years	_____	_____	_____
C. Female, 16 months	_____	_____	_____
D. Male, 17 years	_____	_____	_____
E. Male, 6 years	_____	_____	_____
F. Yourself (_____)	_____	_____	_____
G. Your Patient (_____)	_____	_____	_____

Student _____ Date _____

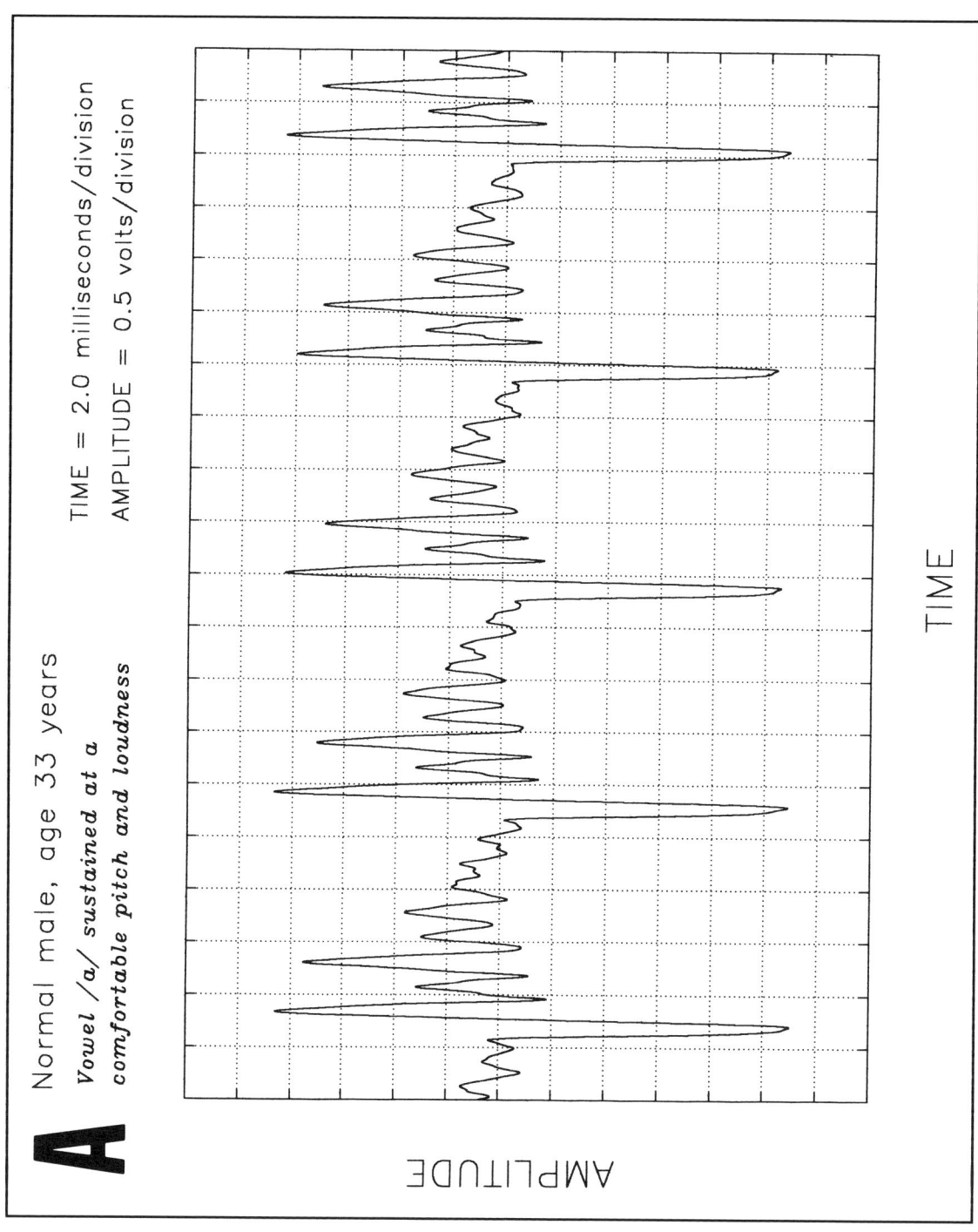

A Normal male, age 33 years
Vowel /a/ sustained at a comfortable pitch and loudness

TIME = 2.0 milliseconds/division
AMPLITUDE = 0.5 volts/division

Student _____ Date _____

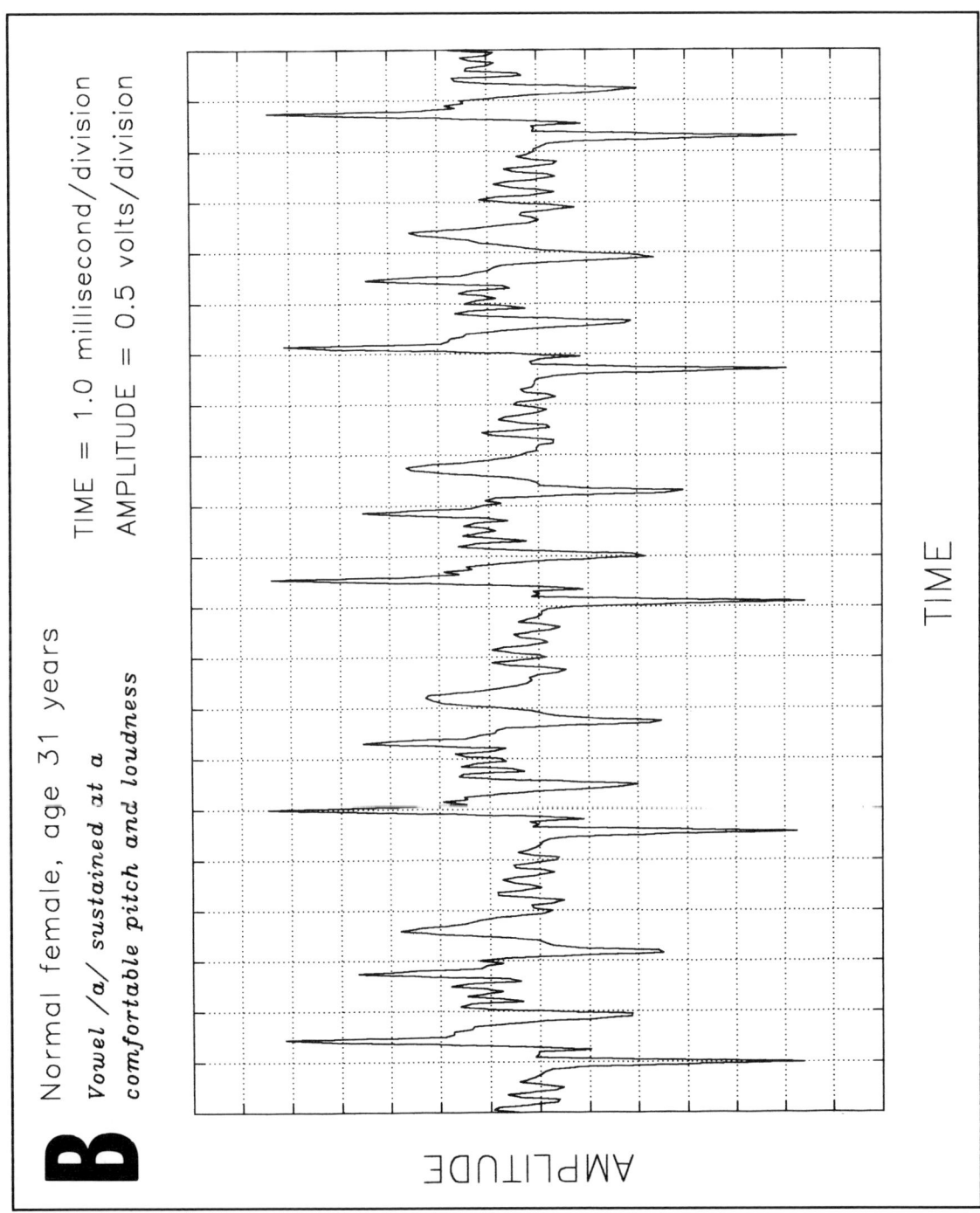

READING OSCILLOGRAMS 109
Copyright © 1993 Singular Publishing Group, Inc. All rights reserved.

Student   Date

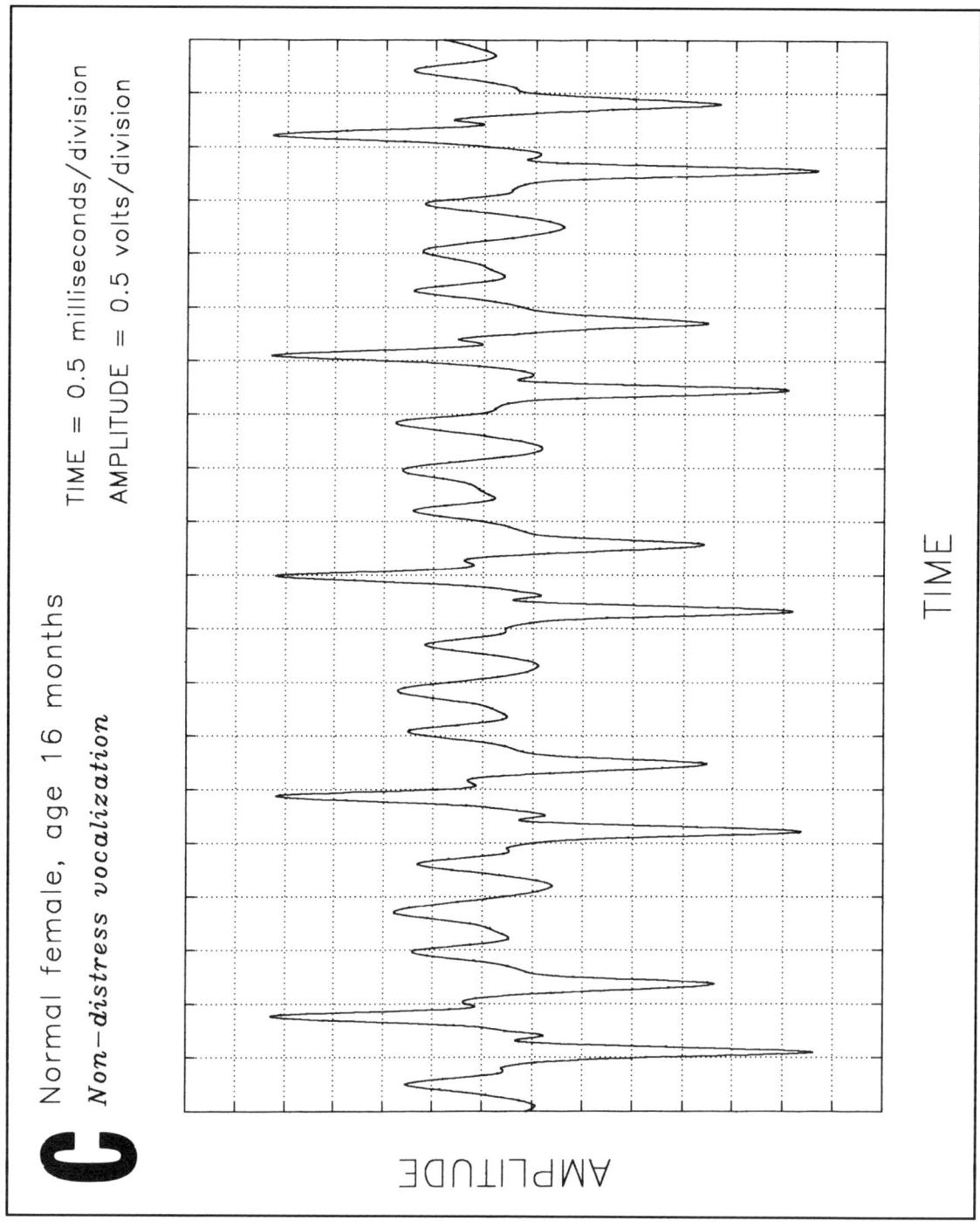

Student   Date

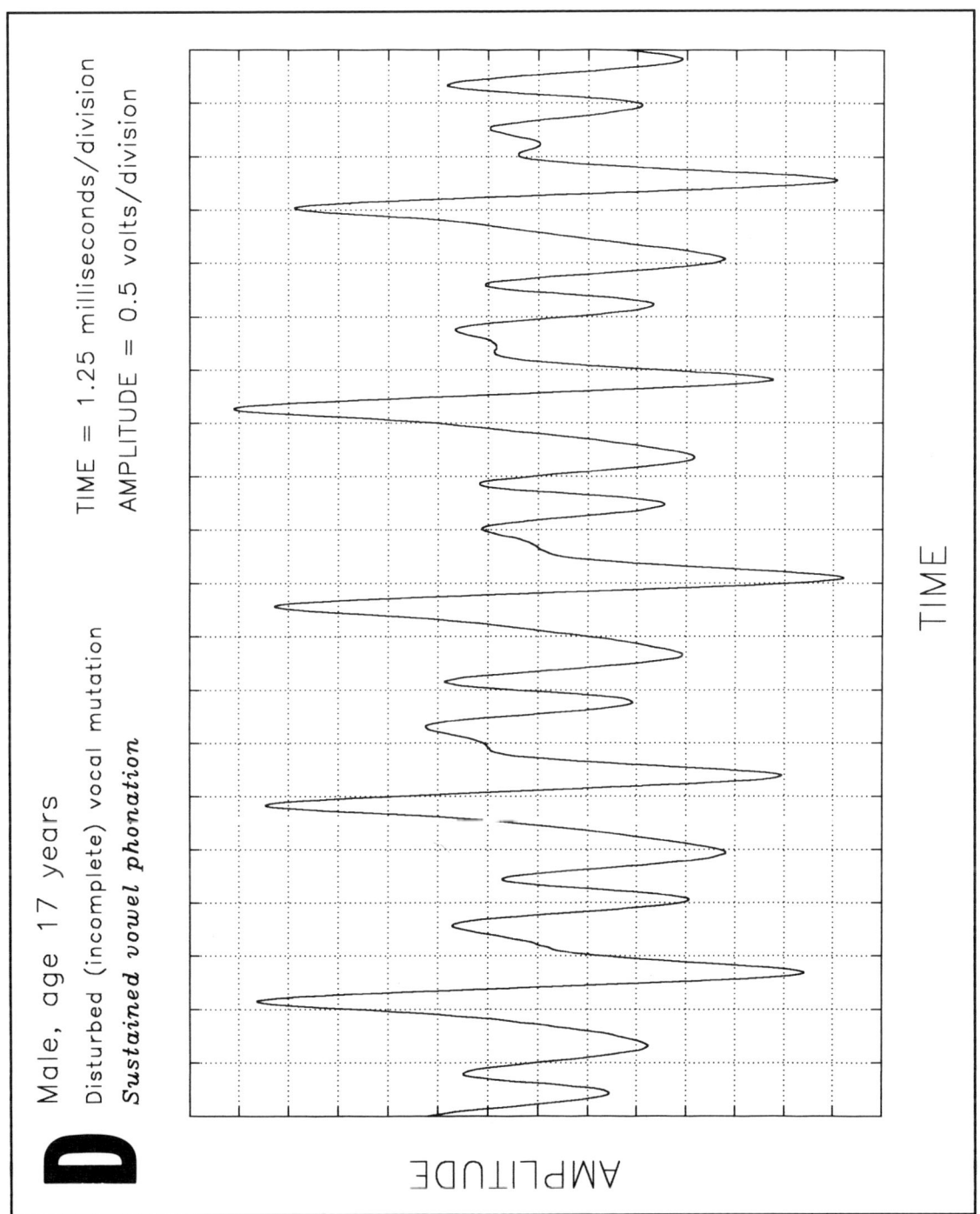

Student _____ Date _____

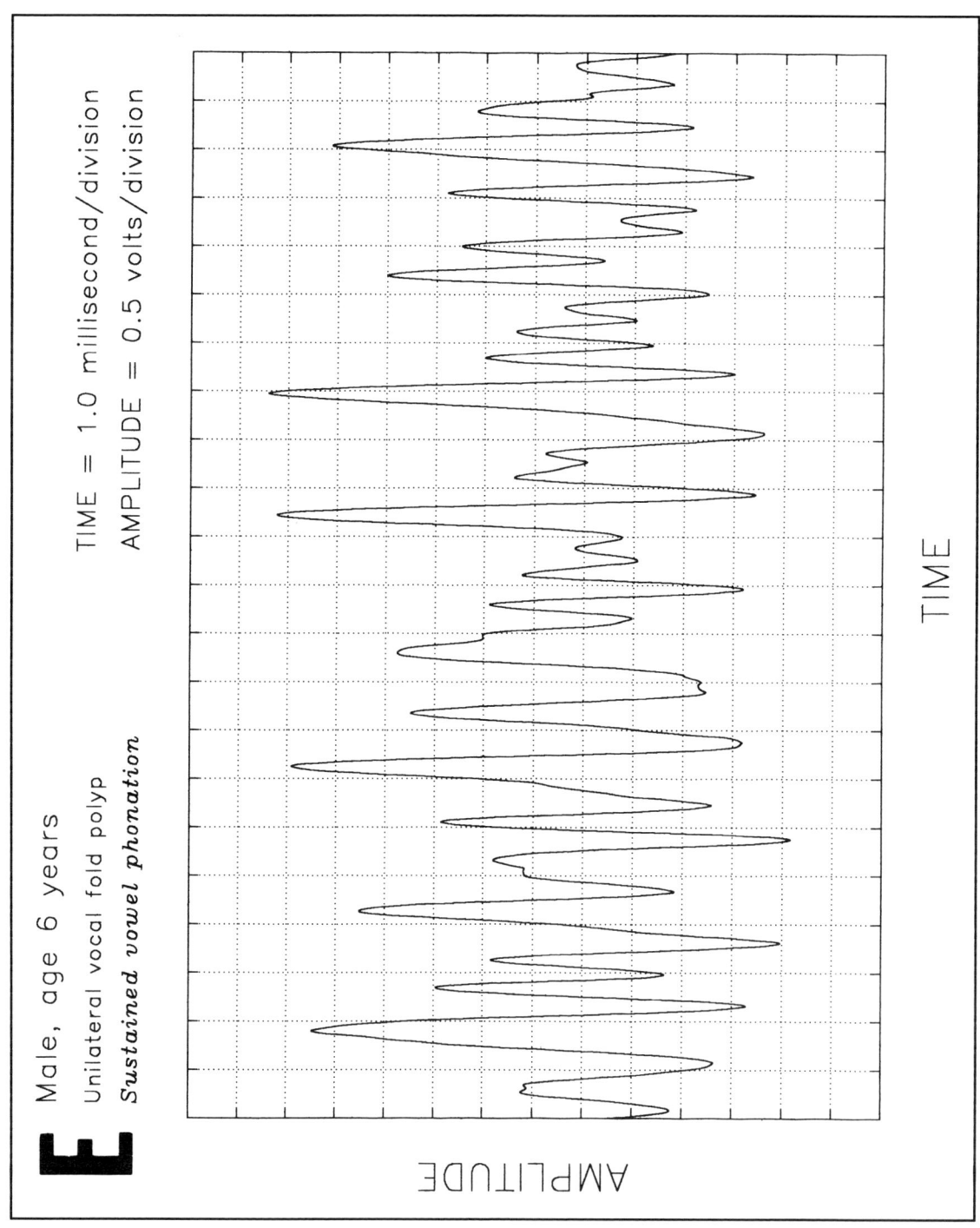

Student _____ Date _____

ATTACH YOUR OSCILLOGRAMS TO THIS PAGE

Speaker F: _____

Time Scale: _____ Vertical Scale: _____

Speaker G: _____

Time Scale: _____ Vertical Scale: _____

Student _____ Date _____

2. Difficulty in data extraction: _____

_____

_____

_____

_____

3. Patient D, assessment of F_0: _____

_____

_____

_____

_____

_____

_____

_____

_____

Source of normative data: _____

4. Comparison of speakers F and G: _____

_____

_____

_____

_____

_____

Student   Date

II. SPEECH

1. a–f. Below is an oscillogram of a simple utterance produced by a normal adult male.

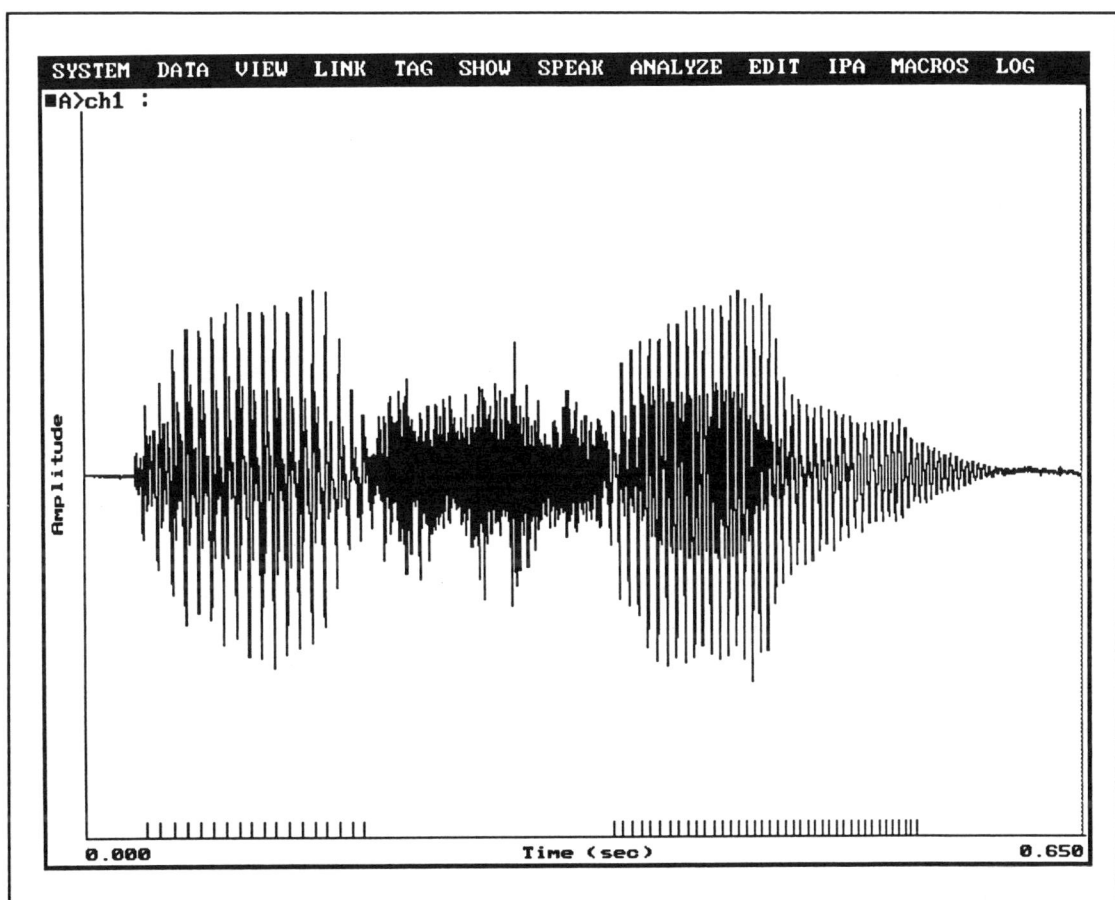

e. _____

_____

_____

_____

_____

_____

_____

Student   Date

2. a. Below is an oscillogram of the word "apples" spoken relatively slowly and deliberately by a normal adult male.

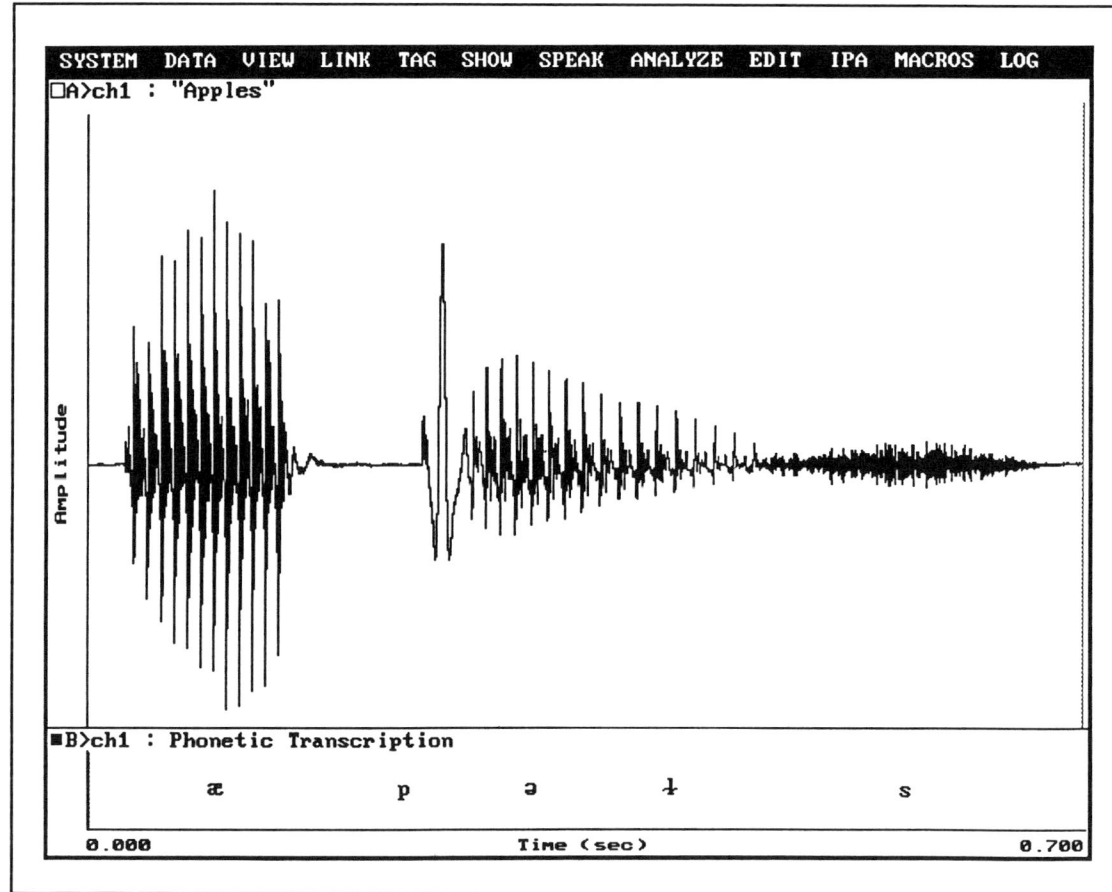

b. Location of speech sounds: _____

_____

_____

_____

_____

c. Which syllable was stressed? _____

Explain: _____

_____

Student _____   Date _____

3. Attach your oscillogram below.

```
┌─────────────────────────────────────────────────────┐
│                                                     │
│                                                     │
│                                                     │
│                                                     │
│                                                     │
│                                                     │
│                                                     │
│  Oscillogram: "Say apples again"                    │
│                                                     │
│  Time Scale: _____ Vertical Scale: _____│
└─────────────────────────────────────────────────────┘
```

Comparison/assessment: _____

_____

_____

_____

_____

_____

_____

_____

_____

_____

Basic Skills: Calibration

All of our instruments produce outputs, but it is unusual for that output to be numerically equal to the quantity that the transducer is sensing, especially in the units in which we are interested. That is, on a chart showing intraoral pressure, a peak 9 *cm* high might, or might not, indicate a pressure of 9 *cm H_2O*. A *voltage* output of 12.15 from an airflow measurement system may, or may not, represent a nasal flow of 12.15 liters/s. An analog-to-digital converter reports that the spirometer contains a volume of "1021." What on earth does that signify?

Calibration is the process of determining the equivalence between the output of a system and standard units of measurement. Calibration might determine, for instance, that 1 cm on a chart equals 0.5 cm H_2O of pressure. So our pressure peak of 9 *cm* really shows 4.5 cm H_2O. Calibrating the airflow system might have indicated that 1 volt of output is equivalent to a flow of 0.11 liters/s. So the airflow reading of 12.15 *volts* translates to an actual airflow of 1.3 *L/s*. The relationship between the digital representation of spirometer volume and the actual volume might be determined to be: "Volume in milliliters = 0.629 (A-to-D value) + 121." This means, then, that the computer's *1021* really stands for a spirometer volume of *763 mL*.

All instrumentation arrays need to be calibrated before we can obtain quantitative information from them. Even commercial instruments that report final values in conventional units (such as Hz, cm H_2O, and dB) need to be calibrated periodically to be certain that they are "telling us the truth." A measurement can be no better than the calibration with which it is associated.

Purpose: In this exercise you will become comfortable with the basic concepts of calibration and develop skill in applying the appropriate arithmetic.

Equipment: A hand calculator with statistical (regression) functions.

General preparation: Review the basic concepts and methods of correlation and regression (see Unit 4 "Descriptive Statistics"). If necessary, review solutions of simple algebraic equations with one unknown.

To calibrate a system we provide it with a known quantity (of airflow, pressure, volume, or whatever is appropriate) and measure its output. For instance, we might use a large syringe to inject 500 mL of air into a spirometer and note how far the spirometer's recording pen moves. If the 500 mL of air caused the pen to move 4 cm, then we have established the equivalence "4 cm = 500 mL." Simple reasoning lets us extend this equivalence to a more universal rule for the spirometer. If 4 cm = 500 mL, how much volume does 1 cm of pen motion represent? We establish a proportion: "4 cm is to 500 mL as 1 cm is to ? mL." Algebraically,

$$\frac{4 \text{ cm}}{500 \text{ mL}} = \frac{1 \text{ cm}}{?}$$

Solving the equation reveals, of course that ? = 125 mL. So we know that, for this spirometer, 1 cm of pen motion represents a 125-mL change in volume. We can now read any chart that the spirometer produces in terms of actual volumes because we have a calibration that tells us that the output is "125 mL per cm." We have provided a scale for the spirometer record.

Exercises

Provide your answers to the following questions on the hand-in sheet.

1. A pneumotachograph system provides an output of 4.67 volts for a flow of 3.5 L/s (liters per second). What is the calibration of this system (expressed in L/s per volt)?

2. A chest wall magnetometer system causes an oscilloscope trace to deflect 1.8 screen divisions when the rib cage is expanded by 2 cm. What is the calibration of the magnetometer?

The proportionality method obviously can be used to determine the value of an output even if we haven't established a separate statement of calibration. For example, suppose we use a pressure system to evaluate the peak intraoral pressure (P_{io}) generated by a dyspraxic child during production of /bu/. It has earlier been determined that the pressure system produces 4.2 volts when the pressure input is 1.8 cm H_2O. The peak pressure during the child's /bu/ is represented by 8.1 volts. How much pressure has the child used?

We know that 1.8 cm H$_2$O is to 4.2 V as "P$_{io}$" is to 8.1 V. Therefore,

$$\frac{1.8 \text{ cm H}_2\text{O}}{4.2 \text{ V}} = \frac{P_{io}}{8.1 \text{ V}}$$

Solving for P$_{io}$ gives us:

$$P_{io} = 8.1 \, (1.8/4.2)$$
$$P_{io} = 3.47 \text{ cm H}_2\text{O}$$

We have determined the child's actual intraoral pressure, even though we don't know how much 1 V output represents. (Of course we could have determined that too!)

3. A frequency meter produces 9.7 volts when the fundamental frequency (F_0) of a test signal is 120 Hz. Using the same frequency meter, you find that phonation at a comfortable frequency by your patient produces an output of 8.2 V. What is your patient's comfortable F_0?

4. With respect to the same frequency meter,

   a. What would the output voltage be if a patient used an F_0 of 190 Hz?; and

   b. How great a frequency increase does an output change of 1 V represent? (That is, what is the calibration of the frequency meter?)

There is a problem with the proportionality method as we have described it thus far: it assumes that an output of 0 units (volts, centimeters, etc.) represents an input of 0 units (Hz, cm H$_2$O, mL/s, etc.). This might not be (and often is not) the case. To deal with this, it is important that we calibrate by checking at least *two* outputs of a system. (It is generally convenient to check the output of the system at 0 input as well as the output at some real value.) Some simple algebra will then give us all the calibrating information we need.

Be this as it may, the best way to calibrate a system is to generate a regression equation. What we really need to do is to determine the output of the measurement system for several different known inputs. We can then take the input-output data pairs and derive an equation that specifies the calibration of the instrumentation.

For example, suppose that we have a computer record the output of an airflow system. The computer, of course, uses its analog-to-digital converter to translate the voltage output into a series of numbers. To know what the digital values mean, we would calibrate the system by providing it with known flows and recording the A-to-D values associated with each. We might generate a table such as the following:

Input Flow (L/s)	A-to-D Value
0.00	−1173
1.00	68
1.50	690
1.75	999
2.00	1310
2.25	1619
2.50	1931
3.00	2552

What we want is an equation that states:

$$\text{Flow} = \text{gain} \times (\text{A-to-D value}) + \text{intercept}.$$

That is, we want a regression equation of the general form $y = mx + b$, where y is the flow and x is the A-to-D value. Using a hand calculator we can easily derive such an equation. For the data tabled above it turns out that:

$$\text{Flow} = 0.0008 \, (\text{A-to-D value}) + 0.945.$$

There are important hidden advantages to calibrating by using several values to derive a regression equation. One is that small errors in the precision of the input quantities (was it really a flow of 1.0 L/s, or was it perhaps 1.05 L/s?) are "averaged out," leaving a better estimate of the overall relationship. (The more input values we use, the more accurate our calibration becomes.) But even more importantly, we can assess the *linearity* of the system.

By linearity we mean that the output change really is the same for equal changes in the input anywhere in the valid range of the system. For example, as airflow increases from 1.00 to 2.00 L/s, the A-to-D output changes by 1242. And as the flow changes from 2.00 to 3.00 L/s, the A-to-D output again changes by 1242. This means that the linearity of the system is good. Another way to assess linearity is by computing the correlation coefficient (r) for the input and output. (This, too, is easily accomplished with a hand calculator.) The higher the correlation, the better the linearity of the system. (In the airflow example above, $r = 0.999$.)

5. A transducer system is designed to measure the movement of the jaw. The output is connected to a computer, which stores jaw position as a set of analog-to-digital values. By definition, position 0 means jaw closure (molars in contact). Opening of the jaw (downward motion) is designated by negative numbers. The system is calibrated by moving the sensor known distances. Calibration data are as follows:

Jaw Position (cm)		A-to-D Value
0.0	(molar contact)	−2000
−1.0		−1249
−1.5		−846
−2.0		−462
−2.5		−79
−3.0		+318
−5.0		+1821

a. What is the regression equation that describes this relationship?

b. Does the system show good linearity? (Justify your opinion.)

6. The figure on the next page shows the record of calibration of a pressure transducer. At the start of the calibration, there is no pressure, and the pen trace is lined up with a major grid line. The tracing then shows plateaus as various test pressures were applied to the transducer and maintained for short periods. Complete the table (on the hand-in sheet) and derive a calibration equation for this pressure system. (Hint: use "number of chart divisions from the bottom" as the "output" value.)

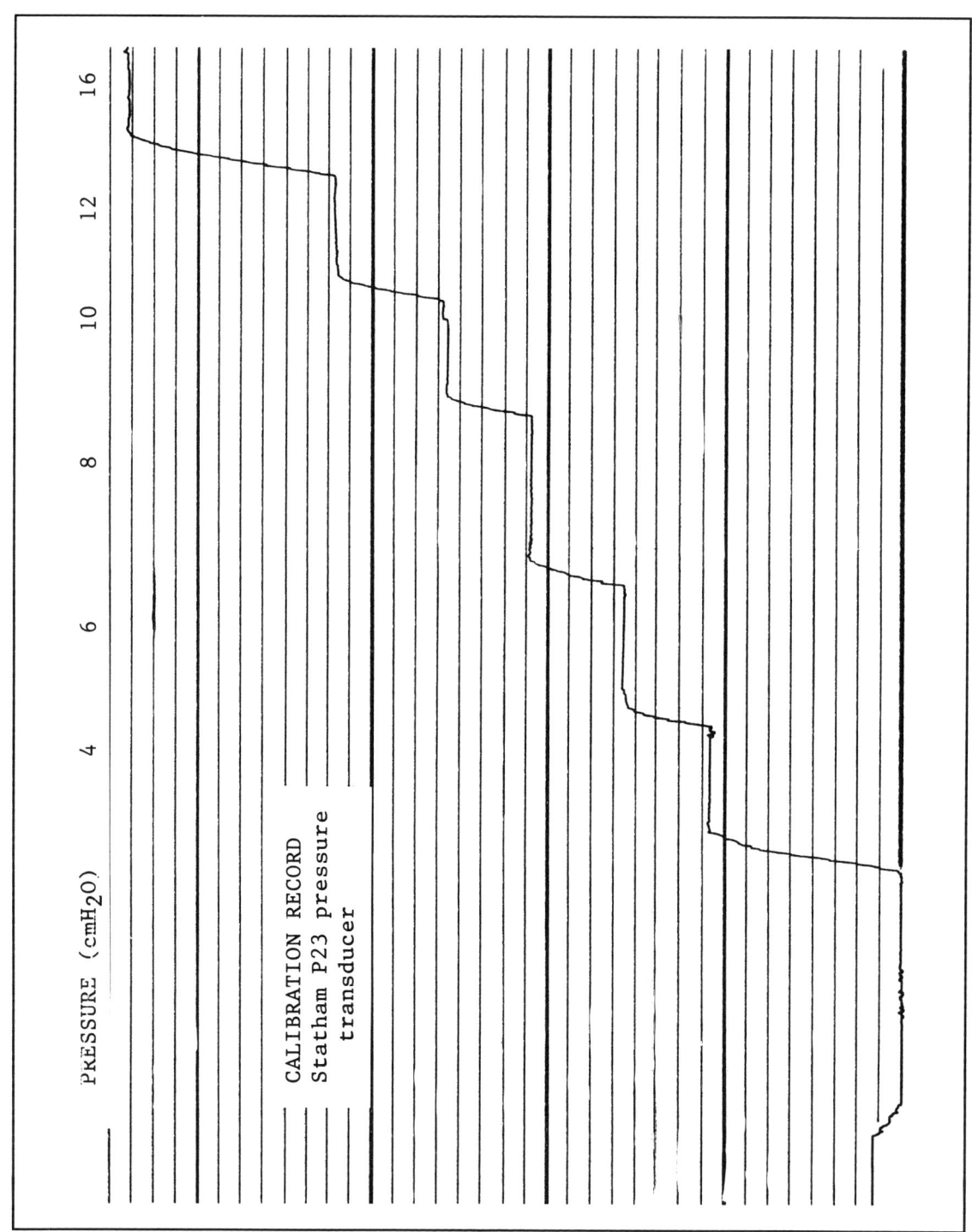

Student _____   Date _____

CALIBRATION

Be sure to show your arithmetic along with your answers.

1. Pneumotachograph calibration: _____

   _____

2. Magnetometer calibration: _____

   _____

3. Patient's comfortable F_0: _____

4. a. At 190 Hz the output would be: _____

   _____

   b. 1 volt represents a frequency change of: _____

   _____

5. a. Jaw position (in cm) = _____

   _____

   b. Linearity? _____

   _____

Student   Date

6. Calibration data for pressure transducer:

Applied Pressure (cm H$_2$O)	System Output (Graph divisions above baseline)
0	_____
4	_____
6	_____
8	_____
10	_____
12	_____
16	_____

Calibration (regression) equation: _____

Correlation coefficient: _____

Estimate of linearity: _____

VOCAL FUNDAMENTAL FREQUENCY

UNIT 12

Clinical Application: Vocal Fundamental Frequency

Abnormal pitch characteristics are commonly associated with many communication disorders. The perception of vocal pitch is related in very complex ways to the intensity and spectral characteristics of the voiced sound. But the vocal *fundamental frequency* (F_0), which is determined by the rate of vocal fold vibration, is the most important contributor to the perceived pitch. Of all clinical speech data, F_0 measures are perhaps the most common since they are easy to obtain with modern computer-interfaced instrumentation and may provide valuable information about vocal fold behavior and status.

Purpose: In this exercise you will use acoustic waveforms and derived fundamental frequency data to obtain measures of maximum phonational frequency range, mean speaking fundamental frequency, and pitch sigma. Although these measures are typically obtained by computer-assisted data extraction, you will analyze short acoustic samples by hand to gain insight into the nature of these measures and to recognize some of the limitations of these techniques.

Equipment: A microphone and a means of generating a printed oscillogram and/or frequency trace (for example, an oscilloscope and camera, visicorder/oscillograph, or automated system such as the Visi-Pitch™ or PM Pitch Analyzer™).

General preparation: Review basic measurement of vocal period and frequency and the principles of semitone scaling (see Unit 10 "Reading Oscillograms" and Unit 7 "Semitones"). Be sure to read the instruction manual(s) thoroughly for the instrumentation you will be using to complete this exercise.

I. MAXIMUM PHONATIONAL FREQUENCY RANGE

As defined by Hollien, Dew, and Philips (1971), a speaker's *maximum phonational frequency range* (MPFR) is that range of vocal fundamental frequencies extending from the lowest sustainable[1] modal-register tone to the highest tone that may be sustained in the falsetto (or loft) register (see Baken, 1987, pp. 162–166). Although many of the frequencies within the range are not typically used in running speech, a restriction of the MPFR may indicate vocal pathology, as a reflection of diminished adjustability of the vocal mechanism.

1. The oscillograms below show a portion of the acoustic signal obtained while an adult male speaker sustained the vowel /ɑ/ at his lowest modal-register pitch (A, above) and then at his highest possible pitch (B, below).

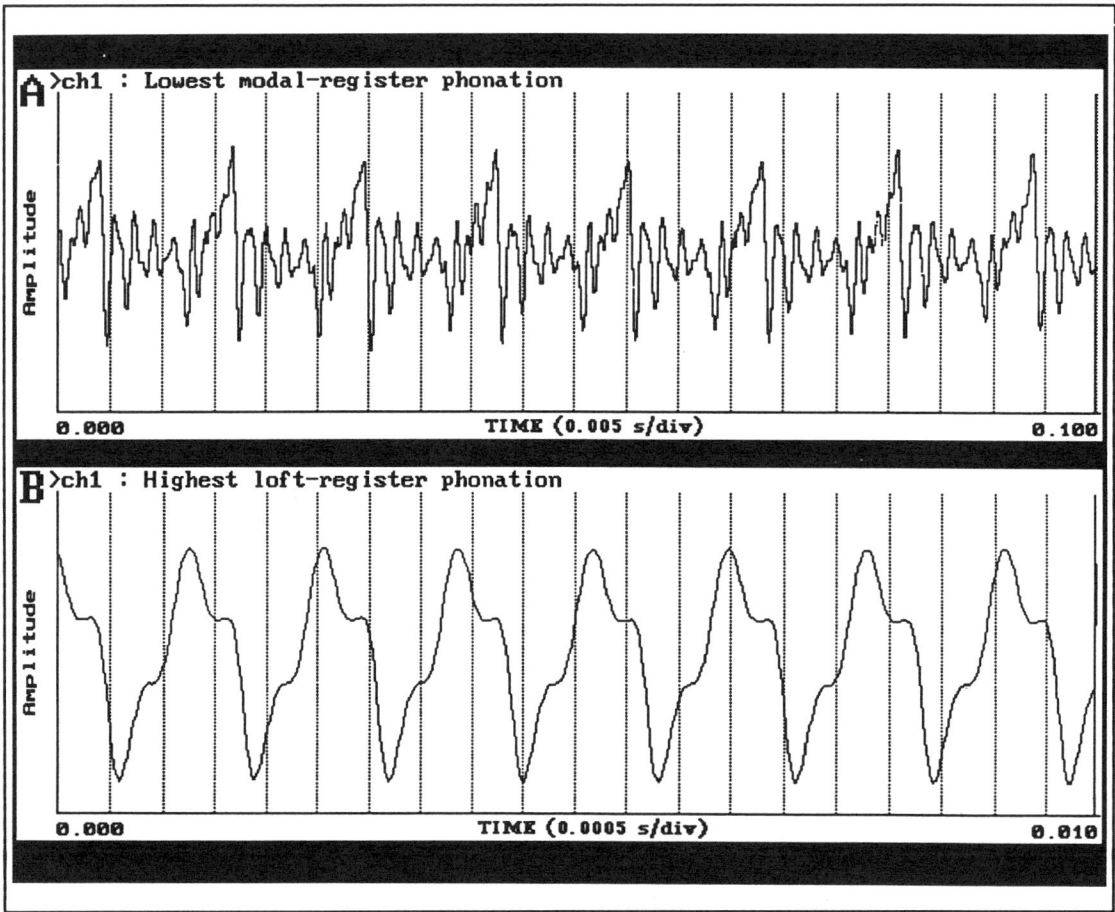

---

[1] Even normal speakers cannot sustain a constant vocal F_0 (see Unit 13 "Fundamental Frequency Perturbation"), especially at the extremes of the frequency range. For instance, an apparently steady 143-Hz phonation may include one disparate 112-Hz cycle, the lowest F_0 value in the sample. The speaker, however, may not be able to *sustain* such a low-frequency tone. Thus the lowest (and highest) sustainable frequency must, by necessity, be represented by an average. Unfortunately, there is no standard sample length from which to derive this average F_0 value. As a clinical rule-of-thumb, a fairly stable 1-s sample will probably suffice.

From these records determine:

a. His mean lowest F_0;

b. His mean highest F_0;

c. His MPFR (in hertz); and

d. His MPFR (in semitones).

e. Is this MPFR "within normal limits" for a young adult man? Cite your source of normative data.

2. The figure below shows two frequency traces (F_0 over time) as displayed on a computer-interfaced Visi-Pitch™ screen.[2] These data were derived from phonations of the vowel /ɑ/ at the lowest modal-register pitch (A, above) and highest falsetto pitch (B, below) that an adult female speaker could sustain. Calculations and comparisons provided by the Visi-Pitch software are also shown. Vertical cursors mark the 1-s sample used for analysis.

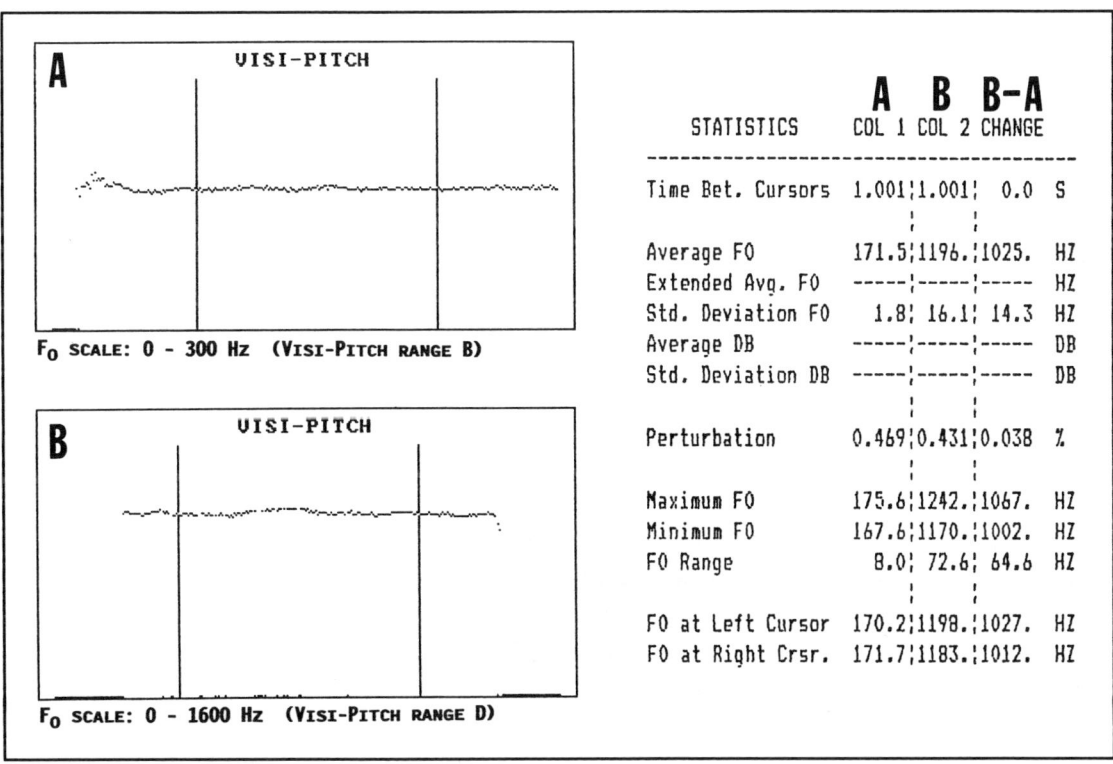

Using the Visi-Pitch data, determine:

a. Her MPFR (in hertz); and

b. Her MPFR (in semitones).

---
[2] Visi-Pitch IBM/PC® Interface, Model 6097, Kay Elemetrics Corporation, Pine Brook, NJ.

c. Is this a normal range for a young adult woman? According to whom?

3. Compare this speaker's MPFR to what you had measured earlier for the male speaker. Who has the larger phonational frequency range? Explain.

4. Obtain your own MPFR (in Hz and ST) using either acoustic waveforms or derived F_0 traces via an acoustic analysis system. How does your semitone range compare to those measured above?

5. Obtain a valid and reliable MPFR measure from a dysphonic speaker.

a. Describe the nature of this speaker's dysphonia.

b. What is the speaker's MPFR (in Hz and ST)?

6. With regard to your measurement procedure:

a. How was this measure influenced by a poor (that is, noisy) voice quality?

b. How did you ensure that the speaker produced his or her lowest (or highest) possible frequency?

c. How did you distinguish between the speaker's lowest modal- and highest pulse-register phonation?

II. FUNDAMENTAL FREQUENCY CONTOURS

During speech, vocal F_0 varies significantly throughout the utterance. Much of this variation is deliberate and linguistically driven, although some frequency characteristics are clearly a consequence of normal physiological factors. In disorder, disrupted speech and voice physiology may impair the speaker's ability to effect a normal or appropriate *intonation contour*. Dysprosody is a common speech symptom that may substantially degrade a speaker's intelligibility. In general, normal intonation contours are associated with an appropriate range of frequencies, a gradually falling frequency (F_0 declination), and local frequency peaks used to signal lexical or syllabic stress.

1. The figure on the facing page shows an oscillogram for a normal adult male saying the word "evil!" below which is the frequency contour derived from the acoustic waveform.[3]

---

[3] The length of each vocal period, as determined by the Kay Elemetrics Corp. CSL™ voicing analysis software, is represented by the "voicing marks" shown directly beneath the oscillogram.

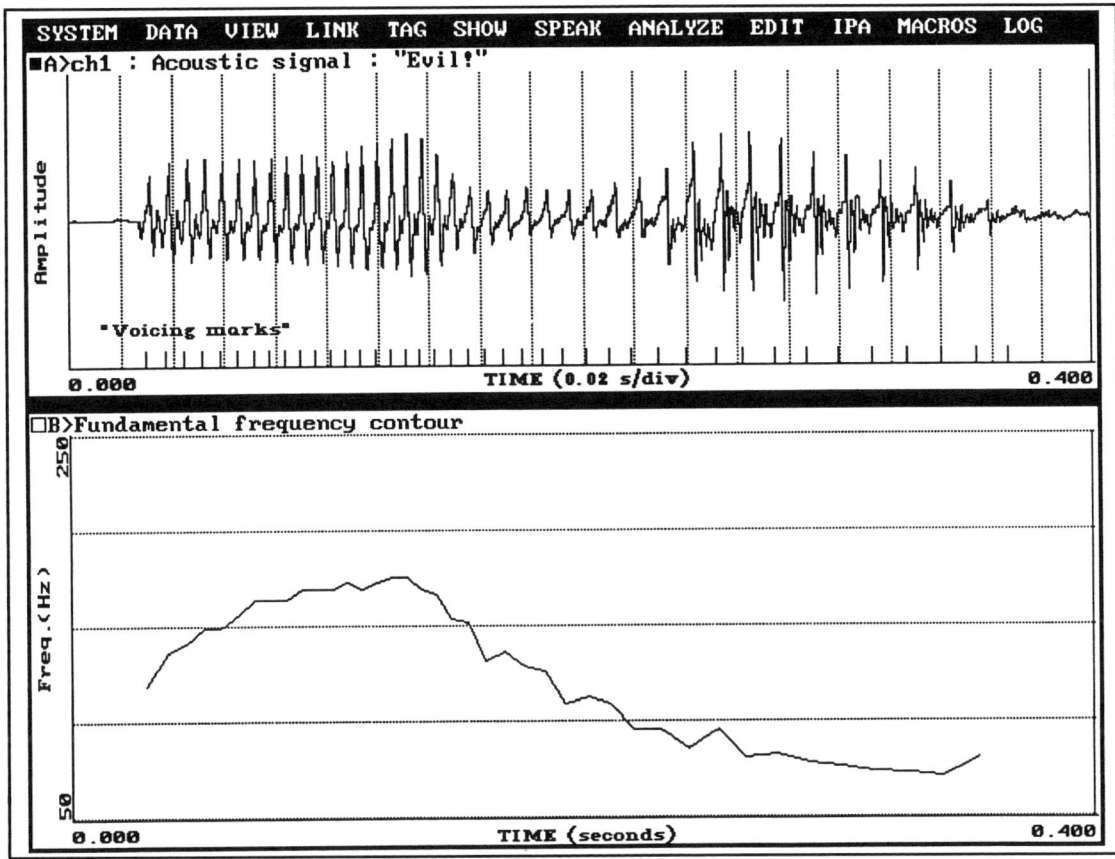

Use these data to determine:

a. The lowest F_0 used in the utterance; and

b. The highest F_0 used in the itterance.

c. Describe the F_0 contour.

2. On the following page is a similar display of a normal adult male producing a CVC (consonant-vowel-consonant) utterance.

Use these data to determine:

a. The lowest F_0 used in the utterance; and

b. The highest F_0 used in the utterance.

c. What is the likely manner of articulation of the middle consonant? Explain.

d. Why isn't the contour a continuous trace?

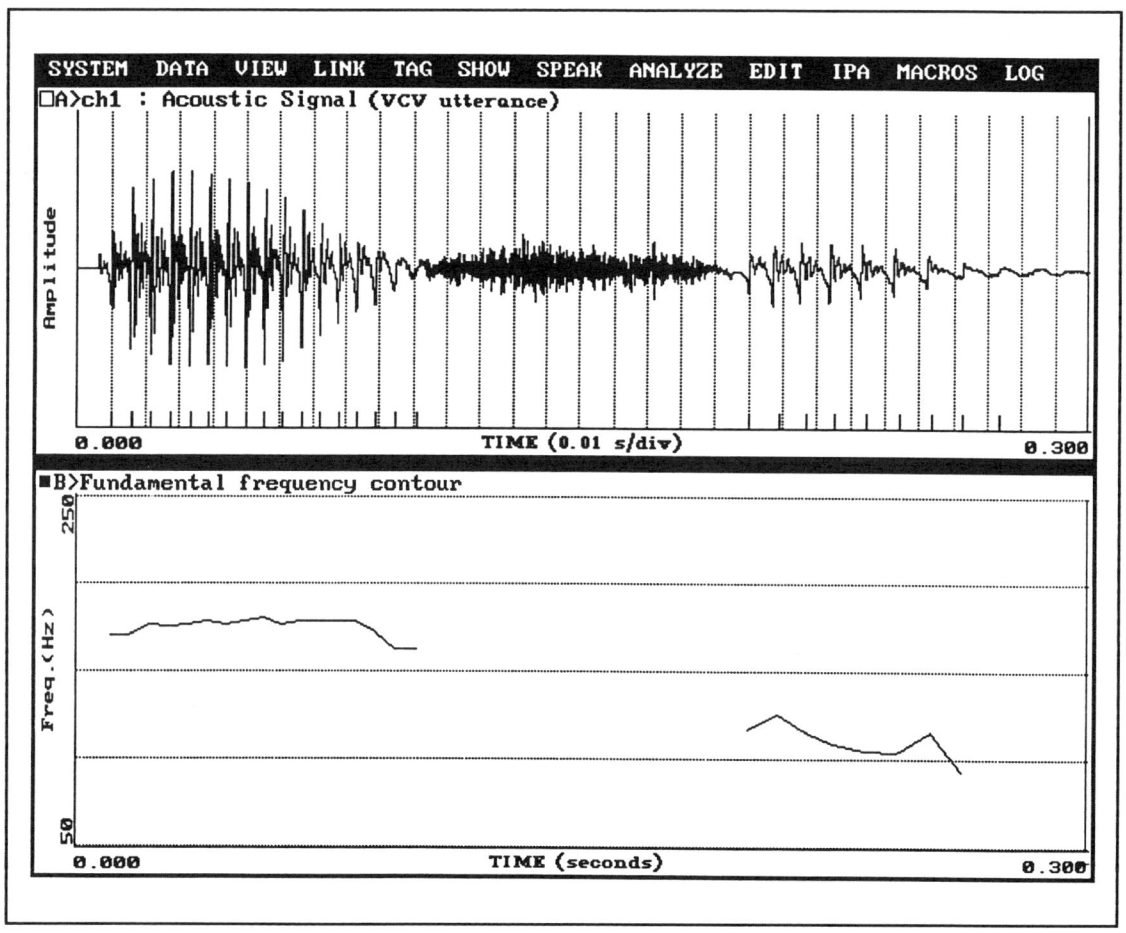

3. Obtain a printed oscillogram or frequency trace of the following utterances. For each, determine the lowest and highest F_0s used and describe the frequency contour.

   a. "*You* are going to the game."

   b. "*Are* you going to the game?"

   c. "*Why* are you going to the game?"

   Be sure to attach your data records to your lab report.

III. SPEAKING FUNDAMENTAL FREQUENCY

The typical use of the phonatory system is reflected in a speaker's *mean speaking fundamental frequency* (mean SF_0), the arithmetic average of all F_0s used in an utterance. Pitch sigma (pitch σ), the standard deviation of these F_0 data, is one measure of the extent to which F_0 is made to vary. Thus a pitch sigma that is abnormally high or low indicates that the speaker does not adjust phonation appropriately when talking. An individual with an abnormal mean SF_0 may be perceived to have an unnatural or unacceptable "habitual pitch," while a deviant pitch sigma may be associated with perceived so-called "monopitch" or, at the other extreme, "tremulousness." Obviously, the length and nature of the speech sample will affect the accuracy, if not the validity, of the pitch sigma and SF_0 estimates (see Baken, 1987, pp. 148–162). Because most of the available normative data have been accumulated using all or part of Fairbank's (1960) "Rainbow Passage" (Appendix D) this probably represents the most useful material for clinical SF_0 measurement.

1. On the hand-in sheet is an oscillogram of a VCV utterance spoken by an adult male at a relatively low pitch and loudness. Note that, not uncommon in such low-frequency/low-amplitude productions, the utterance begins and ends in pulse register. Mark the waveform, identifying the vocalic and nonvocalic portions.

   Sequential frequency data derived from this oscillogram are shown in the following table:

Cycle	F_0	Cycle	F_0	Cycle	F_0
1	63.8	12	98.4	23	98.1
2	75.7	13	105.8	24	92.8
3	77.3	14	92.6	25	88.0
4	72.9	15	110.9	26	77.3
5	68.0	16	100.1	27	62.2
6	67.1	17	98.0	28	51.0
7	56.7	18	105.3	29	49.0
8	51.3	19	110.2	30	35.1
9	52.6	20	107.5	31	37.5
10	58.9	21	109.3	32	29.2
11	125.3	22	101.0	33	28.7

2. Using these data, determine:

   a. The mean speaking fundamental frequency (SF_0) for this sample; and

   b. The sample pitch sigma (σ, in Hz).

3. Describe the intonation contour.

4. Why would it not be valid to use these data to estimate this speaker's (typical) vocal frequency use?

5. Below are fundamental frequency traces (A, B, and C) obtained for three speakers while they read the Rainbow Passage. Vertical "cursors" mark the beginning and end of the passage's second sentence. All frequency measures shown have been determined by Visi-Pitch software for all vocalic segments between the cursors.

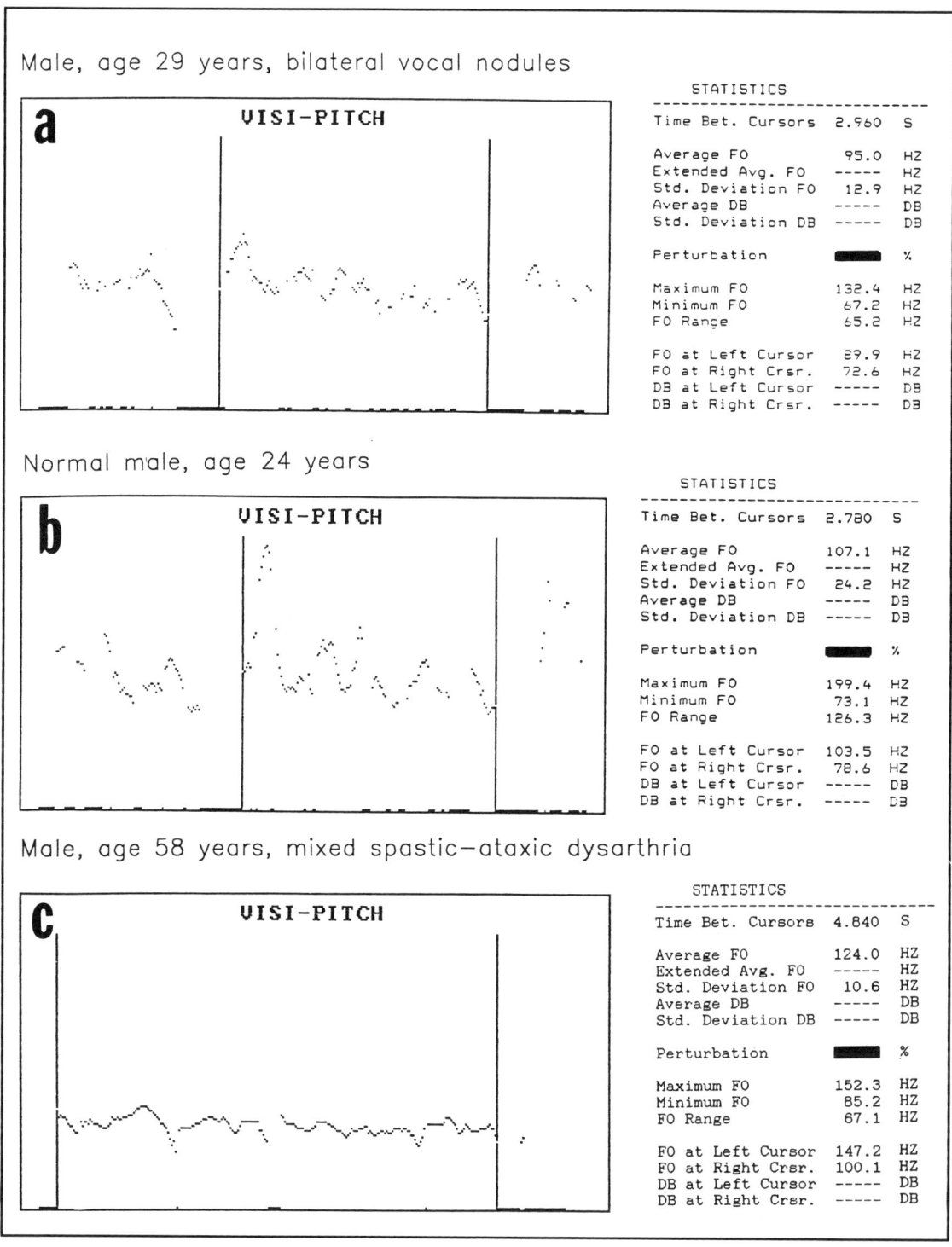

a. Use the data for each trace to complete the table on the hand-in sheet for speakers A–C.

b. How do these values compare with normative data?

c. Are the shapes (that is, contours) of the F_0 traces very different? Explain.

d. What other important differences (or similarities) can you describe?

6. Obtain an oscillogram or frequency trace while a normal *female* speaker reads the Rainbow Passage. Extracting the second sentence as above, attach a printed copy of these data to your lab report.

a. Include this speaker's data in the hand-in table for "Speaker D." Be sure to indicate the speaker's age.

b. How would the expression of pitch sigma in semitones facilitate comparison between this speaker's F_0 variation and those of the first three speakers, or when comparing such data to norms in the literature?

7. Obtain a similar sample for a dysprosodic patient and attach his or her data to your lab report.

a. Include these in the hand-in table for "Speaker E," providing some descriptive information as well (age, sex, disorder).

b. How does this patient compare with the previous speakers? In what way(s) was this speaker similar?

READ MORE ABOUT IT!

Anderson, S. W., & Cooper, W. E. (1986). Fundamental frequency patterns during spontaneous picture description. *Journal of the Acoustical Society of America, 79,* 1172–1174.

Atkinson, J. E. (1976). Inter- and intraspeaker variability in fundamental voice frequency. *Journal of the Acoustical Society of America, 60,* 440–445.

Baken, R. J. (1987). *Clinical measurement of speech and voice.* Boston: Little, Brown.

Baken, R. J., & Orlikoff, R. F. (1988). Changes in vocal fundamental frequency at the segmental level: Control during voiced fricatives. *Journal of Speech and Hearing Research, 31,* 207–211.

Bennett, S. (1983). A 3-year longitudinal study of school-aged children's fundamental frequencies. *Journal of Speech and Hearing Research, 26,* 137–142.

Canter, G. J. (1965). Speech characteristics of patients with Parkinson's disease: II. Physiological support for speech. *Journal of Speech and Hearing Disorders, 30,* 44–49.

Coleman, R. F., & Markham, I. W. (1991). Normal variations in habitual pitch. *Journal of Voice, 5,* 173–177.

Collier, R. (1975). Physiological correlates of intonation patterns. *Journal of the Acoustical Society of America, 58,* 249–255.

Cooper, W. E., & Sorensen, J. (1981). *Fundamental frequency in sentence production.* New York: Springer-Verlag.

Curry, E. T., & Snidecor, J. C. (1961). Physical measurement and pitch perception in esophageal speech. *Laryngoscope, 71,* 415–423.

Fitch, J. L., & Holbrook, A. (1970). Modal vocal fundamental frequency of young adults. *Archives of Otolaryngology, 92,* 379–382.

Gilbert, H. R., & Campbell, M. I. (1980). Speaking fundamental frequency in three groups of hearing-impaired individuals. *Journal of Communication Disorders, 13,* 195–205.

Healey, E. C. (1982). Speaking fundamental frequency characteristics of stutterers and nonstutterers. *Journal of Communication Disorders, 15,* 21–29.

Hollien, H. (1974). On vocal registers. *Journal of Phonetics, 2,* 125–143.

Hollien, H., Dew, D., & Philips, P. (1971). Phonational frequency ranges of adults. *Journal of Speech and Hearing Research, 14,* 755–760.

Hollien, H., & Jackson, B. (1973). Normative

Hollien, H., & Paul, P. (1969). A second evaluation of the speaking fundamental frequency characteristics of post-adolescent girls. *Language and Speech, 12,* 119–124.

Hollien, H., & Shipp, T. (1972). Speaking fundamental frequency and chronologic age in males. *Journal of Speech and Hearing Research, 15,* 155–159.

Horii, Y. (1975). Some statistical characteristics of voice fundamental frequency. *Journal of Speech and Hearing Research, 18,* 192–201.

Horii, Y. (1983). Automatic analysis of voice fundamental frequency and intensity using a Visi-Pitch. *Journal of Speech and Hearing Research, 26,* 467–471.

Hudson, A., & Holbrook, A. (1982). Fundamental frequency characteristics of young black adults: Spontaneous speaking and oral reading. *Journal of Speech and Hearing Research, 25,* 25–28.

Hufnagle, J., & Hufnagle, K. (1984). An investigation of the relationship between speaking fundamental frequency and vocal quality improvement. *Journal of Communication Disorders, 17,* 95–100.

Keating, P., & Buhr, R. (1978). Fundamental frequency in the speech of infants and children. *Journal of the Acoustical Society of America, 63,* 567–571.

Laguaite, J. K., & Waldrop, W. F. (1964). Acoustic analysis of fundamental frequency of voices before and after therapy. *Folia Phoniatrica, 16,* 183–192.

Leder, S. B., & Spitzer, J. B. (1993). Speaking fundamental frequency, intensity, and rate of adventitiously profoundly hearing-impaired adult women. *Journal of the Acoustical Society of America, 93,* 2146–2151.

Lehiste, I., & Peterson, G. E. (1961). Some basic considerations in the analysis of intonation. *Journal of the Acoustical Society of America, 33,* 419–425.

Michel, J. F., Hollien, H., & Moore, P. (1966). Speaking fundamental frequency characteristics of 15, 16, and 17 year-old girls. *Language and Speech, 9,* 46–51.

Montague, J. C., Jr., Hollien, H., Hollien, P. A., & Wold, D. C. (1978). Perceived pitch and fundamental frequency comparisons of institutionalized Down's syndrome children. *Folia Phoniatrica, 30,* 245–256.

Murphy, C., & Doyle, P. (1987). The effects of cigarette smoking on voice fundamental frequency. *Otolaryngology-Head and Neck Surgery, 4,* 376–380.

Murry, T. (1978). Speaking fundamental frequency characteristics associated with voice pathologies. *Journal of Speech and Hearing Disorders, 43,* 374–379.

Mysak, E. D. (1959). Pitch and duration characteristics of older males. *Journal of Speech and Hearing Research, 2,* 46–54.

Neeley, J., Edison, S., & Carlile, L. (1968). Speaking voice fundamental frequency of mentally retarded adults and normal adults. *American Journal of Mental Deficiency, 72,* 944–947.

Przybyla, B. D., Horii, Y., & Crawford, M. H. (1992). Vocal fundamental frequency in a twin sample: Looking for a genetic effect. *Journal of Voice, 6,* 261–266.

Robb, M. P., & Saxman, J. H. (1985). Developmental trends in vocal fundamental frequency of young children. *Journal of Speech and Hearing Research, 28,* 421–427.

Saxman, J. H., & Burk, K. W. (1967). Speaking fundamental frequency characteristics of middle-aged females. *Folia Phoniatrica, 19,* 167–172.

Shadle, C. (1985). Intrinsic fundamental frequency of vowels in sentence context. *Journal of the Acoustical Society of America, 78,* 1562–1567.

Stoicheff, M. L. (1981). Speaking fundamental frequency characteristics of nonsmoking female adults. *Journal of Speech and Hearing Research, 24,* 437–441.

Stone, R. E., Jr., & Sharf, D. J. (1973). Vocal change associated with the use of atypical pitch and intensity levels. *Folia Phoniatrica, 25,* 91–103.

Student _____ Date _____

VOCAL FUNDAMENTAL FREQUENCY

Be sure to show your arithmetic along with your answer(s).

I. MAXIMUM PHONATIONAL FREQUENCY RANGE (MPFR)

1. Adult male speaker:

   a. Mean lowest F_0: _____ Hz

   b. Mean highest F_0: _____ Hz

   c. MPFR = _____ Hz

   d. MPFR = _____ ST

   e. Normal? _____

   Source of normative data: _____

2. Adult female speaker:

   a. MPFR = _____ Hz

   b. MPFR = _____ ST

   c. Normal? _____

   Source of normative data: _____

3. Comparison of male and female speaker: _____

   _____

   _____

   _____

   _____

Student _____ Date _____

4. Yourself (_____):

   MPFR = _____ Hz

   MPFR = _____ ST

   Comparison of ST range: _____
   _____

5. Dysphonic patient

   a. Description: _____

   b. MPFR : _____ Hz

   MPFR = _____ ST

6. a. Voice quality influence(s): _____
   _____
   _____
   _____

   b. Lowest and highest frequency? _____
   _____
   _____
   _____

   c. Modal vs. pulse register: _____
   _____
   _____
   _____
   _____

Student _____   Date _____

II. FUNDAMENTAL FREQUENCY CONTOURS

1. a. Lowest F_0 used: _____ Hz

   b. Highest F_0 used: _____ Hz

   c. F_0 contour: _____
   _____
   _____

2. a. Lowest F_0 used: _____ Hz

   b. Highest F_0 used: _____ Hz

   c. Likely manner of articulation: _____
   _____
   _____
   _____

   d. Discontinuous trace? _____
   _____
   _____

3. a. "*You* are going to the game." _____
   _____
   _____
   _____

   b. "*Are* you going to the game?" _____
   _____
   _____
   _____

Student _____ Date _____

c. *"Why* are you going to the game?" _____

_____

_____

_____

_____

III. SPEAKING FUNDAMENTAL FREQUENCY (SF$_0$)

1. Mark the following oscillogram to indicate the vocalic and nonvocalic portions:

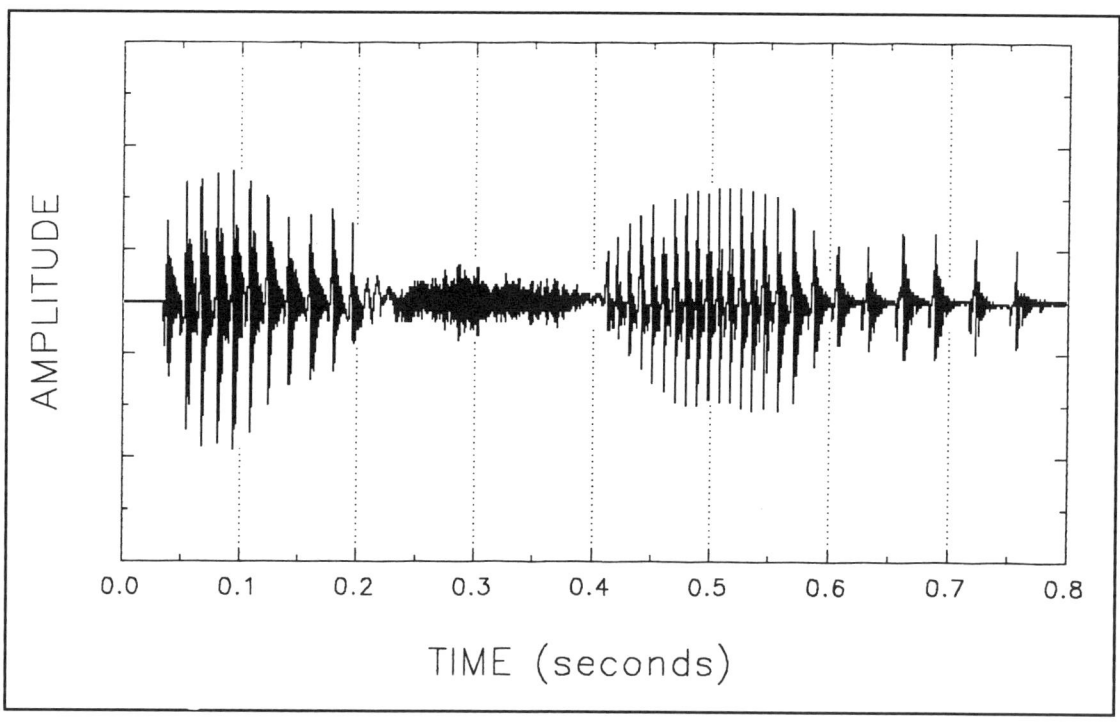

2. a. Mean SF$_0$: _____ Hz

   b. Pitch sigma: _____ Hz

3. Intonation contour: _____

_____

_____

Student _____ Date _____

_____
_____
_____
_____
_____

4. Typical? _____
_____
_____
_____
_____
_____
_____
_____
_____
_____

5. a. Complete the following table using the frequency traces provided in this exercise.

Speaker	Highest F_0 Used	Lowest F_0 Used	Mean SF_0 (in Hz)	Pitch σ (in Hz)
A. Male, 29 years	_____	_____	_____	_____
B. Male, 24 years	_____	_____	_____	_____
C. Male, 58 years	_____	_____	_____	_____
D. Female (_____)	_____	_____	_____	_____
E. Your Patient (_____)	_____	_____	_____	_____

VOCAL FUNDAMENTAL FREQUENCY

Student _____   Date _____

b. Comparison of mean SF_0 and pitch sigma for speakers A, B, and C:

_____
_____
_____
_____
_____
_____

Source(s): _____

c. Comparison of F_0 contours: _____
_____
_____
_____
_____
_____
_____

d. Other differences/similarities: _____
_____
_____
_____
_____
_____
_____

Student _____   Date _____

6. b. Pitch sigma in semitones: _____

_____

_____

_____

_____

7. b. Analysis/comparison of your patient's F_0 contour, mean SF_0 and pitch sigma: _____

_____

_____

_____

_____

_____

_____

_____

_____

_____

_____

_____

UNIT 13

Clinical Application: Fundamental Frequency Perturbation (Vocal Jitter)

Even when trying to sustain as steady a pitch as possible, the frequency of a normal speaker's voice will vary from one cycle to the next. This apparently random period variability is known as *frequency perturbation* or *vocal jitter*. It tends to increase in vocal pathology, and is, in part, responsible for the perception of a harsh, hoarse, or rough voice quality. Jitter measures are used as an index of vocal stability. As a general rule of thumb, a mean cycle-to-cycle period difference under 100 microseconds (0.0001 s) is characteristic of a controlled, sustained phonation produced by the normal speaker. However, research has indicated that this *absolute* jitter is influenced by the mean F_0 of the speaker's phonation (Horii, 1979; Orlikoff & Baken, 1990). For this reason, several *relative* jitter measures have been proposed. Despite the diversity of such measures, it is generally expected that normal voices are associated with an F_0 variation that is less than 1% of the mean phonatory frequency (or period). Below are brief descriptions of the more common indices of frequency perturbation (see Baken, 1987, or Pinto and Titze, 1990, for more detailed reviews):[1]

Mean Absolute Jitter. This is simply the mean absolute difference between sequential vocal periods measured during a sustained phonation.[2] Absolute jitter may be reported in seconds, but is more commonly expressed in milliseconds or microseconds.

Mean Percent Jitter and Jitter Ratio. These measures are obtained by taking the mean absolute jitter and dividing it by the mean vocal period used

---

[1] Mathematical definitions are provided in Appendix E.
[2] Jitter is measured exclusively from sustained phonations during which the speaker attempts to maintain as steady a pitch and loudness as possible. The volitional frequency changes associated with spoken utterances contaminate the measurement and confound clinical interpretation.

during the phonation. This proportion is then multiplied by 100 to yield a percentage. If the proportion is multiplied by 1000, the index is called the jitter ratio (JR), and is dimensionless.

Mean Jitter Factor. This is the mean absolute difference between sequential vocal F_0s (in Hz) divided by the mean frequency of the phonation. This proportion is then multiplied by 100. The mean jitter factor (JF) is the frequency equivalent of mean percent jitter.

Relative Average Perturbation. Relative average perturbation (RAP) is a relative jitter measure that additionally attempts to "desensitize" the measure to long-term fundamental frequency changes (Koike, 1973). Such long-term effects might be associated with a gradually "drifting" (falling or rising) F_0 or with relatively regular upward and downward variations as associated with tremor. RAP employs a mathematical technique called linear smoothing or averaging; in particular, the RAP measure uses 3-point averaging. The absolute difference between a given period and the mean of that period and the two adjacent periods is determined for each cycle in the sample. The average difference is then divided by the mean period. Recently it has become common to report the RAP in percent (that is, the RAP proportion is multiplied by 100). A similar measure, the *frequency perturbation quotient* (FPQ), typically employs 5-point averaging.

Purpose: In these exercises you will become familiar with the uses and calculation of various commonly used F_0 perturbation measures: (a) mean absolute jitter, (b) mean percent jitter, (c) jitter factor, and (d) relative average perturbation. Although the precise computer-assisted analysis of many hundreds of vocal periods is usually necessary for valid and reliable jitter measurement, you will do hand analysis of short samples in this exercise to gain insight into the nature of these measures.

Equipment: A microphone and a means of generating a printed oscillogram.

General preparation: Review basic measurement of vocal period and frequency (see Unit 10 "Reading Oscillograms" and Unit 12 "Vocal Fundamental Frequency").

Exercises

Patient A

On the hand-in sheet is a sound pressure oscillographic waveform for a dysphonic child prolonging a phonation at a comfortable pitch and loudness. The interval from the 50th to the 98th millisecond has been enlarged for measurement.

1. Delineate and number the periods on the record (the first two have been done for you).

2. Fill in the remainder of the table on the hand-in sheet.

3. What is the mean vocal period and mean fundamental frequency?

4. What is the mean absolute vocal jitter?

5. What is the mean percent jitter?

6. Compare the jitter measurements obtained for #4 and #5 above. How do you interpret them?

Patient B

On the hand-in sheet is another acoustic record obtained from an adult dysphonic. Using this sample:

1. Delineate and number the periods on the record.

2. Fill in the corresponding table on the hand-in sheet.

3. What is the mean vocal period and mean fundamental frequency?

4. What is the mean absolute vocal jitter?

5. What is the mean percent jitter?

6. What is the mean jitter factor?

7. How are percent jitter and jitter factor related? Explain.

Patient C

The third acoustic record on the hand-in sheet is from an adult woman whose dysphonia results in a fry-like phonation. As you did for the first two samples:

1. Delineate and number the periods on the record.

2. Fill in the corresponding data table.

3. What is the mean vocal period and mean fundamental frequency?

4. What is the mean absolute vocal jitter?

5. What is the mean percent jitter?

6. Compare the jitter measurements obtained for #4 and #5 above. How do you interpret them?

Normal Child D

The acoustic record on the facing page was obtained from a child with no speech or voice pathology sustaining a comfortable phonation. It is clear, especially from the complete excerpt, that there is a gradually falling fundamental frequency.

Sequential period data (as numbered on the oscillogram) are shown in the table below along with their absolute differences.

Cycle No. (n)	Period (t, in ms)	$\lvert t_n - t_{n+1} \rvert$ (jitter, in ms)
1	4.49	
		0.08
2	4.57	
		0.13
3	4.70	
		0.08
4	4.78	
		0.08
5	4.86	
		0.03
6	4.89	
		0.11
7	5.00	
		0.05
8	5.05	
		0.01
9	5.06	
		0.05
10	5.11	
		0.07
11	5.18	
		0.01
12	5.19	

1. From this data table determine this child's mean absolute and mean relative (percent) jitter.

2. The same period data are provided in a table on the hand-in sheet along with the three-point average of each.

   a. Complete this table; and

   b. Use these data to determine the relative average perturbation for this sample.

3. Compare the jitter measurements obtained for #1 and #2 above. How do you interpret them?

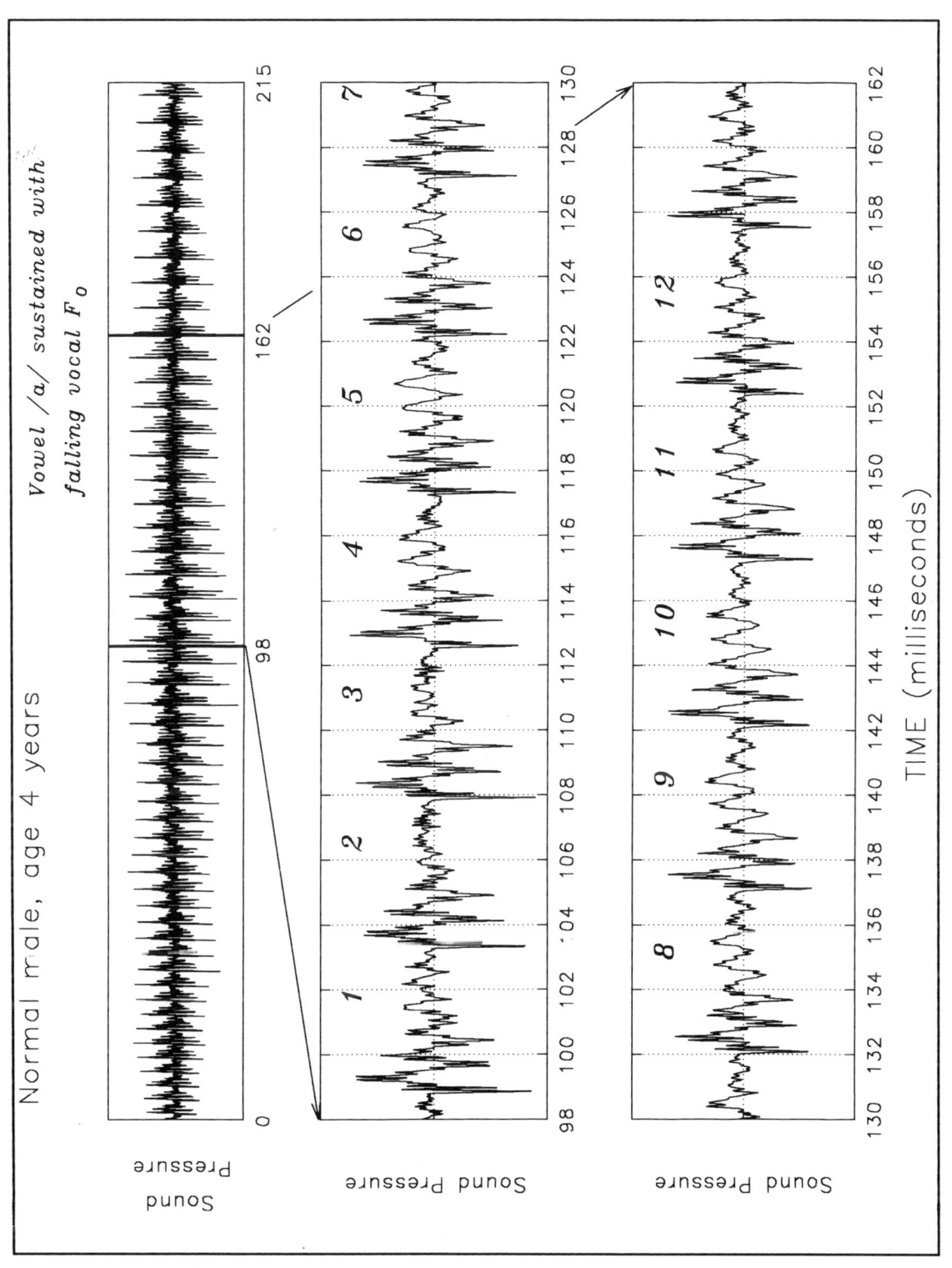

Self-Measurement E

Measure your own absolute and relative jitter using either an oscillogram or analysis system. How do these measurements relate to available normative data? Compare your measurements to those obtained from a similar phonation sustained by a dysphonic speaker.

READ MORE ABOUT IT!

Baer, T. (1981). An investigation of the phonatory mechanism. *ASHA Reports, 11,* 38–47.

Baken, R. J. (1987). *Clinical measurement of speech and voice* (pp. 166–188). Boston: Little, Brown.

Cavallo, S. A., Baken, R. J., & Shaiman, S. (1984). Frequency perturbation characteristics of pulse register phonation. *Journal of Communication Disorders, 17,* 231–243.

Glaze, L. E., Bless, D. M., Milenkovic, P., & Susser, R. D. (1988). Acoustic characteristics of children's voice. *Journal of Voice, 2,* 312–319.

Heiberger, V. L., & Horii, Y. (1982). Jitter and shimmer in sustained phonation. In N. J. Lass (Ed.), *Speech and language: Advances in basic research and practice* (Vol. 7, pp. 299–332). New York: Academic Press.

Hillenbrand, J. (1988). Perception of aperiodicities in synthetically generated voices. *Journal of the Acoustical Society of America, 83,* 2361–2371.

Hollien, H., Michel, J. F., & Doherty, E. T. (1973). A method for analyzing vocal jitter in sustained phonation. *Journal of Phonetics, 1,* 85–91.

Horii, Y. (1979). Fundamental frequency perturbation observed in sustained phonation. *Journal of Speech and Hearing Research, 22,* 5–19.

Horii, Y. (1982). Jitter and shimmer differences among sustained vowel phonations. *Journal of Speech and Hearing Research, 25,* 12–14.

Horii, Y. (1985). Jitter and shimmer differences in sustained vocal fry phonation. *Folia Phoniatrica, 37,* 81–86.

Koike, Y. (1973). Application of some acoustic measures for the evaluation of laryngeal dysfunction. *Studia Phonologica, 7,* 17–23.

Koike, Y., Takahashi, H., & Calcaterra, T. C. (1977). Acoustic measures for detecting laryngeal pathology. *Acta Otolaryngologica, 84,* 105–117.

Laver, J., Hiller, S., & Beck, J. M. (1992). Acoustic waveform perturbations and voice disorders. *Journal of Voice, 6,* 115–126.

Linville, S. E., & Fisher, H. B. (1985). Acoustic characteristics of women's voices with advancing age. *Journal of Gerontology, 40,* 324–330.

Linville, S. E., & Korabic, E. W. (1987). Fundamental frequency stability characteristics of elderly women's voices. *Journal of the Acoustical Society of America, 81,* 1196–1199.

Ludlow, C. L., Coulter, D.C., & Gentges, F. (1983). The differential sensitivity of measures of fundamental frequency perturbation to laryngeal neoplasms and neuropathologies. In D. M. Bless & J. H. Abbs (Eds.), *Vocal fold physiology: Contemporary research and clinical issues* (pp. 381–392). San Diego: College-Hill Press.

Moore, P., & Thompson, C. L. (1965). Comments on physiology of hoarseness. *Archives of Otolaryngology, 81,* 97–102.

Murry, T., & Doherty, E. T. (1980). Selected acoustic characteristics of pathologic and normal speakers. *Journal of Speech and Hearing Research, 23,* 361–369.

Orlikoff, R. F. (1989). Vocal jitter at different fundamental frequencies: A cardiovascular-neuromuscular explanation. *Journal of Voice, 3,* 104–112.

Orlikoff, R. F. (1990). The relationship of age and cardiovascular health to certain acoustic characteristics of male voices. *Journal of Speech and Hearing Research, 33,* 450–457.

Orlikoff, R. F., & Baken, R. J. (1990). Consideration of the relationship between the fundamental frequency of phonation and vocal jitter. *Folia Phoniatrica, 42,* 31–40.

Orlikoff, R. F., & Kahane, J. C. (1991). Influence of mean sound pressure level on jitter and shimmer measures. *Journal of Voice, 5,* 113–119.

Pinto, N. B., & Titze, I. R. (1990). Unification of perturbation measures in speech signals.

Journal of the Acoustical Society of America, 87, 1278–1289.

Ramig, L. A., & Ringel, R. L. (1983). Effects of physiological aging on selected acoustic characteristics of voice. *Journal of Speech and Hearing Research, 26,* 22–30.

Sorensen, D., & Horii, Y. (1983). Frequency and amplitude perturbation in the voices of female speakers. *Journal of Communication Disorders, 16,* 57–61.

Takahashi, H., & Koike, Y. (1975). Some perceptual dimensions and acoustical correlates of pathologic voices. *Acta Oto-laryngologica, Suppl. 338,* 1–24.

Titze, I. R., Horii, Y., & Scherer, R. C. (1987). Some technical considerations in voice perturbation measurements. *Journal of Speech and Hearing Research, 30,* 252–260.

Wendahl, R. (1966). Some parameters of auditory roughness. *Folia Phoniatrica, 18,* 26–32.

Student   Date

VOCAL JITTER

PATIENT A

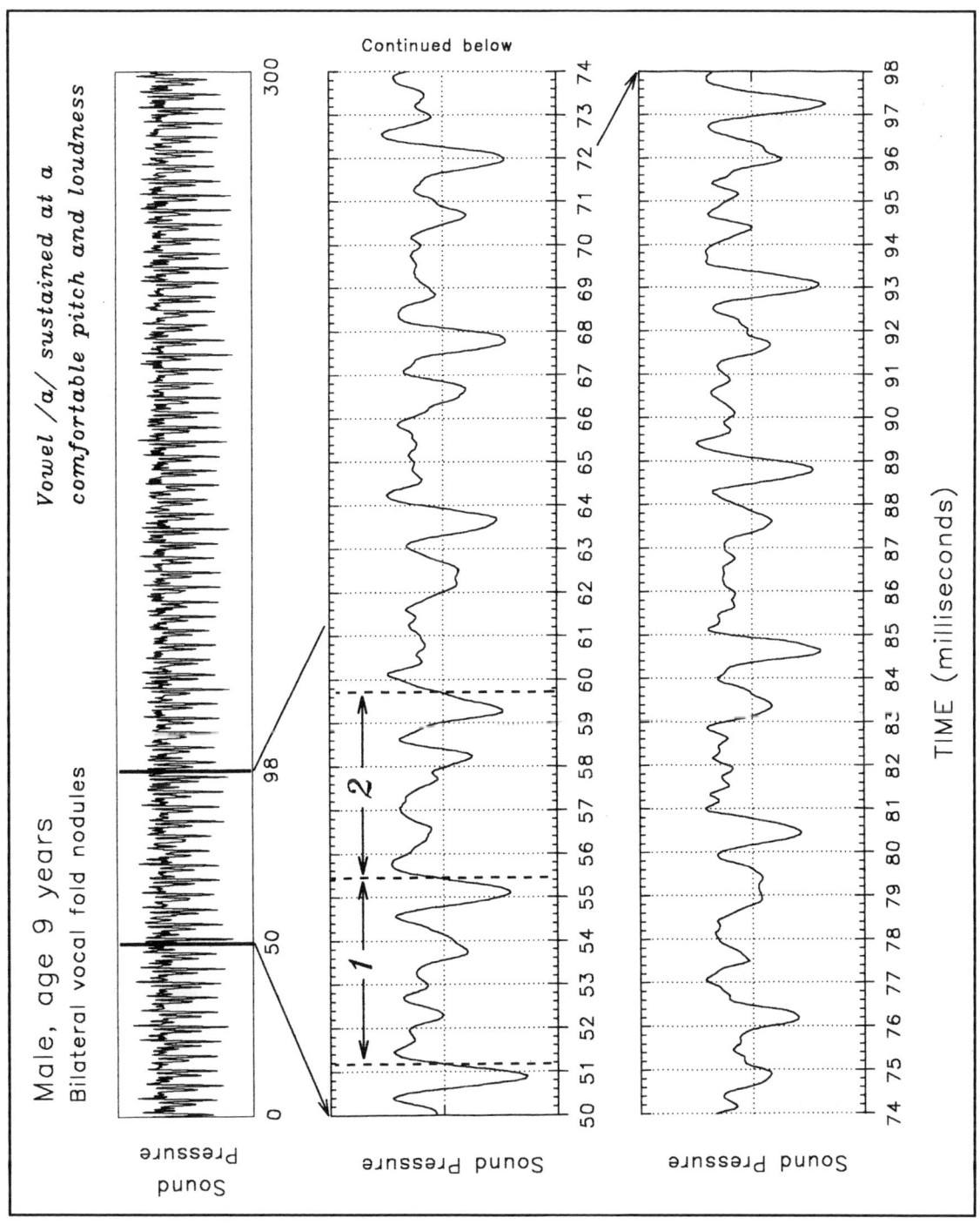

Student _____   Date _____

2. Complete the following table for Patient A:

Cycle No. (n)	Period (t, in ms)	$\|t_n - t_{n+1}\|$ (jitter, in ms)
1	4.20	
		0.08
2	4.28	
3	_____	_____
4	_____	_____
5	_____	_____
6	_____	_____
7	_____	_____
8	_____	_____
9	_____	_____
10	_____	_____
11	_____	

3. Mean period: _____

   Mean F_0: _____

4. Mean absolute jitter: _____

5. Mean percent jitter (show arithmetic): _____
_____

6. Comparison between absolute and percent jitter: _____
_____
_____

Student Date

PATIENT B

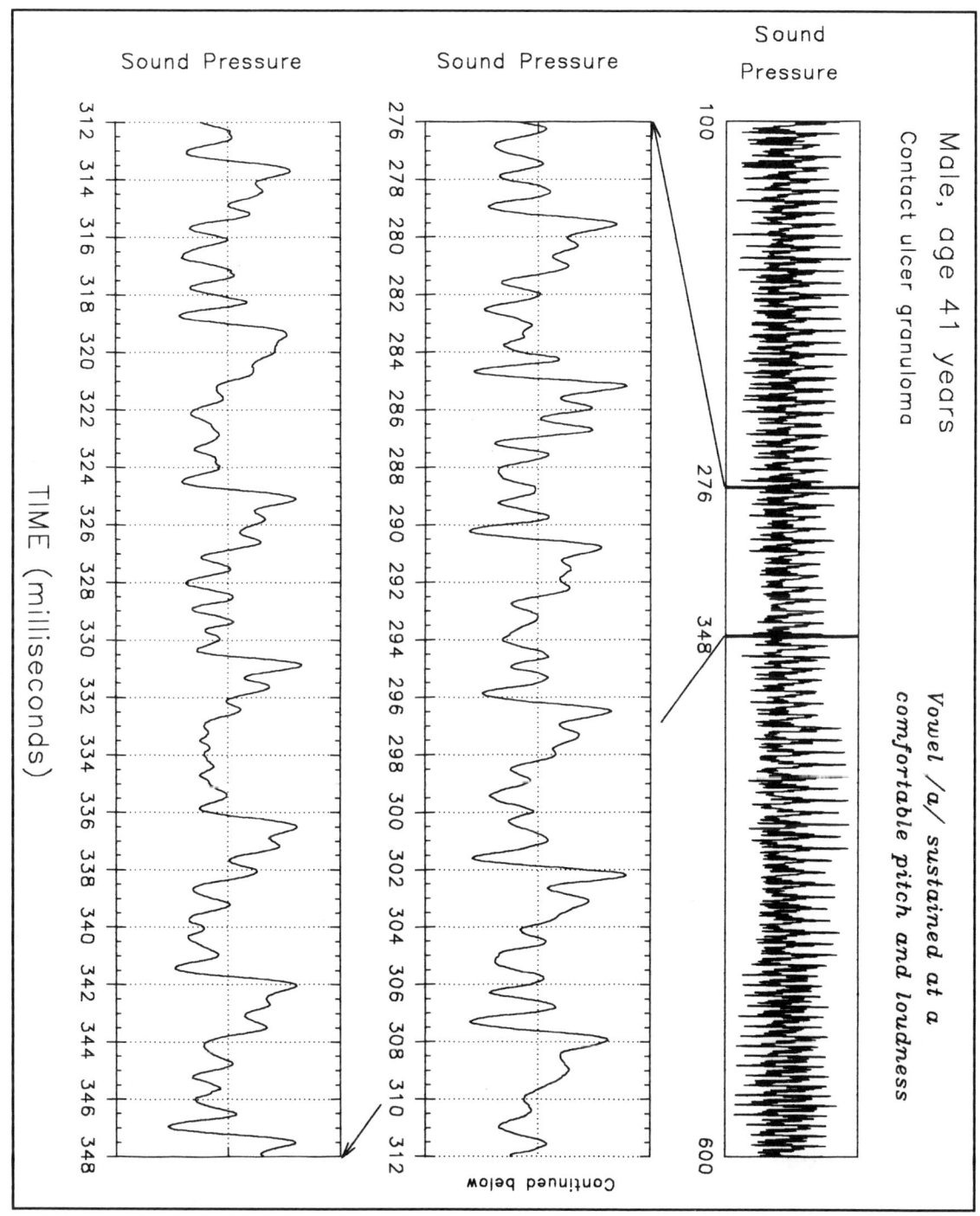

Student _____ Date _____

2. Complete the following table for Patient B:

Cycle No. (n)	Period (t, in ms)	Jitter (in ms)	Frequency (F_0)	Jitter (in Hz)
1	5.64		177.30	
2	5.59	0.05	178.89	1.59
3	____	____	____	____
4	____	____	____	____
5	____	____	____	____
6	____	____	____	____
7	____	____	____	____
8	____	____	____	____
9	____	____	____	____
10	____	____	____	____
11	____	____	____	____
12	____	____	____	____

3. Mean period: _____

Mean F_0: _____

4. Mean absolute jitter: _____

5. Mean percent jitter (show arithmetic): _____

_____

6. Mean jitter factor (show arithmetic): _____

_____

7. Percent jitter vs. jitter factor: _____

_____

Student Date

PATIENT C

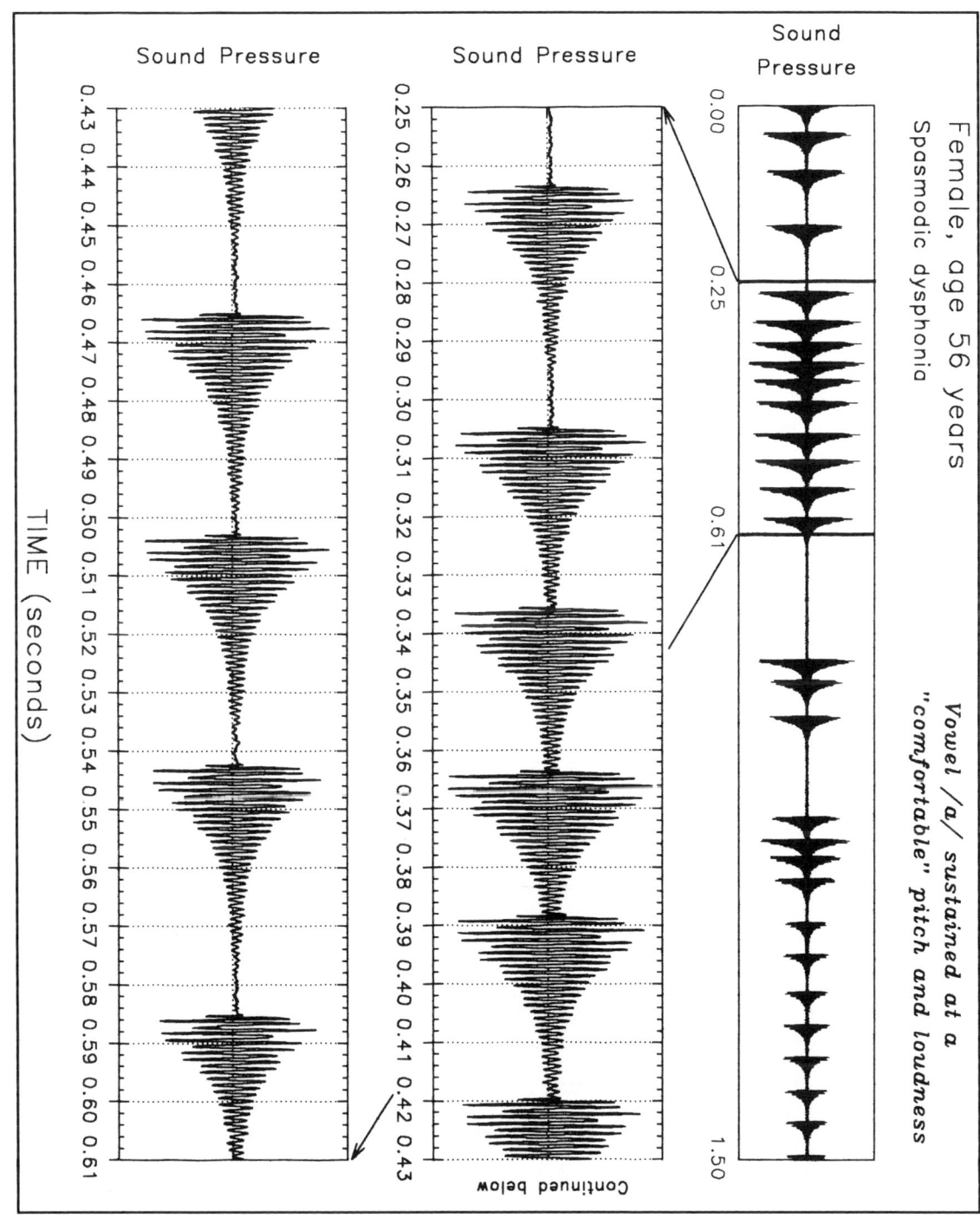

Student _____ Date _____

2. Complete the following table for Patient C:

Cycle No. (n)	Period (t, in ms)	$\|t_n - t_{n+1}\|$ (jitter, in ms)
1	40.62	
		10.50
2	30.12	
		_____
3	_____	
		_____
4	_____	
		_____
5	_____	
		_____
6	_____	
		_____
7	_____	
		_____
8	_____	
		_____
9	_____	

3. Mean period: _____

Mean F_0: _____

4. Mean absolute jitter: _____

5. Mean percent jitter (show arithmetic): _____

_____

6. Comparison between absolute and percent jitter: _____

_____

_____

_____

Student _____ Date _____

NORMAL CHILD D

1. a. Mean absolute jitter: _____

  b. Mean percent jitter (show arithmetic): _____

_____

2. a. Complete the following table:

Cycle Number (n)	Period (t, in ms)	$\dfrac{t_{n-1} + t_n + t_{n+1}}{3}$	$\left\lvert \dfrac{t_{n-1} + t_n + t_{n+1}}{3} - t_n \right\rvert$
1	4.49	[no t_{n-1}]	
2	4.57	4.59	0.02
3	4.70	4.68	_____
4	4.78	4.78	_____
5	4.86	4.84	_____
6	4.89	4.92	_____
7	5.00	4.98	_____
8	5.05	5.04	_____
9	5.06	5.07	_____
10	5.11	_____	_____
11	5.18	_____	_____
12	5.19	[no t_{n+1}]	

  b. Relative Average Perturbation (show arithmetic): _____

_____

3. Comparison of RAP and mean absolute and percent jitter: _____

_____

Student _____   Date _____

_____
_____
_____
_____

SELF-MEASUREMENT E

Measurement and evaluation of your mean absolute and relative jitter: _____

_____
_____
_____
_____
_____
_____
_____
_____
_____

(If a data printout is available, attach it to this page)

VOCAL INTENSITY

Clinical Application: The Sound Level Meter, Vocal Intensity, and the Voice Range Profile

Vocal fundamental frequency (F_0) and intensity are each normally adjustable over a considerable range. Although to a large extent one can change one while holding the other constant, F_0 and intensity are not totally independent: At extremes of F_0 the intensity range is considerably reduced. The vocal intensity range, considered as a function of vocal F_0, is generally considered a meaningful indicator of the competence of the larynx for voice production.

The most commonly accepted, and most nearly standardized way of evaluating the vocal F_0 and intensity capabilities of the larynx is by the *voice range profile*, until recently called the *phonetogram*. The voice range profile shows, in graphic form, all of the combinations of F_0 and intensity at which a speaker can phonate.

Purpose: These exercises will teach you how to measure the voice range profile. You will learn how to determine the appropriate stimulus frequencies, to obtain simultaneous measurements of F_0 and vocal intensity, and how to plot the results on a standard form. This exercise will also familiarize you with the operation of a sound level meter and the measurement of vocal intensity.

Equipment: For delivering stimuli you will need a square wave generator with a frequency range that encompasses the F_0 range of the human voice, together with an amplifier and earphones. A frequency counter should be connected to the square wave generator so you can be certain of the F_0 of the stimulus signal you are providing. You will also require an instrument to measure F_0, a sound level meter for recording vocal intensity, and a meter stick for establishing an appropriate mouth-to-microphone distance.

General preparation: Review semitone scaling (see Unit 7 "Semitones") and the techniques of F_0 measurement (see Unit 12 "Vocal Fundamental Frequency"). Study the principles of the sound level meter (see Baken, 1987, pp. 99–101) and read the manual for the sound level meter you will be using. Familiarize yourself with the norms for frequency and intensity ranges of the human voice (see Baken, 1987, pp. 106–108 and 163–166). Study the recommended techniques for obtaining the voice range profile (see Schutte & Seidner, 1983). You may also need to brush up on your data-plotting skills (see Unit 6 "Plotting Data").

I. MEASURING VOCAL INTENSITY

Vocal intensity is most often measured with a sound level meter. Familiarize yourself with its use by doing the following:

1. Examine the sound level meter you will be using. Locate each of the following controls on your instrument. Indicate the location of the controls on the outline of a sound level meter provided on the hand-in sheet.

    a. On/off (power) switch

    b. Response (fast/slow) selector

    c. Weighting selector

    d. dB range selector

    e. Sound level indicator dial

    f. Microphone

2. Describe the function of the following:

    a. Response (fast/slow) selector

    b. Weighting selector.

3. Set the dB range control to about 110 dB, the weighting selector to "linear," and the response speed to "fast." Turn the instrument on.

4. Point the microphone toward a source of continuous and variable sound. (A radio speaker is a good choice, or have someone read for you.) The microphone should be about 30 cm from the sound source.

5. Carefully change the dB range control until you get a reading on the instrument's dial. [Note: The sound intensity in dB is the value shown on the dB range control PLUS the value shown by the instrument's dial.]

6. While monitoring the same sound source, change the response speed to "slow" and watch the instrument's dial.

7. What effect does the response-speed setting have on your ability to obtain a sound level reading? Under which circumstances would you use each setting?

8. Hold the sound level meter so that the microphone points toward a speaker's mouth at a distance of 30 cm. Set the instrument for a *slow* response and **linear** weighting.

   a. Have your subject sustain /ɑ/ at an intensity of 70 dB. Then quickly change the weighting selector to **A** weighting. What reading does the meter now show?

   b. Reset the weighting to linear and again have your subject phonate at a sound pressure of 70 dB. Now switch quickly to **B** weighting. What reading do you get?

   c. Finally, do a reading on another sustained /ɑ/, this time switching from **linear** to **C** weighting. What reading do you get now?

Tabulate your findings in the table on the hand-in sheet. What conclusions can you draw about the effect of weighting?

II. VOICE RANGE PROFILE: ESTABLISHING STIMULUS FREQUENCIES

To generate the voice range profile, you will have to determine your patient's maximal and minimal vocal intensity across his entire phonational frequency range. It is, of course, impossible to test at every frequency within this range, so you will have to establish a reasonable number of "sample frequencies" to be tested. The samples should be spaced in a rational way, and the best procedure is to separate all the sample points by an equal number of semitones (ST). (A sample speaker's data are already tabulated on the hand-in sheet to guide you in determining *your* patient's stimulus frequencies.)

1. First you will establish the highest and lowest frequency at which your patient can sustain phonation for a minimum of 1 or 2 seconds (see Unit 12 "Vocal Fundamental Frequency").

a. Use your F_0-measuring instrumentation to determine the F_0 of your patient's phonation. Beginning at a comfortable F_0, have your patient sing /ɑ/, moving down the musical scale until the lowest possible modal-register frequency is reached. Pulse register (or "vocal fry") phonation is not included in the voice range profile. Note on the hand-in sheet the lowest frequency that your patient can sustain.

b. Allow a short rest period (1 minute should be adequate), and, beginning again at a comfortable F_0, have your patient sing up the musical scale until he reaches the highest frequency he can sustain for at least a second or two. Enter this frequency on the hand-in sheet.

c. Determine the ST range encompassed by these two frequencies. (That is, how many STs is the highest frequency above the lowest frequency.) Enter the ST range that you have calculated on the hand-in sheet.

2. You will take 10 samples (above the level of the lowest F_0) for the voice range profile.

   a. Divide the ST range by 10. This establishes the separation (in ST units) between your sample points. Enter this value on the hand-in sheet. (We will call it the sample "distance.")

   b. Now you can determine the actual frequencies you will test at. The first frequency, of course, will be the minimal frequency that you measured directly. Enter it into the table as "ST level 0" on the hand-in sheet.

   c. The next highest frequency that you will test is the one that is "distance" semitones above the lowest. Calculate that frequency and enter it on the hand-in sheet.

   d. Repeat this calculation for the rest of the sample frequencies. They will be (2 × "distance") ST, (3 × "distance") ST, (4 × "distance") ST, . . . (10 × "distance") ST above the lowest frequency. If your calculations are correct, the frequency that is 10 × "distance" semitones above the lowest should be equal (within rounding error) to your patient's maximum vocal F_0. (If it is not, you have done something wrong; Check your calculations and method and try again.) You now have a table of the 11 frequencies at which you will test your patient.

III. THE NORMAL VOICE RANGE PROFILE

Now you are ready to determine the voice range profile of a "patient" who has no known vocal disorder.

1. If your F_0-measuring system has a separate microphone as its input, carefully tape it to the microphone on the sound level meter so that they both point in the same direction and their front surfaces are in the same plane. (The idea is to allow you to pick up the voice signal for both F_0 and sound pressure measurement at the same time!)

2. Carefully tape a meter stick to the underside of the sound level meter. The end of the meter stick should be exactly 30 cm from the microphone(s). When testing, you can hold the end of the meter stick against your patient's chin to ensure that the mouth-microphone distance is always 30 cm. Hold the apparatus so that it is directly in front of your patient, at the same level as his mouth.

3. Set the sound level meter for **A** weighting and a slow response speed.

4. Begin with the sample frequency in the middle of your test-frequency list. (It should be semitone level 5.) Use the frequency meter connected to your square wave generator and adjust the latter to produce a signal of the appropriate frequency. Let your patient listen to this tone, and adjust the loudness to a comfortable level for him.

5. Have your patient sustain /ɑ/, matching the pitch of this stimulus tone at comfortable loudness. He should then phonate more and more softly until he can no longer sustain phonation for at least a second. Record the sound pressure reading on the sound level meter and the F_0 on the F_0-measuring system at the softest phonation your patient can sustain. Enter these values on the hand-in sheet.

6. Now do the same for the ST levels below 5 in descending order. Enter the data on the hand-in sheet.

7. Allow a brief rest period before resuming testing. This time, test the ST levels in ascending order from the center (level 5) value up to the 10-ST level. Enter the data in the table. When you are done you should have a table of the minimum sound pressure levels that your patient can sustain across his F_0 range.

8. Repeat steps 4 through 7, but have your patient increase vocal intensity until his maximum is reached at each frequency. Enter your data in the table. These data show your patient's maximum vocal intensity across his F_0 range.

9. Plot your data points on the graph provided on the hand-in sheet. (It conforms to the standard proposed by the Union of European Phoniatricians. See Schutte and Seidner, 1983.)

10. On the basis of your plot, what can you say about your patient's ability to vary vocal intensity at different points of his F_0 range? What happens to the intensity range at very high and very low frequencies?

11. Look at the curve for maximum intensity. Is there a "notch" in it? If so, where is it and what explanation for it does the research literature offer?

IV. VOCAL PATHOLOGY

Vocal frequency and sound pressure data obtained from a dysphonic patient is provided below:

Sex: Male   Lowest F_0: 86 Hz

Age: 28 years   Highest F_0: 346 Hz

Diagnosis: Vocal nodules F_0 Range: 24.1 ST

Semitone Level	Stimulus Frequency	Patient Response F_0	Sound Pressure Minimum	Sound Pressure Maximum
0	86 Hz	89 Hz	53 dB	62 dB
1	99 Hz	96 Hz	54 dB	72 dB
2	119 Hz	119 Hz	49 dB	78 dB
3	133 Hz	133 Hz	56 dB	79 dB
4	153 Hz	153 Hz	56 dB	80 dB
5	169 Hz	169 Hz	59 dB	77 dB
6	204 Hz	204 Hz	62 dB	71 dB
7	226 Hz	226 Hz	61 dB	74 dB
8	275 Hz	275 Hz	63 dB	79 dB
9	294 Hz	294 Hz	68 dB	80 dB
10	350 Hz	350 Hz	71 dB	83 dB

1. Plot these F_0 and SPL data on the voice range profile form (graph) provided on the hand-in sheet and comment on this patient's performance in terms of his "vocal flexibility."

2. Repeat the voice range profile procedure you just learned, but this time test a patient with a known vocal disorder. Enter your data on the hand-in sheet and comment on your findings. Compare this patient's performance with that of the normal speaker you tested.

READ MORE ABOUT IT!

Airainer, R., & Klingholz, F. (1993). Quantitative evaluation of phonetograms in the case of functional dysphonia. *Journal of Voice, 7,* 136–141.

Awan, S. N. (1991). Phonetographic profiles and F_0-SPL characteristics of untrained versus trained vocal groups. *Journal of Voice, 5,* 41–50.

Baken, R. J. (1987). *Clinical measurement of speech and voice.* Boston: Little, Brown.

Coleman, R. F., & Motto, J. B. (1978). Fundamental frequency and sound pressure level profiles of young female singers. *Folia Phoniatrica, 30,* 94–102.

Coleman, R. F., Mabis, J. H., & Hinson, J. K. (1977). Fundamental frequency-sound pressure level profiles of adult male and female voices. *Journal of Speech and Hearing Research, 20,* 197–204.

Cudahy, E. (1988). *Introduction to instrumentation in speech and hearing* (pp. 64–73). Baltimore: Williams & Wilkins.

Damsté, H. (1970). The phonetogram. *Practica Oto-Rhino-Laryngologica, 32,* 185–187.

Decker, T. N. (1990). *Instrumentation: An introduction for students in the speech and hearing sciences* (pp. 87–97). New York: Longman.

Gelfer, M. P. (1989). Stability in phonational frequency range. *Journal of Communication Disorders, 22,* 181–192.

Gramming, P. (1991). Loudness and frequency capabilities of the voice. *Journal of Voice, 5,* 144–157.

Gramming, P., & Akerlund, L. (1988). Phonetograms for normal and pathological voices. In P. Gramming (Ed.), *The phonetogram: An experimental and clinical study* (pp. 117–132). Malmö, Sweden: University of Lund.

Gramming, P., Gauffin, J., & Sundberg, J. (1986). An attempt to improve the clinical usefulness of phonetograms. *Journal of Phonetics, 14,* 421–427.

Gramming, P., & Sundberg, J. (1988). Spectrum factors relevant to phonetogram measurement. *Journal of the Acoustical Society of America, 83,* 2352–2360.

Gramming, P., Sundberg, J., & Akerlund, L. (1991). Variability of phonetograms. *Folia Phoniatrica, 43,* 79–92.

Gramming, P., Sundberg, J., Ternstrom, S., Leanderson, R., and Perkins, W. H. (1988). Relationship between changes in voice pitch and loudness. *Journal of Voice, 2,* 118–126.

Isshiki, N. (1964). Regulatory mechanism of vocal intensity variation. *Journal of Speech and Hearing Research, 7,* 17–29.

Komiyama, S., Watanabe, H., & Ryu, S. (1984). Phonographic relationship between pitch and intensity of the human voice. *Folia Phoniatrica, 36,* 1–7.

Linville, S. E. (1987). Maximum phonational frequency range capabilities of women's voices with advancing age. *Folia Phoniatrica, 39,* 297–301.

Linville, S. E., Skarin, B. D., & Fornatto, E. (1989). The interrelationship of measures related to vocal function, speech rate, and laryngeal appearance in elderly women. *Journal of Speech and Hearing Research, 32,* 323–330.

Murry, T., Bone, R. C., & von Essen, C. (1974). Changes in voice production during radiotherapy for laryngeal cancer. *Journal of Speech and Hearing Disorders, 39,* 194–201.

Pabon, J. P. H. (1991). Objective acoustic voice-quality parameters in the computer phonetogram. *Journal of Voice, 5,* 203–216.

Pabon, J. P. H., & Plomp, R. (1988). Automatic phonetogram recording supplemented with acoustical voice-quality parameters. *Journal of Speech and Hearing Research, 31,* 710–722.

Pedersen, M. F., & Boberg, A. (1973). Examination of voice function of patients with paralysis of the recurrent nerve. *Acta Otolaryngologica, 75,* 372–374.

Peppard, R. C., Bless, D. M., & Milenkovic, P. (1988). Comparison of young adult singers and nonsingers with vocal nodules. *Journal of Voice, 2,* 250–260.

Reich, A. R., Mason, J. A., Frederickson, R. R., & Schlauch, R. S. (1989). Factors influencing fundamental frequency range estimates in children. *Journal of Speech and Hearing Disorders, 54,* 429–438.

Schutte, H. K., & Seidner, W. (1983). Recommendation by the Union of European Phoniatricians (UEP): Standardizing voice area measurement/phonetography. *Folia Phoniatrica, 35,* 286–288.

Stone, R. E., Jr., Bell, C. J., & Clack, T. D. (1978). Minimum intensity of voice at selected levels within pitch range. *Folia Phoniatrica, 30,* 113–118.

Stone, R. E., Jr., & Ferch, P. A. K. (1982). Intrasubject variability in F_0-SPL_{min} voice profiles. *Journal of Speech and Hearing Disorders, 47,* 123–134.

Titze, I. R. (1992). Acoustic interpretation of the voice range profile (phonetogram). *Journal of Speech and Hearing Research, 35,* 21–34.

Student _____ Date _____

THE SOUND LEVEL METER, VOCAL INTENSITY AND THE VOICE RANGE PROFILE

I. MEASURING VOCAL INTENSITY

1. Use the schematic illustration below to show the location of the controls on your sound level meter.

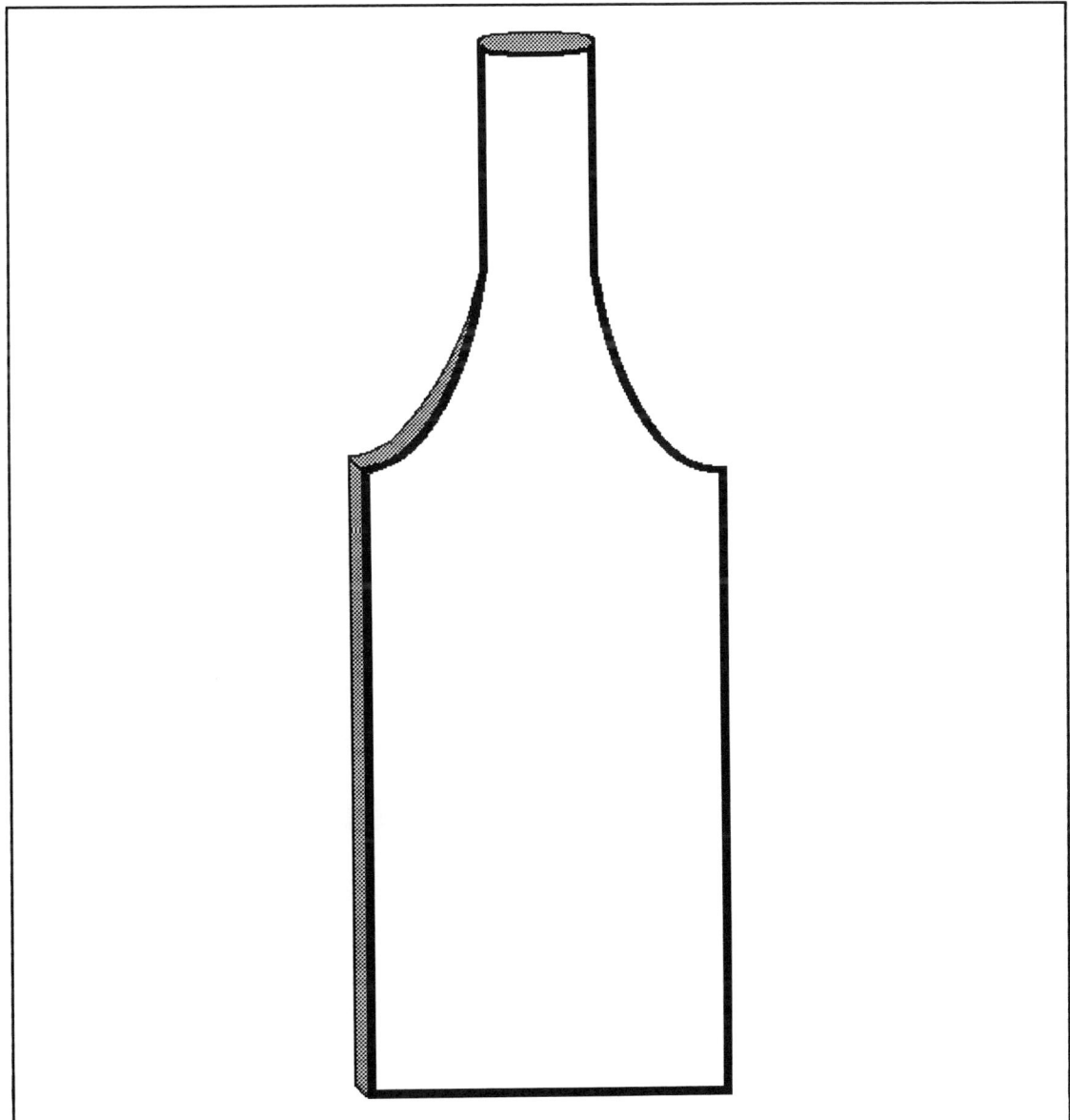

VOICE RANGE PROFILE **173**
Copyright © 1993 Singular Publishing Group, Inc. All rights reserved.

Student _____   Date _____

2. Describe the function of the following:

  a. Response (fast/slow) selector: _____

  _____

  _____

  _____

  _____

  _____

  b. Weighting selector: _____

  _____

  _____

  _____

  _____

  _____

7. Effect of the response-speed setting: _____

  _____

  _____

  _____

  _____

Student _____   Date _____

8. Sound level for similar phonations with different meter weightings:

Weighting	Meter Reading
Linear	_____ dB
A	_____ dB
B	_____ dB
C	_____ dB

Effect of weighting: _____

_____

_____

_____

_____

_____

Student _____ Date _____

II. VOICE RANGE PROFILE: ESTABLISHING STIMULUS FREQUENCIES

A Sample Patient		My Patient	
Sex: Male	Age: 33 years	Sex: _____	Age: _____
Lowest F_0	74 Hz	Lowest F_0	_____ Hz
Highest F_0	612 Hz	Highest F_0	_____ Hz
F_0 range	36.6 ST	F_0 range	_____ ST
"Distance"	3.66 ST	"Distance"	_____ ST

ST Level	ST above Lowest F_0	Stimulus Frequency	ST Level	ST above Lowest F_0	Stimulus Frequency
0	0 ST	74 Hz	0	_____ ST	_____ Hz
1	3.7 ST	78 Hz	1	_____ ST	_____ Hz
2	7.3 ST	113 Hz	2	_____ ST	_____ Hz
3	11.0 ST	140 Hz	3	_____ ST	_____ Hz
4	14.6 ST	172 Hz	4	_____ ST	_____ Hz
5	18.3 ST	213 Hz	5	_____ ST	_____ Hz
6	22.0 ST	264 Hz	6	_____ ST	_____ Hz
7	25.6 ST	325 Hz	7	_____ ST	_____ Hz
8	29.3 ST	402 Hz	8	_____ ST	_____ Hz
9	32.9 ST	495 Hz	9	_____ ST	_____ Hz
10	36.6 ST	612 Hz	10	_____ ST	_____ Hz

III. THE NORMAL VOICE RANGE PROFILE

Sample Patient

Semitone Level	Stimulus Frequency	Patient Response		
		F_0	Sound Pressure	
			Minimum	Maximum
0	74 Hz	72 Hz	45 dB	62 dB
1	78 Hz	81 Hz	43 dB	74 dB
2	113 Hz	110 Hz	50 dB	81 dB
3	140 Hz	144 Hz	52 dB	83 dB
4	172 Hz	167 Hz	51 dB	91 dB
5	213 Hz	217 Hz	50 dB	86 dB
6	264 Hz	254 Hz	52 dB	81 dB
7	325 Hz	333 Hz	56 dB	84 dB
8	402 Hz	394 Hz	58 dB	87 dB
9	495 Hz	507 Hz	59 dB	88 dB
10	612 Hz	604 Hz	60 dB	84 dB

Student _____   Date _____

My Patient

Semitone Level	Stimulus Frequency	Patient Response		
		F_0	Sound Pressure	
			Minimum	Maximum
0	_____ Hz	_____ Hz	_____ dB	_____ dB
1	_____ Hz	_____ Hz	_____ dB	_____ dB
2	_____ Hz	_____ Hz	_____ dB	_____ dB
3	_____ Hz	_____ Hz	_____ dB	_____ dB
4	_____ Hz	_____ Hz	_____ dB	_____ dB
5	_____ Hz	_____ Hz	_____ dB	_____ dB
6	_____ Hz	_____ Hz	_____ dB	_____ dB
7	_____ Hz	_____ Hz	_____ dB	_____ dB
8	_____ Hz	_____ Hz	_____ dB	_____ dB
9	_____ Hz	_____ Hz	_____ dB	_____ dB
10	_____ Hz	_____ Hz	_____ dB	_____ dB

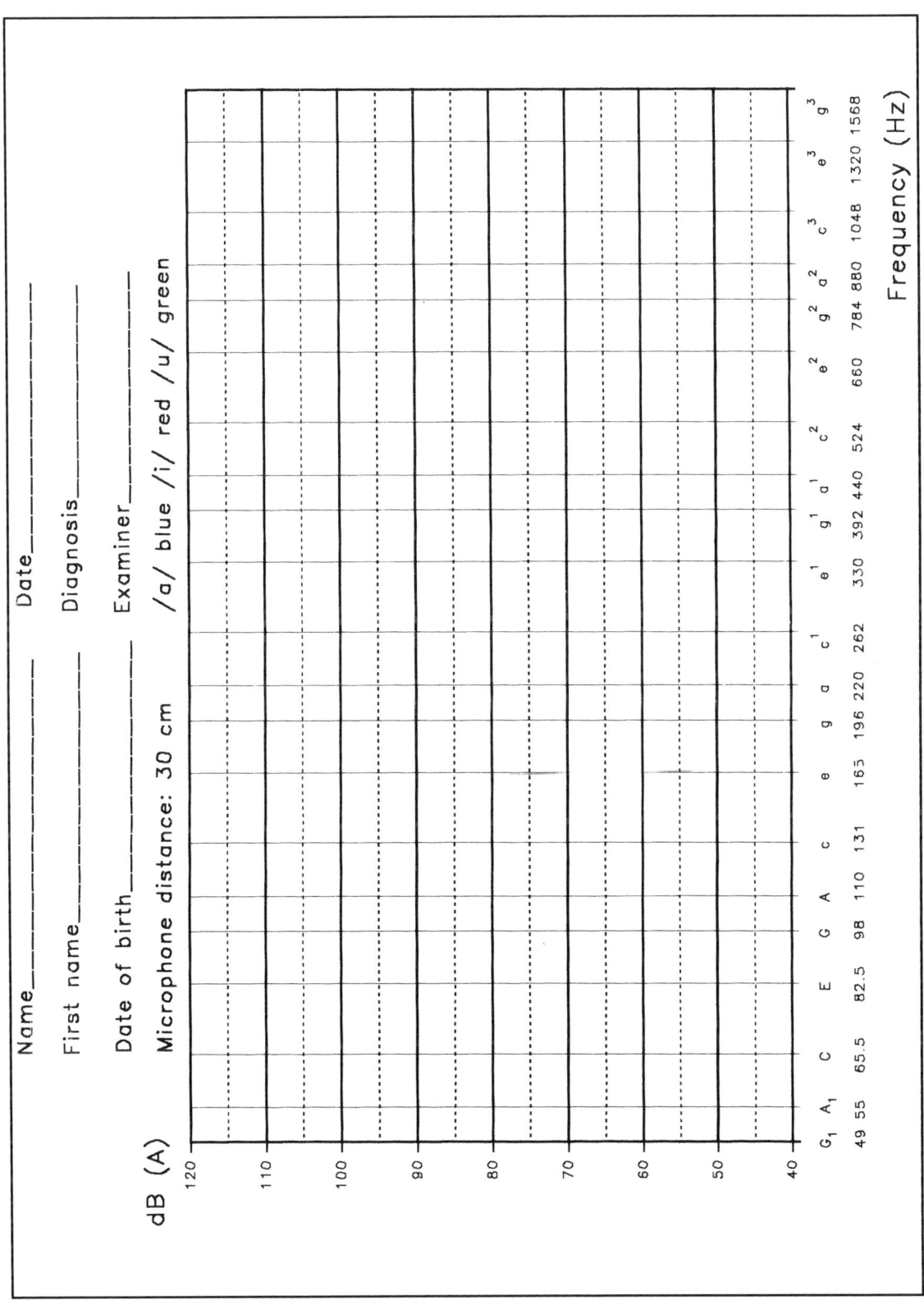

VOICE RANGE PROFILE

Student _____ Date _____

10. Ability to vary intensity at different F_0s: _____

_____

_____

_____

_____

_____

_____

Intensity range at frequency extremes: _____

_____

_____

_____

_____

_____

11. Notch in maximum intensity curve: _____

_____

_____

_____

_____

_____

_____

_____

Student _____ Date _____

IV. VOCAL PATHOLOGY

1. Plot the dysphonic patient's voice range profile on the next page.

Observations and impressions of this patient: _____

_____

_____

_____

_____

_____

_____

_____

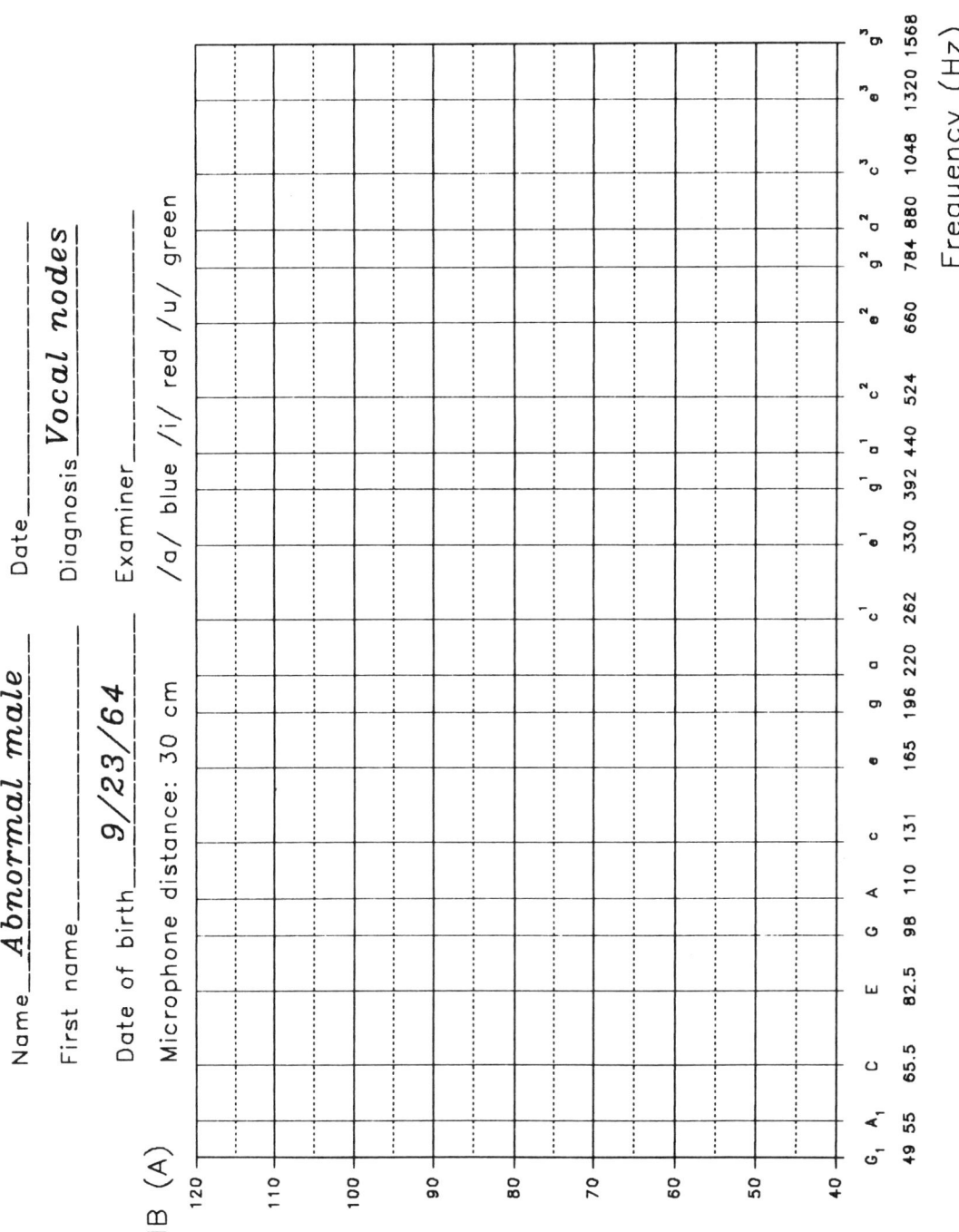

Student _____ Date _____

2. Enter the data obtained from your dysphonic speaker in the table below:

Sex: _____   Lowest F_0: _____ Hz

Age: _____   Highest F_0: _____ Hz

Diagnosis: _____ F_0 Range: _____ ST

Semitone Level	Stimulus Frequency	Patient Response		
		F_0	Sound Pressure Minimum	Sound Pressure Maximum
0	_____ Hz	_____ Hz	_____ dB	_____ dB
1	_____ Hz	_____ Hz	_____ dB	_____ dB
2	_____ Hz	_____ Hz	_____ dB	_____ dB
3	_____ Hz	_____ Hz	_____ dB	_____ dB
4	_____ Hz	_____ Hz	_____ dB	_____ dB
5	_____ Hz	_____ Hz	_____ dB	_____ dB
6	_____ Hz	_____ Hz	_____ dB	_____ dB
7	_____ Hz	_____ Hz	_____ dB	_____ dB
8	_____ Hz	_____ Hz	_____ dB	_____ dB
9	_____ Hz	_____ Hz	_____ dB	_____ dB
10	_____ Hz	_____ Hz	_____ dB	_____ dB

VOICE RANGE PROFILE

Copyright © 1993 Singular Publishing Group, Inc. All rights reserved.

Student _____ Date _____

Name _____ Date _____

First name _____ Diagnosis _____

Date of birth _____ Examiner _____

Microphone distance: 30 cm   /a/ blue /i/ red /u/ green

dB (A): 120, 110, 100, 90, 80, 70, 60, 50, 40

Frequency (Hz):
- G_1 49
- A_1 55
- C 65.5
- E 82.5
- G 98
- A 110
- c 131
- e 165
- g 196
- a 220
- c^1 262
- e^1 330
- g^1 392
- a^1 440
- c^2 524
- e^2 660
- g^2 784
- a^2 880
- c^3 1048
- e^3 1320
- g^3 1568

184 CLINICAL SPEECH AND VOICE MEASUREMENT
Copyright © 1993 Singular Publishing Group, Inc. All rights reserved.

Student _____ Date _____

Observations and impressions of the dysphonic speaker you tested: _____

_____
_____
_____
_____
_____
_____
_____
_____

UNIT 15

Clinical Application: Vocal Rise Time

According to Koike (1967), the vocal rise time is the amount of time it takes from the onset of voice until the amplitude of the acoustic signal (that is, the acoustic envelope) has reached the mean amplitude of the steady portion of the phonation. As such, measures of "rise time" include all amplitude adjustments made prior to the maintenance of a relatively stable vowel amplitude. Several studies have identified abnormal voice initiation characteristics in fluency, voice, or articulatory disorders. Clinicians will commonly examine the onset of comfortably sustained phonations, but occasionally there may be clinical interest in the rise time associated with the patient's softest or fastest voice initiation.

Purpose: In these exercises you will learn to measure vocal rise time from an acoustic record and to provide a basic interpretation of abnormal voice onset characteristics.

Equipment: A microphone and a means of generating a printed oscillogram and/or amplitude trace.

General preparation: Review what is known about normal and abnormal vocal rise time (Koike, 1967; Koike, Hirano, & von Leden, 1967; Baken, 1987, pp. 108–109; see Unit 10 "Reading Oscillograms").

Exercises

On the hand-in sheet are oscillograms obtained from three different patients who sustained a vowel at a "comfortable" pitch and loudness:

Patient A. 22-year-old female with arthritis of the cricoarytenoid joint

Patient B. 26-year-old male stutterer

Patient C. 62-year-old male with spastic dysarthria

Each waveform has been truncated at some point after the speaker's vowel reaches a relatively steady amplitude.

1. Using these samples:

   a. Mark each oscillogram to indicate the initiation of phonation and the end of the vocal rise envelope.
   b. Determine the vocal rise time of each sample and enter these data in the table provided on the hand-in sheet.
   c. Consulting available norms on vocal rise time, provide a brief description/classification of each speaker's vowel onset.

2. Provide a more detailed assessment of each speaker's acoustic onset characteristics. Whose rise time was most difficult to measure? Explain.

3. Obtain acoustic samples of your own fastest and softest vowel onsets and compare those rise times to that obtained for the initiation of a "comfortable" phonation. Place labeled copies of these waveforms in your lab report and enter these values in the table for speaker "D." Provide a brief assessment of each rise time where indicated.

4. Obtain fast, soft, and comfortable vowel samples from a dysphonic patient. Attach these labeled waveforms to your lab report and enter the data in the table for speaker "E," along with some evaluative comments.

5. Compare your comfortable vocal onset and that of your patient to those of speakers A–C. Describe possible reasons for any similarities or differences among them. Comment on any differences between your fast and soft onsets and those of your patient.

READ MORE ABOUT IT!

Adams, M. R., & Hayden, P. (1976). The ability of stutterers and nonstutterers to initiate and terminate phonation during production of an isolated vowel. *Journal of Speech and Hearing Research, 19,* 290–296.

Adams, M. R., Riemenschneider, S., Metz, D., & Conture, E. (1974). Voice onset and articulatory constriction requirements in a speech segment and their relation to the amount of stuttering. *Journal of Fluency Disorders, 1,* 23–29.

Adams, M. R., & Reis, R. (1971). The influence of the onset of phonation on the frequency of stuttering. *Journal of Speech and Hearing Research, 14,* 639–644.

Adams, M. R., & Reis, R. (1974). The influence of the onset of phonation on the frequency of stuttering: A replication and re-evaluation. *Journal of Speech and Hearing Research, 17,* 752–754.

Agnello, J. C. (1975). Voice onset and termination features of stutterers. In L. M. Webster & L. Furst (Eds.), *Vocal tract dynamics and dysfluency* (pp. 40–70). New York: Speech and Hearing Institute.

Baken, R. J. (1987). *Clinical measurement of speech and voice.* Boston: Little, Brown.

Borden, G. J., Baer, T., & Kenney, M. K. (1985). Onset of voicing in stuttered and fluent utterances. *Journal of Speech and Hearing Research, 28,* 363–372.

Cullinan, W., & Springer, M. (1980). Voice initiation and termination times in stuttering and nonstuttering children. *Journal of Speech and Hearing Research, 23,* 344–360.

Flower, R. M. (1959). Voice training in the management of dysphonia. *Laryngoscope, 69,* 940–946.

Koike, Y. (1967). Experimental studies on vocal attack. *Practica Otologica Kyoto, 60,* 663–688.

Koike, Y., Hirano, M., & von Leden, H. (1967). Vocal initiation: Acoustic and aerodynamic investigations of normal subjects. *Folia Phoniatrica, 19,* 173–182.

Lamprecht, A. (1990). Untersuchungen zur Regelung von Stimmschallparametern zu Beginn der Phonation [Studies on the regulation of voice parameters at the beginning of phonation]. *Folia Phoniatrica, 42,* 302–311.

Leeper, H. A., Jr. (1976). Voice initiation characteristics of normal children and children with vocal nodules: A preliminary investigation. *Journal of Communication Disorders, 9,* 83–94.

Peters, H. F. M., Boves, L., & van Dielen, J. C. H. (1986). Perceptual judgment of abruptness of voice onset in vowels as a function of the amplitude envelope. *Journal of Speech and Hearing Disorders, 51,* 299–308.

Rees, M. (1958). Harshness and glottal attack. *Journal of Speech and Hearing Research, 1,* 344–349.

Student _____   Date _____

VOCAL RISE TIME

1. b. Indicate each speaker's vocal rise time; and

   c. provide a brief assessment to complete the following table:

Speaker	Phonatory Condition	Vocal Rise Time (in ms)	Assessment*
A. Female, 22 years	Comfortable	_____	_____
B. Male, 26 years	Comfortable	_____	_____
C. Male, 62 years	Comfortable	_____	_____
D. Yourself (_____)	Fast	_____	_____
	Soft	_____	_____
	Comfortable	_____	_____
E. Your Patient (_____)	Fast	_____	_____
	Soft	_____	_____
	Comfortable	_____	_____

* Source(s) for comparison: _____

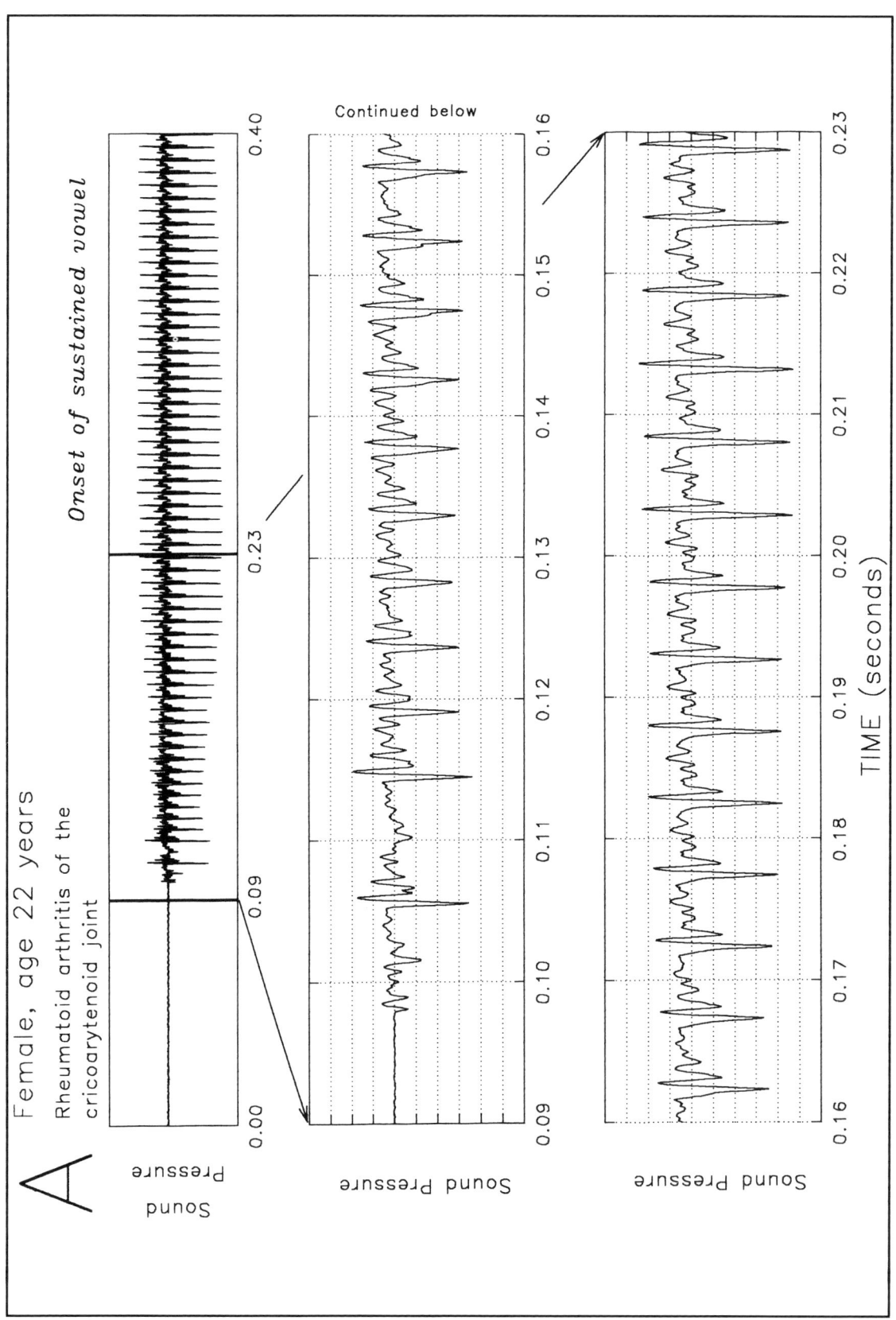

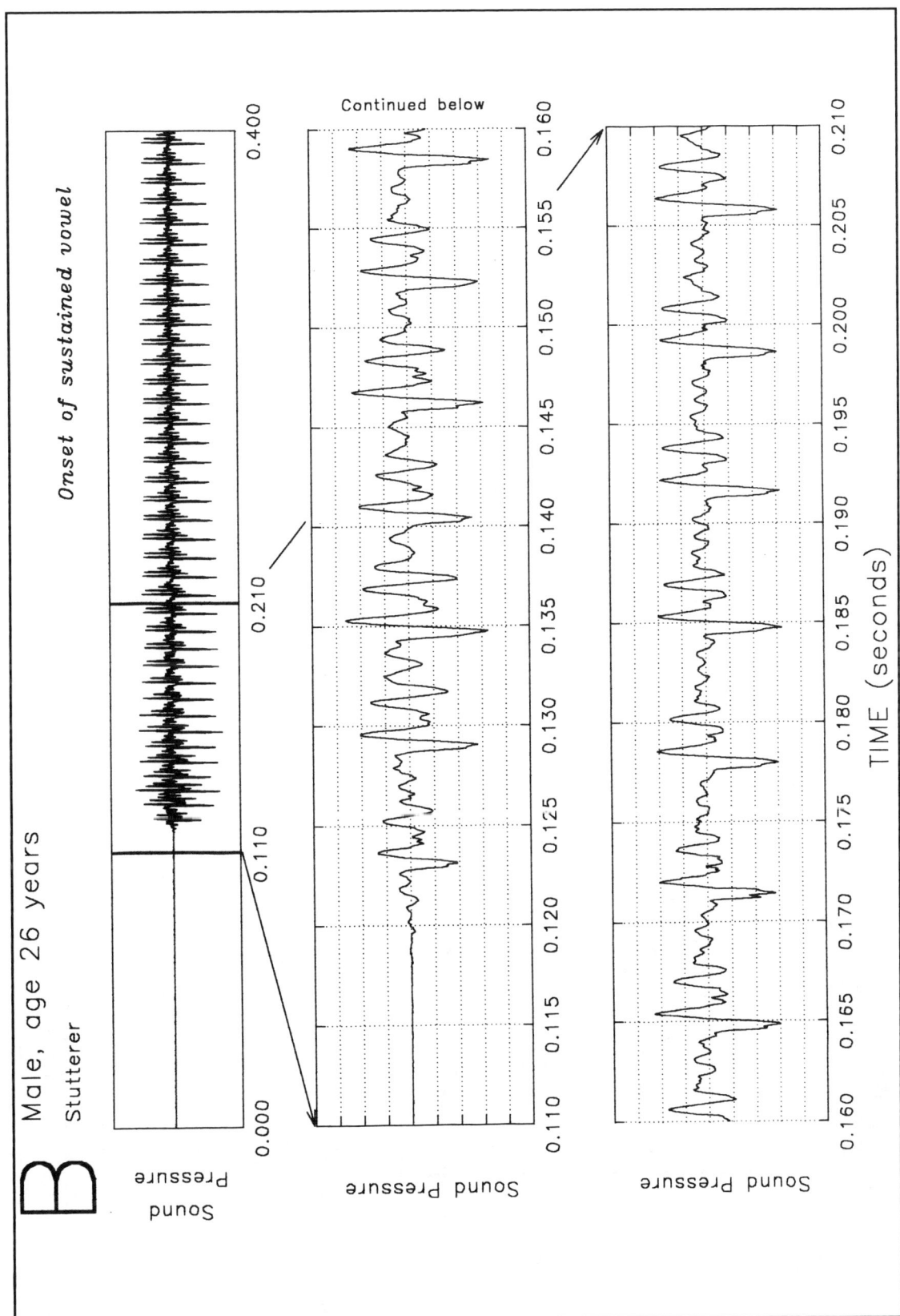

VOCAL RISE TIME

Student   Date

c. The following figure shows the acoustic waveform (a, above) and derived energy (dB SPL) data (b, below) as might be displayed using an acoustic analysis system, such as the Kay Elemetrics CSL™ 4300 used here.

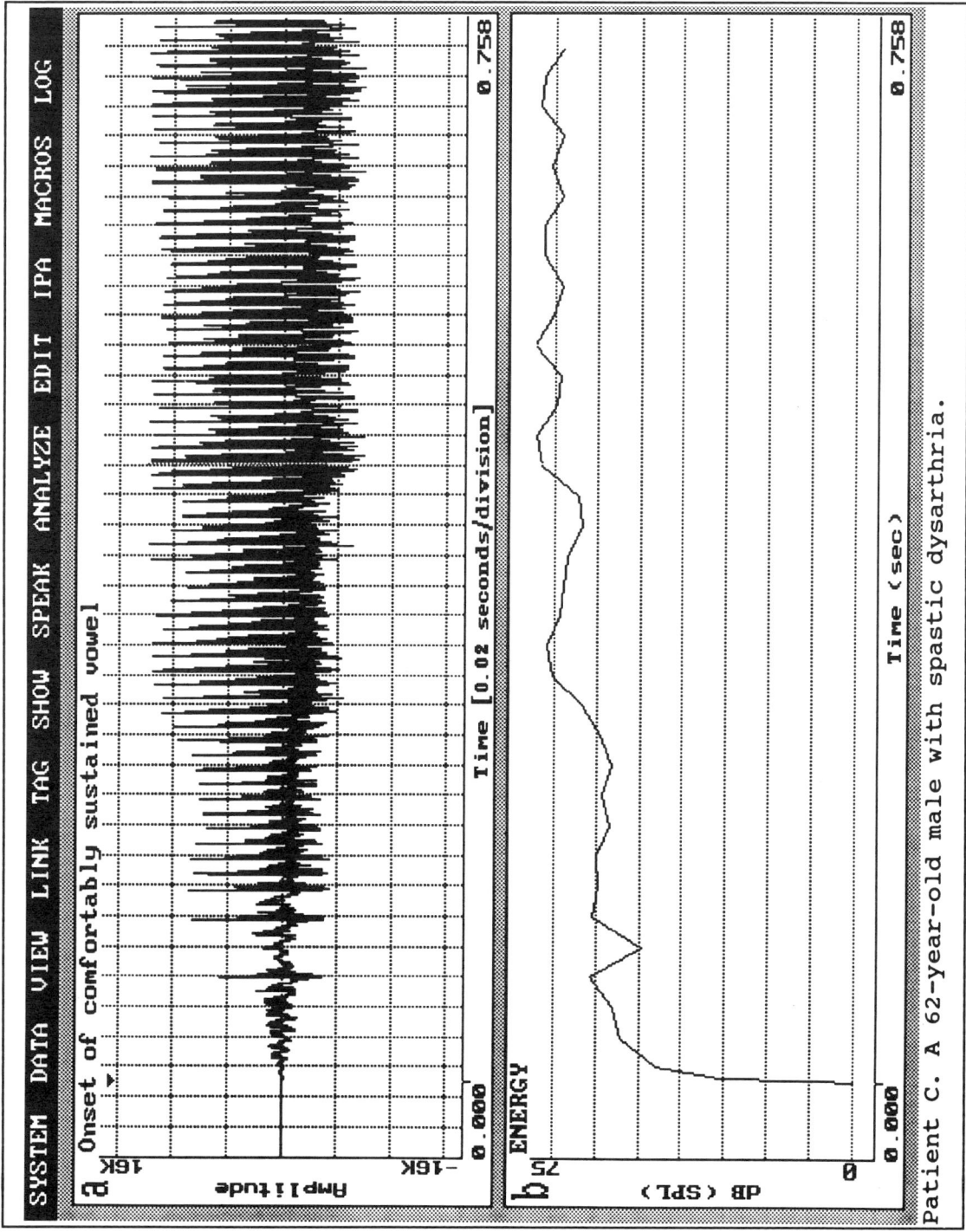

Patient C. A 62-year-old male with spastic dysarthria.

Student _____ Date _____

2. Measurement and assessment of vocal rise time:

Speaker A: _____

_____

_____

Speaker B: _____

_____

_____

Speaker C: _____

_____

_____

Most difficult rise time measure: _____

_____

_____

_____

5. Comparison of comfortable vocal onsets: _____

_____

_____

_____

_____

_____

_____

Student _____   Date _____

_____
_____
_____
_____

Comparison of fast and soft vocal onsets: _____

_____
_____
_____
_____
_____

Attach your data records and those of your patient to this page.

UNIT 16

Clinical Application: Amplitude Perturbation (Vocal Shimmer)

Analogous to frequency perturbation, measures of short-term amplitude perturbation (vocal shimmer) serve as an index of vocal stability. Excessive shimmer, like jitter, has been tied to the perception of hoarseness and some research has indicated that it might be an even more sensitive index of vocal pathology. A mean cycle-to-cycle amplitude difference on the order of 0.7 dB or less or variation less than about 7% of the mean amplitude may be expected in a controlled, sustained phonation produced by a normal speaker. Like jitter, mean shimmer tends to be generally higher in vocal pathology and in normal phonations sustained at low fundamental frequencies and intensities (e.g., Horii, 1980; Orlikoff & Kahane, 1991). Below are brief descriptions of the more common indices of amplitude perturbation (see Baken, 1987, for a more detailed review):[1]

Mean Shimmer in Decibels. This is simply the mean absolute dB (SPL) difference between sequential vocal amplitudes measured during a sustained phonation (see Unit 8 "Decibels").

Mean Shimmer in Percent. Percent shimmer is the mean absolute cycle-to-cycle difference in vocal amplitude (in any arbitrary unit, such as volts) divided by the mean amplitude (in the same unit of measurement). This proportion is then multiplied by 100 to yield a percentage.

Amplitude Perturbation Quotient. Analogous to RAP or FPQ measures of relative jitter, the amplitude perturbation quotient (APQ) attempts to "de-

---
[1] Mathematical definitions are provided in Appendix F.

sensitize" the measure to long-term amplitude changes (Takahashi & Koike, 1975). Again, such long-term effects might be associated with a gradually "drifting" (falling or rising) amplitude or with relatively regular upward and downward variations as associated with tremor. Most commonly, measures of APQ employ 11-point averaging (although 3- and 5-point averaging have also been used). The average cycle-to-cycle amplitude difference from the derived "trend line" is then divided by the mean period. As with RAP, it has become common to report APQ in percent.

Purpose: In this exercise you will become familiar with the uses and calculation of acoustic amplitude perturbation in sustained phonation. As with jitter measurement, the precise analysis of many hundreds of vocal cycles is necessary for valid shimmer measurement. In these exercises hand analysis of relatively short samples will be used for you to gain insight into the nature of these measures.

Equipment: A microphone and a means of generating a printed oscillogram.

General preparation: Review basic measurement of vocal amplitude (see Unit 10 "Reading Oscillograms" and Unit 14 "The Sound Level Meter") and frequency perturbation (see Unit 13 "Fundamental Frequency Perturbation").

> **CLINICAL NOTE:** There are now several commercially available acoustic analysis systems that will provide various measures of vocal noise. Because there are so many indices of frequency and amplitude perturbation, as well as turbulence and waveform (so-called *additive*) noise, it is essential for the clinician to become familiar with the instruction manuals accompanying a given instrument so that the nature of data extraction and calculation are clearly understood.

An example of one such computer-automated analysis is shown on the next page. Here the voicing analysis software of the Kay Elemetrics CSL™ system[2] provides several acoustic voice measures (in this case percent RAP, mean shimmer in dB, and Yumoto's [1983, 1988] spectral harmonics-to-noise ratio. These measures were derived from the acoustic signal (displayed in A, at the top). A normal 36-year-old male sustained the vowel /ɑ/ for approximately 8 seconds while attempting to maintain a comfortable phonation with a maximally steady pitch and loudness. The derived frequency and sound pressure level traces appear in the two lower panels (B and C, respectively). Because vocal instability at the initiation and termination of a sustained vowel is typical even for normal voices, these data have been excluded from the analysis (note the vertical cursors). When assessing pathology, many clinicians select the most stable portion of the sample for voice analysis.

---

[2] Computerized Speech Lab (CSL)™, model 4300, Kay Elemetrics Corporation, Pine Brook, NJ (software version 3.11)

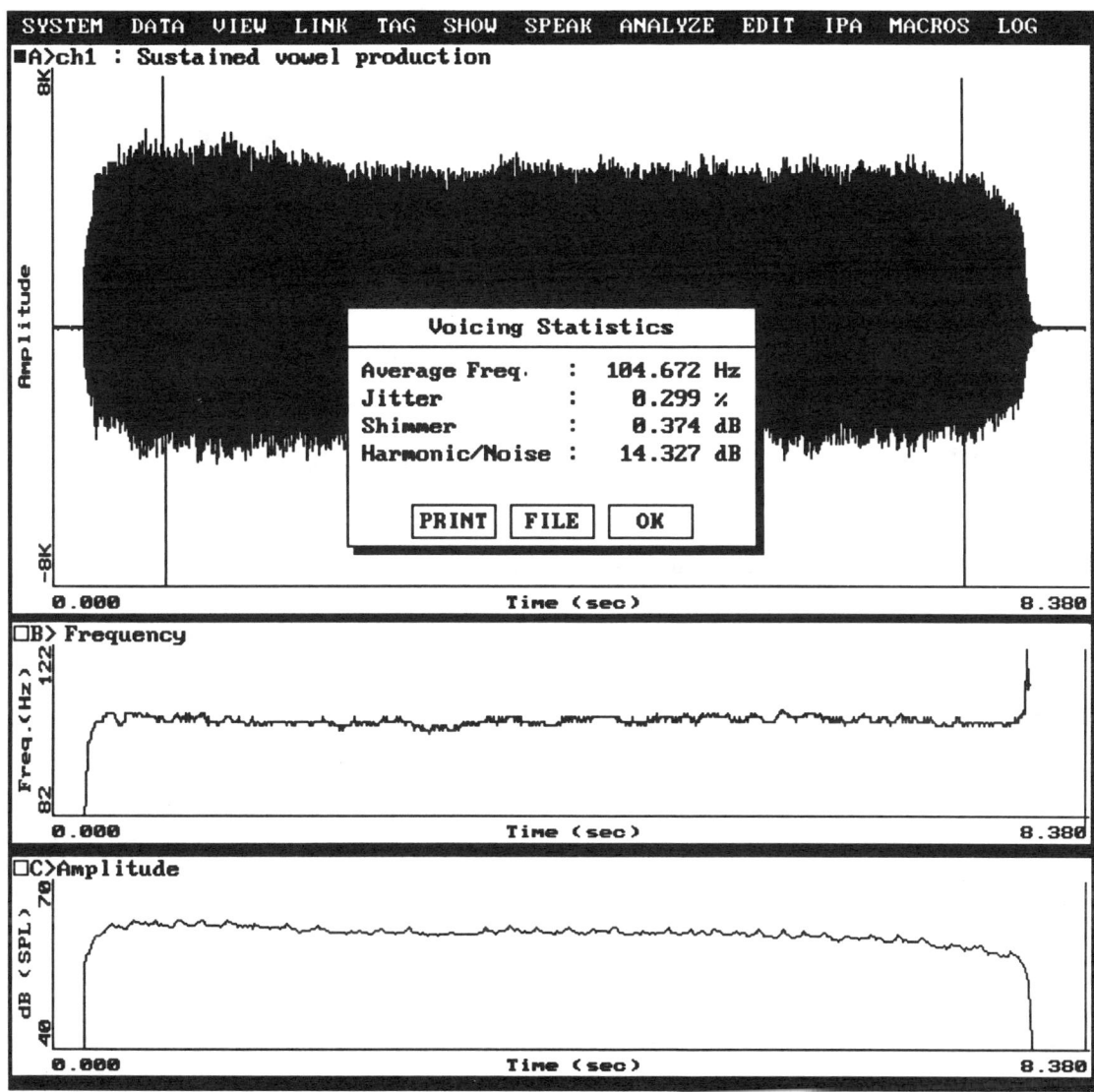

Exercises

Patient A

On the hand-in sheet is a sound pressure (acoustic) waveform obtained while a dysphonic woman prolonged a phonation at a comfortable pitch and loudness. The interval from the 770th to 870th millisecond has been enlarged for more precise measurement.

1. Delineate and number the vocal cycles on the record (the first three have been done for you).

2. Fill in the remainder of the table on the hand-in sheet.

3. Based on the amplitude values entered in the table, what is the mean shimmer (in percent and dB)?

4. Compare these values with available normative data. Be sure to cite your source, also providing a brief assessment.

Patient B

On the hand-in sheet is a similar acoustic record for another dysphonic speaker. Using this sample:

1. Delineate and number the cycles on the record (again, the first three cycles have been done for you).

2. Complete the corresponding table on the hand-in sheet.

3. Using this table, what is the mean shimmer (in percent and dB)?

4. Compare these values with available normative data and provide your assessment as you did for Patient A.

Patient C

The acoustic record on the next page is from an adult woman with organic voice tremor attempting to sustain a steady phonation. It is clear, especially from the complete excerpt, that the acoustic amplitude of the signal gradually rises and falls (at a frequency of about 4.25 Hz).

Sequential amplitude data (numbered on the oscillogram) are shown in the table on page 202 along with their mean absolute differences:

1. From this data table determine the mean percent shimmer.

2. The sample amplitude data are provided in a table on the hand-in sheet along with the five-point average of each.

   a. Complete this table; and

   b. Use these data to determine the amplitude perturbation quotient (APQ, 5-point) for this sample.

3. Compare the shimmer measurements obtained for #1 and #2 above. How do you interpret them?

Female, age 56 years
Essential (organic) voice tremor

Vowel /a/ sustained at a comfortable pitch and loudness

VOCAL SHIMMER

Cycle No. (n)	Amplitude (A, in volts[3])	$\|A_n - A_{n+1}\|$ (shimmer, in volts)
1	1.166	
		0.004
2	1.170	
		0.006
3	1.164	
		0.192
4	1.356	
		0.054
5	1.410	
		0.092
6	1.502	
		0.200
7	1.702	
		0.160
8	1.542	
		0.004
9	1.538	
		0.048
10	1.490	
		0.070
11	1.560	
		0.204
12	1.356	
		0.232
13	1.124	

[3] Because shimmer is a relative measure, vocal amplitude can be measured in any arbitrary unit such as millimeters or simply "horizontal divisions" (see Unit 5 "Relative Measures and Logarithmic Scaling").

Self-Measurement

Measure your own shimmer using either an oscillogram or analysis system (as shown above). How do these measurements relate to available normative data? Compare your measurements to those obtained from a similar phonation sustained by a dysphonic speaker.

READ MORE ABOUT IT!

Baken, R. J. (1987). *Clinical measurement of speech and voice* (pp. 113–119). Boston: Little, Brown.

Glaze, L. E., Bless, D. M., Milenkovic, P., & Susser, R. D. (1988). Acoustic characteristics of children's voice. *Journal of Voice, 2,* 312–319.

Glaze, L. E., Bless, D. M., & Susser, R. D. (1990). Acoustic analysis of vowel and loudness differences in children's voice. *Journal of Voice, 4,* 37–44.

Heiberger, V. L., & Horii, Y. (1982). Jitter and shimmer in sustained phonation. In N. J. Lass (Ed.), *Speech and language: Advances in basic research and practice* (vol. 7, pp. 299–332). New York: Academic Press.

Hillenbrand, J. (1988). Perception of aperiodicities in synthetically generated voices. *Journal of the Acoustical Society of America, 83,* 2361–2371.

Horii, Y. (1980). Vocal shimmer in sustained phonation. *Journal of Speech and Hearing Research, 23,* 202–209.

Horii Y. (1982). Jitter and shimmer differences among sustained vowel phonations. *Journal of Speech and Hearing Research, 25,* 12–14.

Koike, Y., Takahashi, H., & Calcaterra, T. C. (1977). Acoustic measures for detecting laryngeal pathology. *Acta Otolaryngologica, 84,* 105–117.

Laver, J., Hiller, S., & Beck, J. M. (1992). Acoustic waveform perturbations and voice disorders. *Journal of Voice, 6,* 115–126.

Ludlow, C. L., Bassich, C. J., Connor, N. P., Coulter, D. C., & Lee, Y. J. (1987). The validity of using phonatory jitter and shimmer to detect laryngeal pathology. In T. Baer, C. T. Sasaki, & K. S. Harris (Eds.), *Laryngeal function in phonation and respiration* (pp. 492–508). San Diego: Singular Publishing Group.

Orlikoff, R. F. (1990). The relationship of age and cardiovascular health to certain acoustic characteristics of male voices. *Journal of Speech and Hearing Research, 33,* 450–457.

Orlikoff, R. F., & Kahane, J. C. (1991). Influence of mean sound pressure level on jitter and shimmer measures. *Journal of Voice, 5,* 113–119.

Sorensen, D., & Horii, Y. (1983). Frequency and amplitude perturbation in the voices of female speakers. *Journal of Communication Disorders, 16,* 57–61.

Takahashi, H., & Koike, Y. (1975). Some perceptual dimensions and acoustical correlates of pathologic voices. *Acta Oto-laryngologica* (Suppl. 338), 1–24.

Yumoto, E. (1983). The quantitative evaluation of hoarseness. *Archives of Otolaryngology, 109,* 48–52.

Yumoto, E. (1988). Quantitative assessment of the degree of hoarseness. *Journal of Voice, 1,* 310–313.

Student   Date

VOCAL SHIMMER

PATIENT A

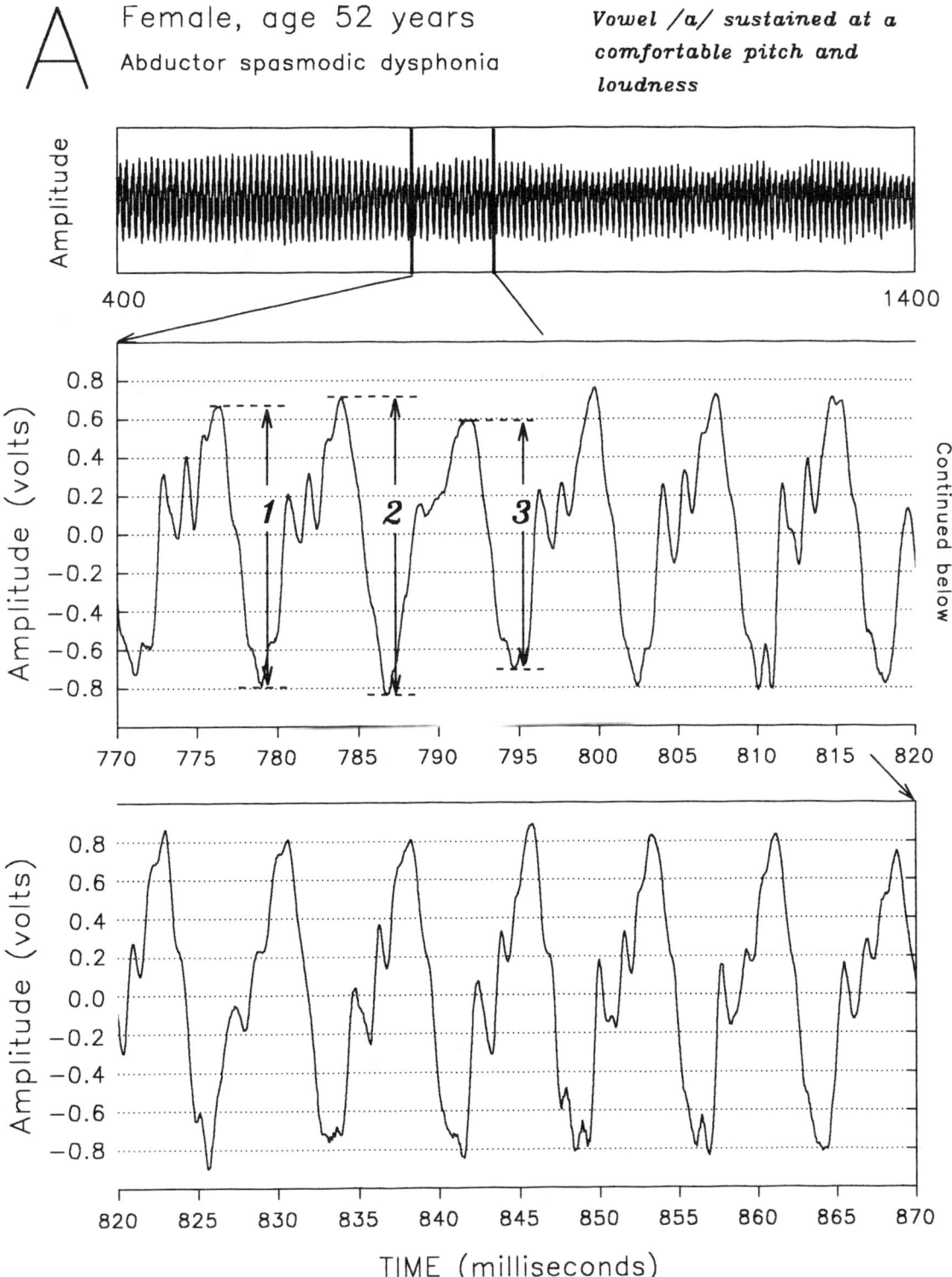

A Female, age 52 years
   Abductor spasmodic dysphonia

Vowel /a/ sustained at a comfortable pitch and loudness

Student _____   Date _____

2. Complete the following table for Patient A.

Cycle No. (n)	Amplitude (A, in volts)	$\|A_n - A_{n+1}\|$ (Shimmer, in volts)	$\|20 \times \log (A_n/A_{n+1})\|$ (Shimmer, in dB)
1	1.440		
2	1.520	0.080	0.473
3	1.287	0.233	1.445
4	_____	_____	_____
5	_____	_____	_____
6	_____	_____	_____
7	_____	_____	_____
8	_____	_____	_____
9	_____	_____	_____
10	_____	_____	_____
11	_____	_____	_____
12	_____	_____	_____

3. Mean shimmer (show arithmetic) —

In percent: _____

_____

In decibels: _____

_____

4. Comparison: _____

_____

_____

Source: _____

3. Complete the following summary table:

Spectrogram Characteristics	Origin
Harmonic line spacing	VOCAL SOUND SOURCE
Noise between harmonics	VOCAL SOUND SOURCE
Decrease of harmonic strength with increasing frequency	VOCAL SOUND SOURCE
Glottal pulses	VOCAL SOUND SOURCE
Movement of harmonic lines	VOCAL SOUND SOURCE
Formant bands	VOCAL TRACT FILTER

4. Complete the following table concerning the effects of various communication disorders/symptoms:

Condition	Origin: Source/Filter	Effect on: Harmonics/Formants
a. Dysphonia (vocal nodules)	SOURCE	HARMONICS
b. Dysarthria	FILTER or BOTH	FORMANTS or BOTH
c. Abnormal vocal mutation	SOURCE	HARMONICS
d. Delayed speech maturation	FILTER	FORMANTS
e. Stuttering	BOTH	BOTH
f. Hypernasality	FILTER	FORMANTS

Student _____   Date _____

2. Complete the following table for Patient B:

Cycle No. (n)	Amplitude (A, in volts)	$\|A_n - A_{n+1}\|$ (Shimmer, in volts)	$\|20 \times \log(A_n/A_{n+1})\|$ (Shimmer, in dB)
1	1.125		
		0.048	0.363
2	1.173		
		0.133	1.045
3	1.040		
4	_____	_____	_____
5	_____	_____	_____
6	_____	_____	_____
7	_____	_____	_____
8	_____	_____	_____
9	_____	_____	_____
10	_____	_____	_____
11	_____	_____	_____
12	_____		

3. Mean shimmer (show arithmetic) —

In percent: _____

_____

In decibels: _____

_____

4. Comparison: _____

_____

_____

Source: _____

Student   Date

PATIENT C

1. Mean percent shimmer (show arithmetic):

2. a. Complete the following table:

Cycle No. (n)	Amplitude (A, in volts)	$\dfrac{A_{n-2} + A_{n-1} + A_n + A_{n+1} + A_{n+2}}{5}$	$\dfrac{A_{n-2} + A_{n-1} + A_n + A_{n+1} + A_{n+2}}{5} - A_n$
1	1.166	[no A_{n-1} or A_{n-2}]	
2	1.170	[no A_{n-2}]	
3	1.164	1.123	0.089
4	1.356	1.320	_____
5	1.410	1.427	_____
6	1.502	1.502	_____
7	1.702	1.539	_____
8	1.542	1.555	_____
9	1.538	1.566	_____
10	1.490	_____	_____
11	1.560	_____	_____
12	1.356	[no A_{n+2}]	
13	1.112	[no A_{n+1} or A_{n+2}]	

b. Amplitude Perturbation Quotient (APQ_5) (show arithmetic):

_____ %

3. Comparison of APQ and percent shimmer: _____

Student _____ Date _____

_____
_____
_____

SELF-MEASUREMENT

Measurement and evaluation of your mean shimmer: _____

_____
_____
_____
_____
_____

Comparison with dysphonic speaker: _____

_____
_____
_____
_____
_____

(If data printouts are available, attach them to this page.)

AIR PRESSURES FOR SPEECH AND VOICE

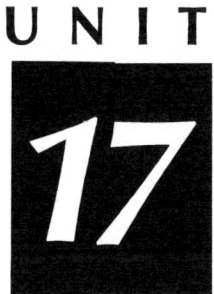

Clinical Application: Intraoral Pressure During Consonant Production

Speech sounds result from the precise use of air pressure generated by the respiratory system. The pressure of air behind a consonantal constriction (the *intraoral pressure*, or P_{io}) can reveal a great deal about articulatory coordination.

Purpose: In these exercises you will

- Become familiar with the instrumentation required to observe intraoral pressure;
- Learn to form an intraoral pressure probe (catheter);
- Learn to obtain valid measures of P_{io} during consonant production;
- Gain some skill in assessing the validity of the data record; and
- Undertake some basic interpretation of the articulatory behavior that produced the intraoral pressure.

Equipment: A pressure transducer and associated electronic support circuits. Catheter tubing is needed for an intraoral pressure probe (together with copper wire and boiling water for shaping it). You will also need a 3-way stopcock, a large-volume hypodermic syringe, and a water (U-tube) manometer. Lastly, you will need a microphone, audio amplifier, and a 2-channel data recording system.

General preparation: Review the general physics of air pressure and the units of its measurement (Baken, 1987, pp. 241–245). Read about P_{io} in children and adults (Arkebauer, Hixon, & Hardy, 1967; Baken, 1987, pp. 254–260; Stathopoulos, 1986).

Examine the pressure transducer that you will be using and study the manual that accompanies it. You should understand the principles upon which it works (Baken, 1987, pp. 245–254) and, in particular, you should be able to specify: (1) The maximum pressure that the transducer can safely measure; (2) The kind of support electronics that your pressure transducer requires; and (3) The sensitivity of the pressure transducer (usually stated in the manual).

I. SETTING UP AND CALIBRATING THE PRESSURE SYSTEM

Before we can do any measurement, the pressure transduction system must be calibrated. That is, we need to know how much output is produced (in terms of volts, or the height of the tracing on a graph) for each unit of pressure sensed by the transducer. We will do this using a water (U-tube) manometer.

1. Prepare a block diagram of the pressure instrumentation array that you will use. Be sure to label each of its parts.

2. Indicate the maximum allowed pressure and the sensitivity of the transducer.

3. Connect the apparatus according to your diagram, and connect the U-tube and syringe (about half-filled with air) as shown in Baken (1987, Fig. 7–4, p. 247) in preparation for calibrating the system (see also Unit 11 "Calibration").

4. Turn on the transducer electronics and the recording system and allow several minutes for them to warm-up and stabilize. [NOTE: Be sure that the transducer amplifier and recording systems are set for a "DC response."]

5. Move the plunger of the syringe so that the U-tube manometer shows 0 pressure. (The pressure in the transducer, in other words, is the same as that of the atmosphere.) If necessary, adjust the trace (pen) position on the data recorder.

6. Activate the paper drive of the recorder system and let it run for a few seconds. You will have produced a trace on the chart that represents zero pressure. Label the line that you made on the chart "0."

7. Now move the syringe's plunger to obtain a pressure of about 12 cm H_2O. Record a couple of seconds at this pressure, and mark the new line on your chart "12." [NOTE: The lines on your recording should extend over about 2/3 of the available vertical range. If you need to, adjust the sensitivity of your transducer amplifier or data recorder and recalibrate.]

8. Repeat #7 using pressures 2, 4, 8, and 10 cm H_2O. Label the resulting lines on your chart recording.

9. Disconnect the U-tube and syringe from the input of your pressure system.

10. Use a ruler to measure, as accurately as possible, the vertical distance from the 0 line to the 12 line. Use this distance to determine the calibration of your chart in terms of "cm height per cm H$_2$O." Indicate the calibration both on the hand-in sheet and on the chart you have made and include it with the materials you submit to your instructor.

> **WARNING:** If you later change any of the settings, either on your transducer amplifier or on your data recorder, your calibration will be invalid and you will have to recalibrate. It is a good idea to carefully put strips of adhesive tape across all adjustment dials on the equipment to remind you not to change anything!

II. MAKING AN ORAL PRESSURE PROBE

Although intraoral pressure can be sensed by passing a catheter through the nasal cavity and velopharyngeal port into the oropharynx, for routine clinical work it is generally more convenient to insert a sensing tube directly into the oral cavity. It is critical, of course, that the tube opening be perpendicular to the airflow. It will also minimize interference with speech production if the sensing tube runs around the last molar and along the buccal side of the maxillary dental arch, to emerge at the corner of the mouth (see Baken, 1987, Fig. 7–11A, p. 256). Achieving this will require shaping a length of medical catheter tubing as an oral pressure probe.

1. Fill a suitable container with water to a depth of about 10 cm and heat it to boiling.

2. Take a 15 cm length of copper wire and insert it into the end of a piece of catheter tubing about 25 cm long. Leave about 1 cm of the wire protruding from the end of the tube. Be sure that the end of the protruding section is not sharp.

3. Seat your patient comfortably, with her head supported and her mouth at about the level of your eyes. Arrange for good illumination of her oral cavity (see Unit 3 "Physical Examination").

4. Insert the wired end of the catheter into your patient's mouth, and gently bend it to assume the shape shown in the diagram on page 216.

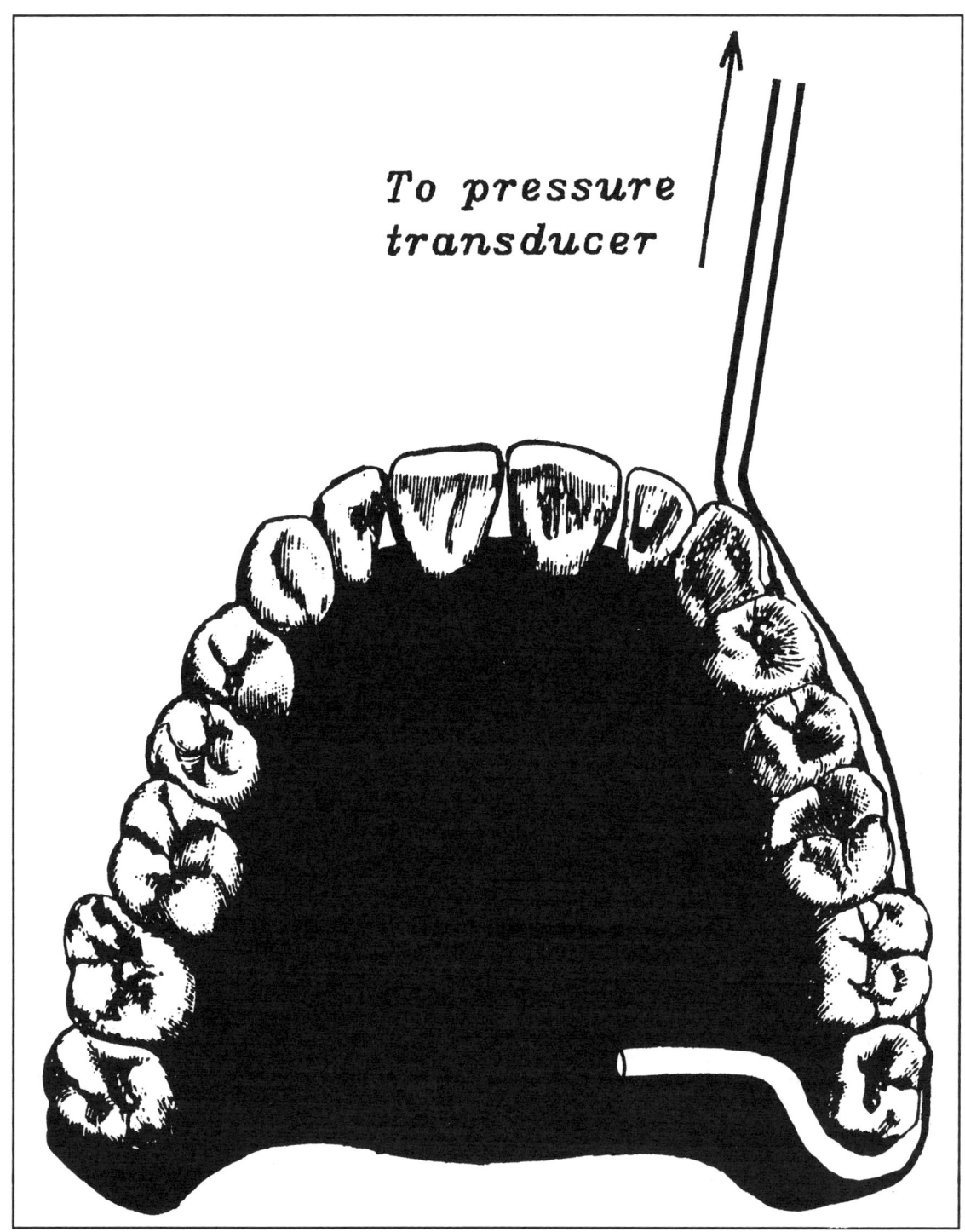

The object is to bend the tube so that its open end points directly at the midline, while the catheter hugs the dental surface as it wraps around the three exposed surfaces of the last molar. The catheter should also lie against the dental arch until it exits at the corner of the mouth. There should be no sharp kinks in the tubing. The purpose of the copper wire is, of course, to hold the shape you have formed. [NOTE: Getting the right shape may take some practice. Keep trying until you have it!]

5. Remove the catheter from you patient's mouth and wash it with detergent and water.

6. Immerse the wired end of the catheter in the boiling water, making certain that you have submerged the entire length of the shaped segment. Keep the catheter in the water for about 1½ minutes. During this time, the plastic should soften.

7. Remove the catheter from the boiling water and, without touching the heated end, cool it to room temperature.

8. Pull on the free end of the wire, removing it from the catheter. If you have done everything correctly, the plastic catheter should retain the shape into which you bent it. [NOTE: If the final shape seems too "loose" you may have to try again. This time, exaggerate the bends that you made after you remove the wired catheter from the mouth but before you heat it. That is, with some catheter materials it may be necessary to overshape the unheated catheter to ensure a tight fit of the final product.]

9. Fit the finished catheter into the patient's mouth to verify that it lies properly in the oral cavity. Make sure that the open end is perpendicular to the midline!

10. To the straight (unmodified) end of the catheter attach a coupler that will allow you to connect it to your pressure transducer.

To store the catheter for later use:

11. Write your patient's name on a piece of adhesive tape and stick this on the coupler end of the tube. The catheter can be coiled and stored in a clean, sealed jar for later use. Always clean and disinfect the catheter before storage.

III. INTRAORAL PRESSURE DURING CONSONANTS

WARNING: Basic considerations of infection control dictate that you never put the catheter directly onto a table top or other surface (see Unit 2 "A Few Technicalities").

1. Attach your catheter to one of the ports of the pressure transducer. To the other port, connect a 3-way stopcock. Then couple a relatively large (20 mL or so) hypodermic syringe to one of the other stopcock connections. There should be one connector on the stopcock with nothing attached (see Baken, 1987, Fig. 7-11B, p. 256).

2. The syringe arrangement allows you to force air through the catheter when it becomes clogged with saliva. Practice moving the stopcock lever to allow you to draw air into the syringe directly from the room (surrounding atmosphere) and then changing the lever position so that you can force the air out through the catheter, into the patient's mouth. You should become fairly comfortable and adept with this maneuver. You should also become familiar with the "closed" position of the stopcock, which disconnects the transducer from either the atmosphere or the syringe. This is the position the stopcock should be in during actual testing. If you later misposition the stopcock lever you may accidentally suck saliva into the pressure transducer. This will not damage the transducer, but you will have to stop and clean it before proceeding.

3. Place a microphone on a stand slightly to the side of your patient's mouth.

4. Place the catheter in your patient's mouth and hold it lightly where it leaves the corner of her mouth. Allow a minute or so for your patient to acclimate to it.

5. Have your patient say the phrase "Tie-dye a zoo suit" using her normal articulation and speech rate. Obtain chart recordings of the intraoral pressure and microphone signals during several repetitions. Keep an eye on the output to be certain that the data are acceptable. [NOTE: A weak or "sluggish" trace might mean that the stopcock is open. Sudden loss of signal amplitude generally means that the end of the tube has filled with saliva. Use the stopcock/syringe arrangement to clear it.]

6. Use the calibration data you obtained earlier to scale your chart recording. Attach your record to the hand-in sheet (a sample record is also provided).

7. Examine your data carefully:

    a. Is the frequency response of your system adequate? How do your know (see Baken, 1987, p. 257)?

    b. On the basis of the audio and pressure data, label the pressure peaks associated with /t/, /d/, /z/, and /s/ on the data record.

    c. What evidence is there in the pressure trace that signals the presence of voicing?

    d. Fill in the table on the hand-in sheet to describe the peak pressure and duration of the pressure event associated with each consonant.

    e. How do the data in your table accord with what is known about the pressure relationships of plosives and fricatives? Voiced and unvoiced phones? Why should voicing make a difference in the oral pressure?

    f. What is there in the shape of the pressure peaks that differentiates a plosive from a fricative?

    g. What can you say about the final /t/ of the utterance?

8. Repeat your pressure observation with a patient who has a clinical disorder affecting articulation. (You will, of course, need to make a new pressure probe.) Assess the differences between the record of this patient and the normal individual you tested.

9. A sample pressure record from a stutterer is shown below. Study it to identify any abnormalities and prepare a report for your instructor.

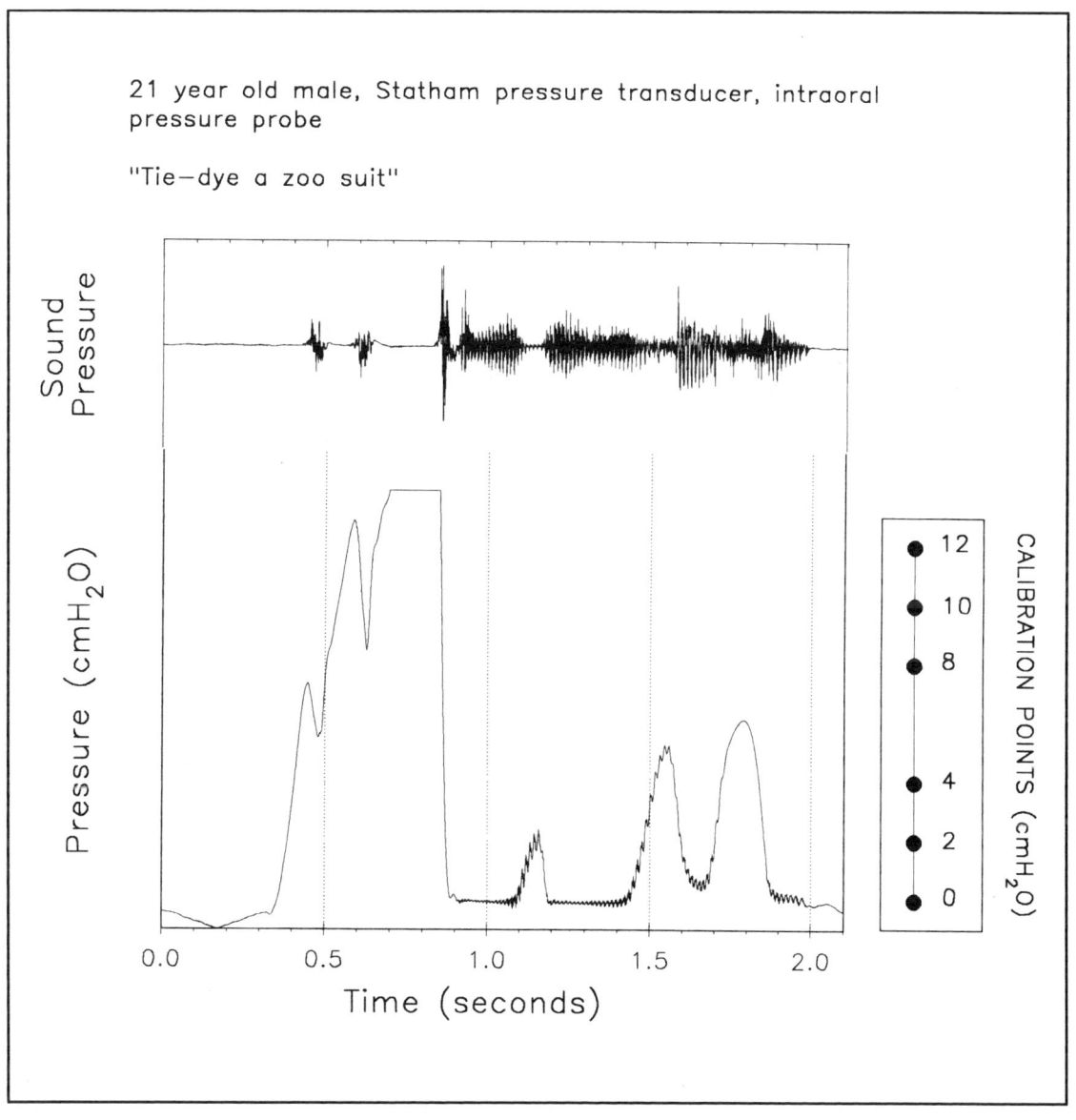

READ MORE ABOUT IT!

Arkebauer, H. J., Hixon, T. J., & Hardy, J. C. (1967). Peak intraoral pressures during speech. *Journal of Speech and Hearing Research, 10,* 196–208.

Baken, R. J. (1987). *Clinical measurement of speech and voice.* Boston: Little, Brown.

Bernthal, J. E., & Beukelman, D. R. (1978). Intraoral air pressure during the production of /p/ and /b/ by children, youths, and adults. *Journal of Speech and Hearing Research, 21,* 361–371.

Brown, W. S., Jr., & McGlone, R. E. (1974). Aerodynamic and acoustic study of stress in sentence productions. *Journal of the Acoustical Society of America, 56,* 971–974.

Brown, W. S., Jr., McGlone, R. E., Tarlow, A., & Shipp, T. (1970). Intraoral pressure associated with specific phonetic positions. *Phonetica, 22,* 202–212.

Flege, J. E. (1983). The influence of stress, position, and utterance length on the pressure characteristics of English /p/ and /b/. *Journal of Speech and Hearing Research, 26,* 111–118.

Leeper, H. A., Jr., & Noll, J. D. (1972). Pressure measurements of articulatory behavior during alterations of vocal effort. *Journal of the Acoustical Society of America, 51,* 1291–1295.

Lisker, L. (1970). Supraglottal air pressure in the production of English stops. *Language and Speech, 13,* 215–230.

Miller, C. J., & Daniloff, R. (1977). Aerodynamics of stops in continuous speech. *Journal of Phonetics, 5,* 351–360.

Müller, E. M., & Brown, W. S., Jr. (1980). Variations in the supraglottal air pressure waveform and their articulatory interpretation. In N. J. Lass (Ed.), *Speech and language: Advances in basic research and practice* (Vol. 4, pp. 317–389). New York: Academic Press.

Murry, T., & Brown, W. S., Jr. (1975). Intraoral air pressure variability in esophageal speakers. *Folia Phoniatrica, 27,* 237–249.

Netsell, R. (1969). Subglottal and intraoral pressures during the intervocalic contrast of /t/ and /d/. *Phonetica, 20,* 68–73.

Scully, C. (1971). A comparison of /s/ and /z/ for an English speaker. *Language and Speech, 14,* 187–200.

Shipp, T. (1973). Intraoral pressure and lip occlusion in midvocalic stop consonant production. *Journal of Phonetics, 1,* 167–170.

Stathopoulos, E. T. (1986). Relationship between intraoral air pressure and vocal intensity in children and adults. *Journal of Speech and Hearing Research, 29,* 71–74.

Stathopoulos, E. T., & Weismer, G. (1985). Oral airflow and air pressure during speech production: A comparative study of children, youths, and adults. *Folia Phoniatrica, 37,* 152–159.

Subtelny, J. D., Worth, J. H., & Sakuda, M. (1966). Intraoral air pressure and rate of flow during speech. *Journal of Speech and Hearing Research, 9,* 498–518.

Warren, D. W. (1976). Aerodynamics of speech production. In N. J. Lass (Ed.), *Contemporary issues in experimental phonetics* (pp. 105–137). New York: Academic Press.

Warren, D. W., Hall, D. J., & Davis, J. (1981). Oral port constriction and pressure-airflow relationships during sibilant productions. *Folia Phoniatrica, 33,* 380–394.

Student _____ Date _____

INTRAORAL PRESSURE DURING CONSONANT PRODUCTION

I. SETTING UP AND CALIBRATING THE PRESSURE SYSTEM

Block Diagram of Your Pressure Instrumentation

Maximum pressure: _____ cm H_2O Sensitivity: _____

Chart calibration: _____ cm vertical height per cm H_2O

(Attach your calibration record to this page.)

Student   Date

III. INTRAORAL PRESSURE DURING CONSONANTS

(Attach your pressure record to this page.)

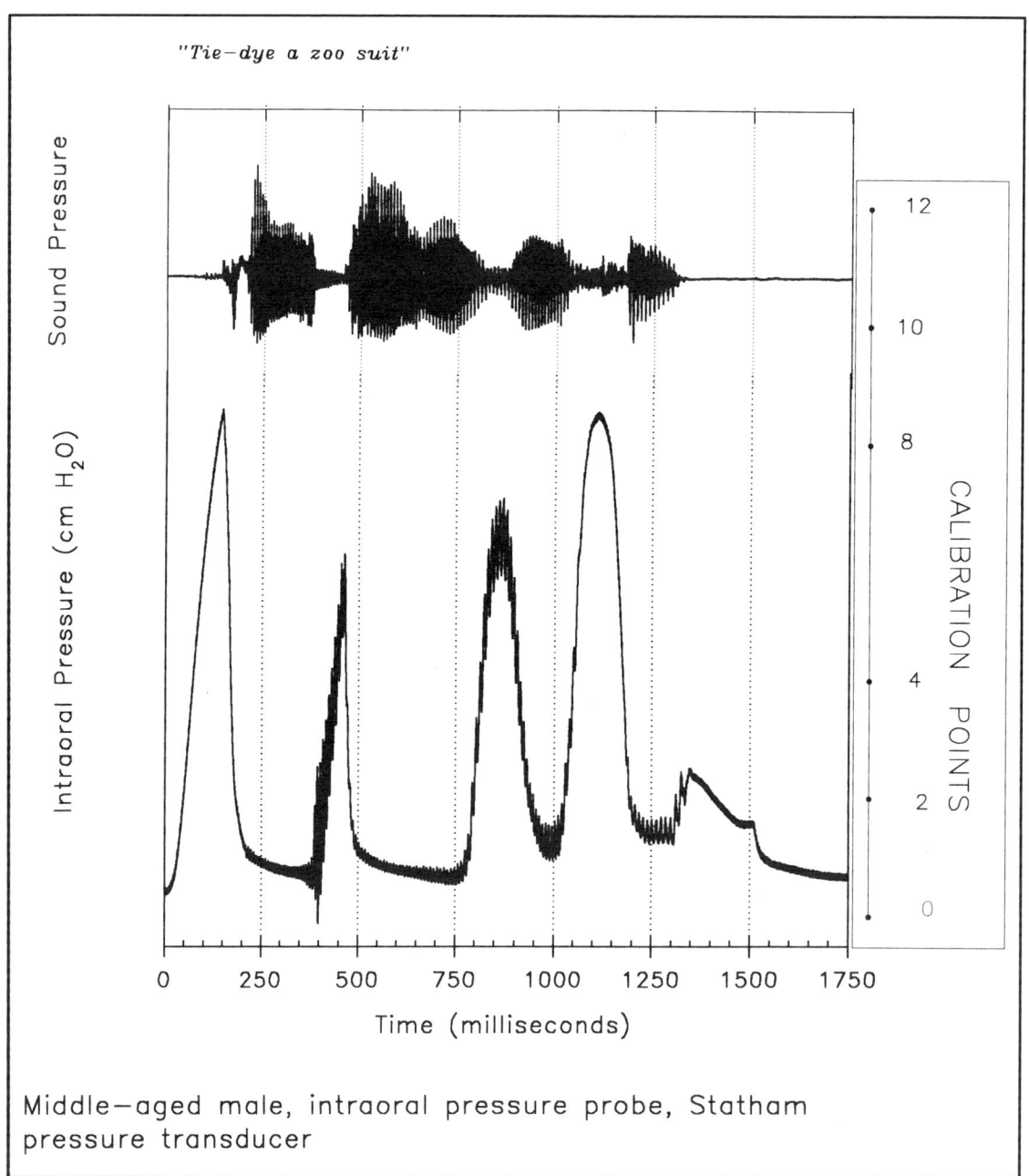

Student _____ Date _____

7. a. Adequacy of frequency response: _____

_____

_____

_____

_____

_____

c. Evidence of voicing in pressure record: _____

_____

_____

_____

_____

_____

d. Complete the following table based on your pressure record:

Phone	Peak Pressure (cm H_2O)	Duration of Pressure Event (milliseconds)
[t]	_____	_____
[d]	_____	_____
[z]	_____	_____
[s]	_____	_____

Student _____ Date _____

e. Characteristics of consonant classes: _____

_____

_____

_____

_____

_____

f. Differences in the shapes of pressure peaks: _____

_____

_____

_____

_____

_____

g. Final /t/ of the utterance: _____

_____

_____

_____

_____

_____

Student _____   Date _____

Attach your patient's labeled data recording to this page.

8. Patient: _____
_____

Assessment: _____
_____
_____
_____
_____
_____
_____
_____
_____
_____
_____
_____
_____
_____
_____
_____
_____
_____
_____
_____

Student _____ Date _____

9. Patient: ___21-year-old male stutterer_____

Assessment: _____

_____

_____

_____

_____

_____

_____

_____

_____

_____

_____

_____

_____

_____

_____

_____

_____

_____

_____

_____

UNIT 18

Clinical Application: Estimating Subglottal Pressure

The pressure of the air in the lungs represents the power available for the fashioning of voice or speech. It is frequently useful to know how well the power supply is "charged," that is, to know the subglottal pressure (P_s).

A precise measurement of P_s requires placing a pressure probe in the subglottal space, a procedure far too invasive for routine practice. Fortunately, there is a noninvasive way of obtaining an estimate that is likely to satisfy the requirements of most clinical examinations.

Purpose: In these exercises you will learn to estimate the subglottal pressure from recordings of intraoral pressure (P_{io}) during the production of the syllable /pi/ and you will examine the relationship of P_{io} to vocal intensity.

Equipment: Instrumentation for the measurement of intraoral pressure (see Unit 17 "Intraoral Pressure During Consonant Production").

General preparation: Review the general physiology of the generation of subglottal pressure (Zemlin, 1988, pp. 83–93) and the several ways in which it can be measured or estimated (Baken, 1987, pp. 260–72).

ESTIMATING SUBGLOTTAL PRESSURE

1. Set up the instrumentation for measuring P_{io} with an intraoral probe tube and calibrate it (see Unit 17 "Intraoral Pressure During Consonant Production"). Prepare a block diagram of your instrumentation array.

2. Obtain intraoral pressure and audio (microphone) records of a patient repeating the syllable /pi/. Instruct your patient to: (a) inhale to about twice normal depth; (b) use normal vocal pitch and loudness; (c) produce all of the syllables on a single breath; and (d) repeat the syllables at a rate of about 1.5 syllables per second.

3. Examine the record of P_{io} during /pi/ that you have produced (a sample record is provided on the hand-in sheet). Mark the record to identify:

   a. The beginning of lip closure for /p/ in the P_{io} record;

   b. The beginning of lip opening in the P_{io} record;

   c. The point of peak P_{io};

   d. Evidence of the release of /p/ in the audio record; and

   e. The waveform of /i/ in the audio record.

4. Explain why the peak intraoral pressure of /p/ is likely to be a good reflection of the subglottal pressure.

5. Ignoring the first two and last two syllables shown in your record, measure the peak pressure of each /pi/ and enter the data in the table on the hand-in sheet.

6. Is the pressure for /p/ the same for all repetitions? If not, what does this imply for the stability of the subglottal pressure?

7. The value of P_s during each /i/ is likely to be somewhere between the P_s of the preceding /p/ and the P_s of the following /p/. We can estimate the probable P_s during an /i/ by drawing a line from the preceding P_{io} peak to the following P_{io} peak. The pressure represented by the height of this line at the middle of the /i/ is the best estimate of P_s during the vowel production. (Technically, drawing a line in this way is a means of deriving a "linear interpolation" of the pressure.)

8. Use the method just outlined to derive the estimated P_s of the /i/ portion of each of the syllables you tabulated. Mark your data sheet to show your interpolations, and enter the data on the hand-in sheet.

9. Why isn't the P_{io} during the vowel a valid estimator of P_s?

II. VOCAL INTENSITY AND SUBGLOTTAL PRESSURE

1. Retest your patient, first with repeated /pi/ produced softly (less loud than normal speech) and then loudly (but not shouted).

2. Mark your data records (samples are provided on the hand-in sheet) and tabulate the results.

3. What conclusion can you draw about the relationship of P_s to vocal intensity in normal speakers?

4. How do the P_s values you have obtained compare to the values generally cited in the literature?

READ MORE ABOUT IT!

Baken, R. J. (1987). *Clinical measurement of speech and voice.* Boston: Little, Brown.

Hixon, T. J., & Smitheran, J. R. (1982). A reply to Rothenberg. *Journal of Speech and Hearing Disorders, 47,* 220–223.

Isshiki, N. (1964). Regulatory mechanism of voice intensity variation. *Journal of Speech and Hearing Disorders, 7,* 17–29.

Kitajima, K., & Fujita, F. (1990). Estimation of subglottal pressure with intraoral pressure. *Acta Otolaryngologica, 109,* 473–478.

Katiajim, K., & Fujita, F. (1992). Clinical report on preliminary data on intraoral pressure in the evaulation of laryngeal pathology. *Journal of Voice, 6,* 79–85.

Ladefoged, P., & McKinney, N. P. (1963). Loudness, sound pressure, and subglottal pressure in speech. *Journal of the Acoustical Society of America, 35,* 454–460.

Löfqvist, A., Carlborg, B., & Kitzing, P. (1982). Initial validation of an indirect measure of subglottal pressure during vowels. *Journal of the Acoustical Society of America, 72,* 633–635.

Netsell, R. (1969). Subglottal and intraoral air pressure during the intervocalic contrast of /t/ and /d/. *Phonetica, 20,* 68–73.

Netsell, R. (1973). Speech physiology. In F. D. Minifie, T. J. Hixon, & F. Williams (Eds.), *Normal aspects of speech, hearing, and language* (pp. 211–234). Englewood Cliffs, NJ: Prentice-Hall.

Netsell, R., Lotz, W. K., DuChane, A. S., & Barlow, S. M. (1991). Vocal tract aerodynamics during syllable productions: Normative data and theoretical implications. *Journal of Voice, 5,* 1–9.

Rothenberg, M. (1982). Interpolating subglottal pressure from oral pressure. *Journal of Speech and Hearing Disorders, 47,* 219–220.

Shipp, T. (1973). Intraoral air pressure and lip occlusion in midvocalic stop consonant production. *Journal of Phonetics, 1,* 167–170.

Smitheran, J. R., & Hixon, T. J. (1981). A clinical method for estimating laryngeal airway resistance during vowel production. *Journal of Speech and Hearing Disorders, 46,* 138–146.

Warren, D. W. (1976). Aerodynamics of speech production. In N. J. Lass (Ed.), *Contemporary issues in experimental phonetics* (pp. 105–137). New York: Academic Press.

Zemlin, W. R. (1988). *Speech and hearing science* (3rd ed.) Englewood Cliffs, NJ: Prentice-Hall.

Student _____   Date _____

SUBGLOTTAL PRESSURE

I. ESTIMATING SUBGLOTTAL PRESSURE

Block Diagram of Your Instrumentation Array

Maximum pressure: _____ cm H_2O Sensitivity: _____

Chart calibration: _____ cm vertical height per cm H_2O

(Attach your calibration record to this page.)

Student   Date

Attach your labeled data recording to this page.

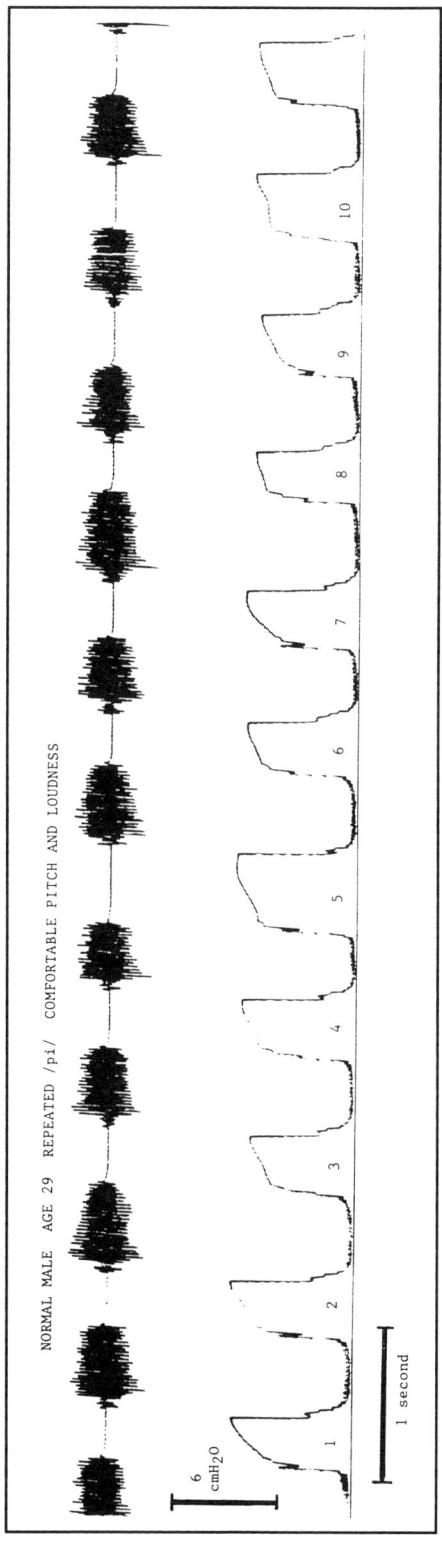

Student _____ Date _____

4. Why is P_{io} during /p/ a good reflection of P_s? _____

_____

_____

_____

_____

_____

_____

5 (and **8**). Complete the following table:

Speaker sex: _____   Speaker age: _____

Syllable Number	Peak P_{io} during /p/ (cm H_2O)	Estimated P_s during /i/ (cm H_2O)
3	_____	_____
4		_____
5	_____	_____
6	_____	_____
7	_____	_____
8	_____	_____
9	_____	_____
10	_____	_____
MEAN	_____	_____
SD	_____	_____

ESTIMATING SUBGLOTTAL PRESSURE

Student _____ Date _____

6. Stability of P_{io} and implication for P_s: _____

_____

_____

_____

_____

_____

_____

_____

9. Invalidity of P_{io} during vowels as an estimator of P_s: _____

_____

_____

_____

_____

_____

_____

_____

Student   Date

II. VOCAL INTENSITY AND SUBGLOTTAL PRESSURE

Attach your labeled data recording to this page.

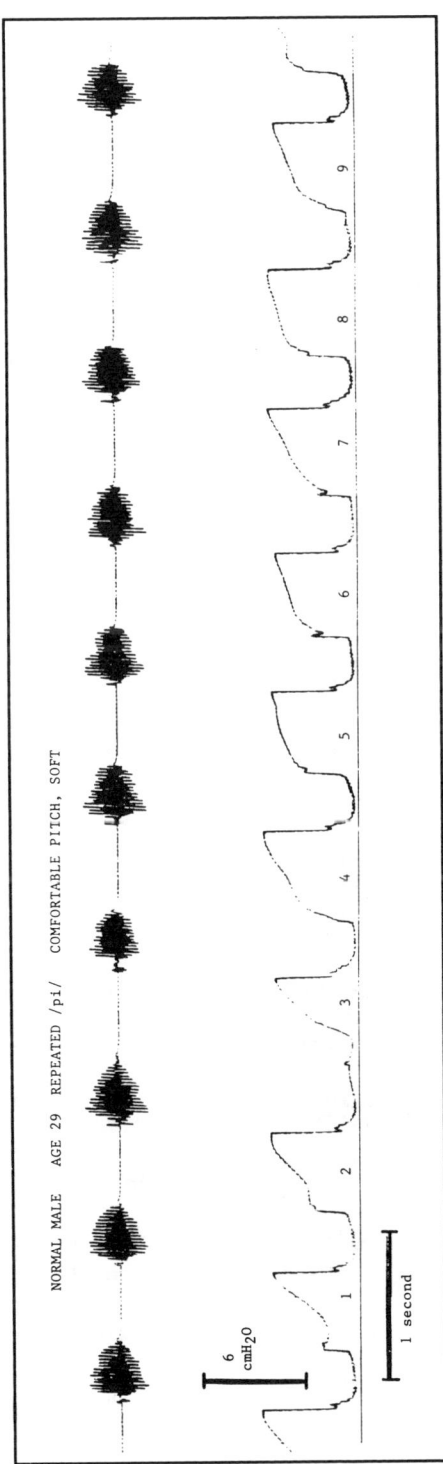

Student   Date

Attach your labeled data recording to this page.

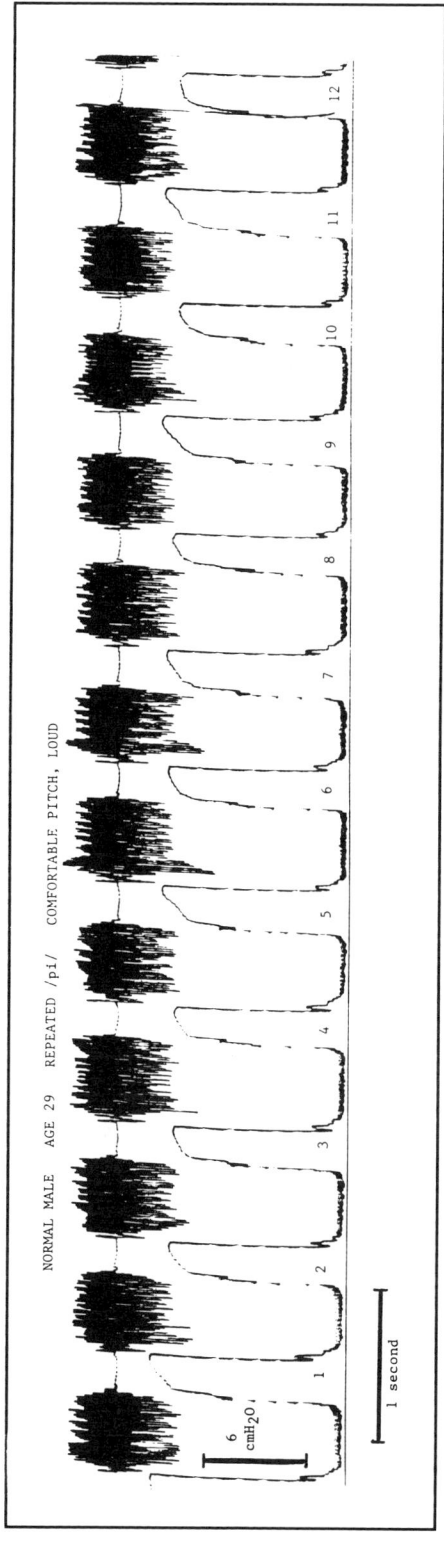

Student   Date

2. Complete the following table:

Syllable Number	Soft Peak P_{io} cm H_2O	Comfortable[1] Peak P_{io} (cm H_2O)	Loud Peak P_{io} (cm H_2O)
3	_____	_____	_____
4	_____	_____	_____
5	_____	_____	_____
6	_____	_____	_____
7	_____	_____	_____
8	_____	_____	_____
9	_____	_____	_____
10	_____	_____	_____
11	_____	_____	_____
12	_____	_____	_____
MEAN	_____	_____	_____
SD	_____	_____	_____

[1] Use data from exercise I.

3. Relationship of P_s to vocal loudness: _____

_____

_____

_____

_____

_____

_____

Student _____ Date _____

4. Comparison to data in the literature: _____

_____

_____

_____

_____

_____

_____

Source(s): _____

_____

AIRFLOWS FOR SPEECH AND VOICE

UNIT 19

Clinical Application: Mean Phonatory Airflow Using a Pneumotachograph

The instrument most commonly used by clinicians to transduce airflow is called the pneumotachograph or pneumotachometer (also known simply as the pneumotach). As part of an airflow system, a pneumotach provides a signal allowing us to precisely measure dynamic flow characteristics associated with speech and voice production. In the absence of severe ventilatory disorder, the measurement of the mean airflow a speaker uses during a sustained phonation has proven to be an effective clinical indicator of laryngeal dysfunction, both in organic and functional dysphonia.

Purpose: In these exercises you will

- Become familiar with the instrumentation required to observe phonatory airflow.
- Learn to obtain valid measures of mean phonatory airflow.
- Provide a rudimentary assessment of the phonatory behavior that produced the airflow data.

Equipment: A heated pneumotachograph, compressed air supply, flow meter (rotameter), differential pressure transducer and associated electronics, and a means of displaying the output signal.

General preparation: Review the general physical principles of airflow and the units of its measurement. Be sure to familiarize yourself with the nature of pneumotachographic systems in particular (Baken, 1987, pp. 277–302; see also Sullivan, Peters, & Enright, 1984). It is important that you also study the manuals accompanying the pneumotach, pressure transducer, and associated electronics you will be using. In particular, you should be able to specify the flow range over which the transducer provides a useful (linear) output and how much ventilatory dead space will be added to the patient's airway. (Answers to these questions should be provided in the manual accompanying the pneumotach.)

I. SETTING UP AND CALIBRATING THE AIRFLOW SYSTEM

1. Prepare a block diagram of the airflow instrumentation array you will use. Be sure to label each of its parts.

2. Indicate the maximum airflow that may be transduced by your system (consult the specifications that accompany your pneumotach). [NOTE: For later exercises you will need a pneumotach that can transduce flows up to 1200 mL/s.]

3. Connect the apparatus according to your diagram, and connect the supply tank to the flowmeter as shown in Baken (1987, Fig. 8–12, p. 295) in preparation for calibrating the flow system (see also Unit 11 "Calibration").

4. Turn on the transducer electronics and the recording system and allow several minutes for them to warm-up and stabilize. [NOTE: Be sure that the transducer amplifier and recording systems are set for a "DC response."]

5. Before releasing air from the tank, adjust the trace position on the data recorder. Activate the paper drive of the recorder system and let it run for a few seconds. You will have produced a trace on the chart that represents zero flow. Label the line that you made on the chart "0."

6. Now adjust the tank's regulator valve to release a small but steady stream of air from the tank. Adjust this valve until the flow rate registers 800 mL/s (48 L/min) on the flowmeter. Record a couple of seconds at this airflow and mark the new line on your chart "800." [NOTE: The lines on your recording should extend over about 2/3 of the available vertical range. If you need to, adjust the sensitivity of your transducer amplifier or data recorder and recalibrate.]

7. Repeat #6 using airflows of 50 mL/s (3 L/min), 100 mL/s (6 L/min), 200 mL/s (12 L/min), and 400 mL/s (24 L/min). Label each line on your chart recording.

8. Disconnect the tank and flowmeter from the input of your airflow system.

9. Measure the vertical distance from the 0 to the 800 line on your chart recording as accurately as you can. Use this distance to determine the calibration in terms of "cm height per L/s." Indicate the calibration both on the hand-in sheet and on the chart you have made and include it with the materials you submit to your instructor.

> **WARNING:** Remember that if any of the transducer or recorder amplifier settings are later changed, the calibration will no longer be valid.

II. MEAN AIRFLOW DURING PHONATION

There are two additional components to the transduction system necessary for valid airflow measurement. First, we need a cushioned face mask which, when fitted snugly against the face, ensures that all air in or out of the vocal tract passes through the pneumotach. The face mask can either be held against the face or strapped on with an adjustable harness. Under some circumstances a mouthpiece used in conjunction with a noseclip can be substituted for the mask; in this case a tight lip seal must be ensured. The second essential component is a heater for the pneumotach. Heating it to just above body temperature prevents condensation from expired air that would invalidate our flow transduction.

> **CLINICAL NOTE:** The mean airflow rate measured during a sustained vowel is necessarily equal to the mean glottal airflow. While the oscillation of the signal is due to glottal pulsing, the waveform does not depict changes in either vocal fold movement or glottal dimensions.[1] Because we are only interested in the *mean* (or average) flow value separate from vocal tract and transducer resonance effects, we typically low-pass filter the transduced flow signal to remove much, if not all, of its oscillatory (A/C) characteristics.

A. On the next page are complete flow records obtained from two different speakers who each prolonged the vowel /ɑ/ at a "comfortable" pitch and loudness. Both airflow signals have been low-pass filtered at 25 Hz and scaled to a prior calibration. Patient *a* (top) is 24-year-old woman and patient *b* (bottom) is a 45-year-old man.

---

[1] Be this as it may, a flow signal that is irregular in its period, amplitude, or waveshape does reflect poor and/or inefficient laryngeal function when ventilatory instability has been ruled out.

Patient a

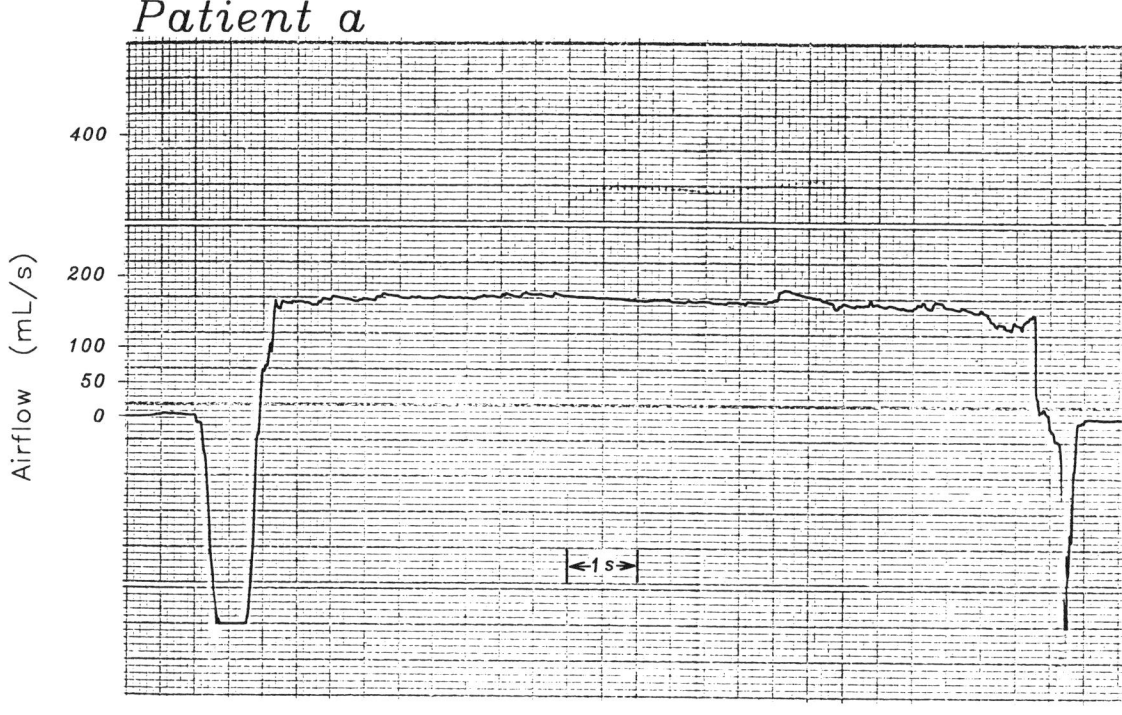

Patient b

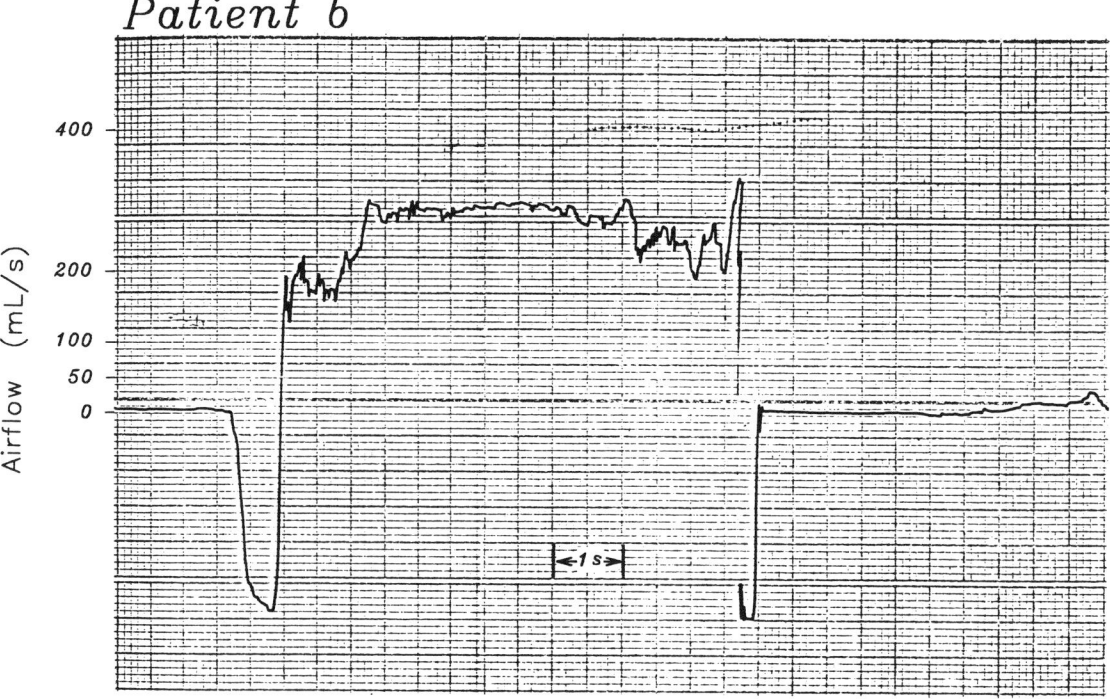

1. What is each speaker's mean phonatory airflow?

2. Are these normal flow rates? Compare patients *a* and *b* to available norms for adult women and men, respectively. Cite your source(s).

3. Compare the onset and offset characteristics of these two patients' flow records.

4. Compare the stability of the two traces during vowel production. What may have contributed to the shortened length of patient *b*'s phonation?

B. Below is a partial 0.1/s flow record obtained while a patient with polypoid degeneration of the vocal fold prolonged the vowel /ɑ/ at his "comfortable" pitch and loudness. The airflow signal has been low-pass filtered at 250 Hz and scaled to a prior calibration. Because the "cut-off frequency" of the filter is higher than the patient's F_0, oscillatory changes are apparent in the flow signal.[2]

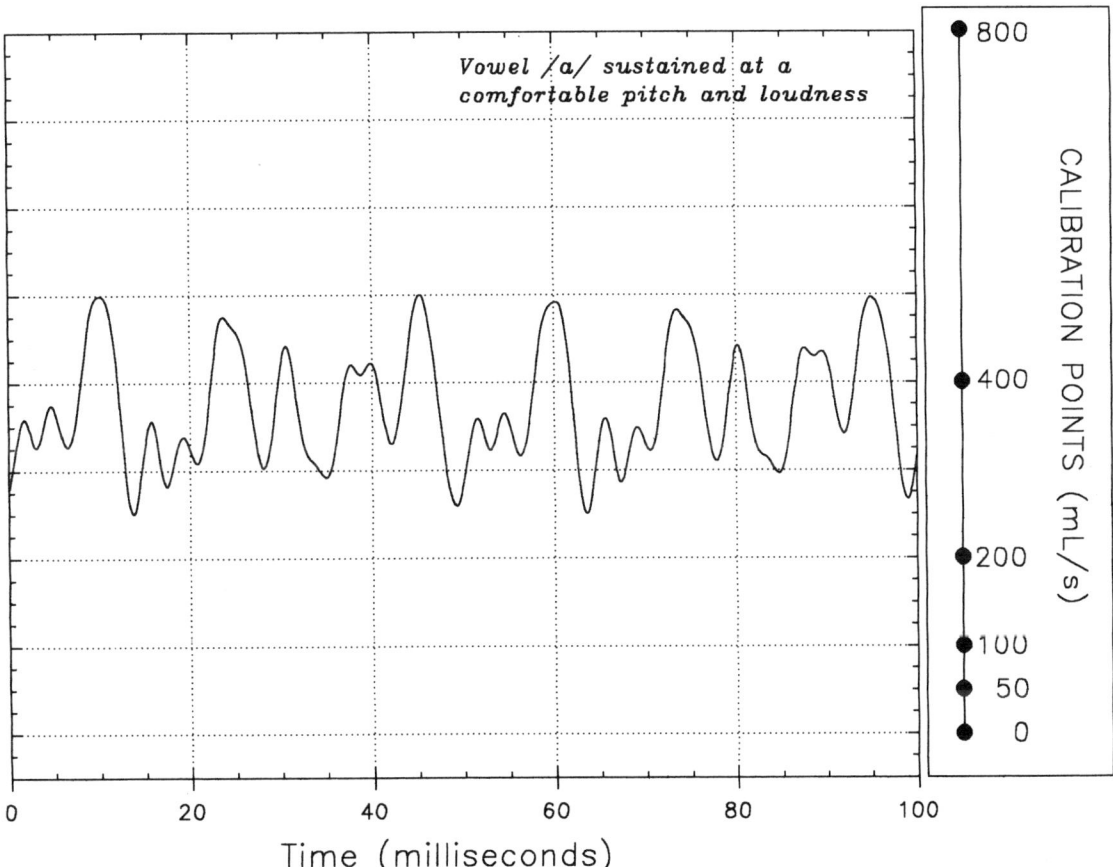

1. Use this recording to estimate this patient's mean airflow during vowel production.[3]

2. Is this a normal flow rate? Compare this airflow to available norms for adult male speakers.

---

[2] In this case the first three harmonics are represented.
[3] The correct (or DC equivalent) airflow of each phonation is correctly the root-mean-square (RMS) amplitude. However, for clinical purposes, estimation of the mean or mid-wave flow may suffice.

3. Provide a brief assessment of the irregularities in this speaker's flow trace.

4. Suppose this patient's vital capacity is 4.3 liters. Based on this information and your reported mean flow rate, what maximum phonation time (MPT) would you expect from this patient?

C. Obtaining flow recordings.

1. Attach a clean, cushioned face mask to in the input of the pneumotachograph.

2. Connect and turn on the heater and allow several minutes for the pneumotach to warm up. [NOTE: Make sure that the pneumotach does not get hot. It should be just slightly warmer than body temperature.]

3. Low-pass filter your signal to remove airflow changes faster than 25 Hz. (Now all evidence of glottal pulsing should be eliminated from your airflow signal.)

4. Place the face mask over your patient's nose and mouth. After making sure that your patient maintains a tight seal, begin your data recording.

> **WARNING:** Guidelines concerning infection control apply to the airflow mask, cushion, and/or mouthpiece during and after use (see Unit 2 "A Few Technicalities").

5. With the mask in place, have your patient prolong the vowel /ɑ/ at a "comfortable" pitch and loudness. Watch the output to be sure that the data are acceptable. Use the calibration data you obtained earlier to scale your chart recording.

6. What is your patient's mean phonatory airflow? Is this flow rate normal? Compare this airflow to available norms for your patient's age and sex.

7. Now low-pass filter your flow trace at 250 Hz. Repeat #5 above and compare your records.

8. Obtain additional airflow traces while your patient sustains /ɑ/ at:

   a. A relatively low pitch, but at the same comfortable loudness;

   b. A relatively high pitch, again at the same comfortable loudness;

   c. A comfortable pitch, but at a "softer than comfortable" loudness; and

   d. A comfortable pitch at a "greater than comfortable" loudness.

9. Scale each of these samples using your calibration data.

10. Examine these data records (or use the ones provided) to determine the mean flow rate of each. Fill in the appropriate data on the hand-in sheet.

11. Describe the observed differences in flow rate for these samples with respect to intensity and vocal F_0.

12. Obtain an airflow record from a dysphonic patient sustaining the vowel /ɑ/ at a comfortable pitch and loudness. Study the record carefully to identify any abnormalities. Determine your patient's mean phonatory airflow and prepare a lab report for your instructor.

READ MORE ABOUT IT!

Baken, R. J. (1987). *Clinical measurement of speech and voice.* Boston: Little, Brown.

Beckett, R. L., Thoelke, W., & Cowan, L. (1971). A normative study of airflow in children. *British Journal of Disorders of Communication, 6,* 13–16.

D'Antonio, L., Lotz, W. K., Chait, D., & Netsell, R. (1987). Perceptual-physiologic approach to evaluation and treatment of dysphonia. *Annals of Otology, Rhinology and Laryngology, 96,* 187–190.

D'Antonio, L., Netsell, R., & Lotz, W. K. (1988). Clinical aerodynamics for the evaluation and management of voice disorders. *Ear, Nose and Throat Journal, 67,* 394–399.

Gordon, M. T., Morton, M., & Simpson, I. C. (1978). Air flow measurements in diagnosis, assessment, and treatment of mechanical dysphonia. *Folia Phoniatrica, 30,* 161–174.

Hirano, M. (1981). *Clinical examination of voice.* New York: Springer-Verlag.

Hirano, M., Koike, Y., and von Leden, H. (1968). Maximum phonation time and air usage during phonation. *Folia Phoniatrica, 20,* 185–201.

Isshiki, N. (1965). Vocal intensity and air flow rate. *Folia Phoniatrica, 17,* 92–104.

Isshiki, N., Okamura, H., & Morimoto, M. (1967). Maximum phonation time and air flow rate during phonation: Simple clinical tests for vocal function. *Annals of Otology, Rhinology and Laryngology, 76,* 998–1007.

Isshiki, N., & von Leden, H. (1964). Hoarseness: Aerodynamic studies. *Archives of Otolaryngology, 80,* 206–213.

Isshiki, N., Yanagihara, N., & Morimoto, M. (1966). Approach to the objective diagnosis of hoarseness. *Folia Phoniatrica, 18,* 393–400.

Iwata, S., von Leden, H., & Williams, D. (1972). Air flow measurement during phonation. *Journal of Communication Disorders, 5,* 67–79.

Kelman, A. W., Gordon, M. T., Simpson, I. C., & Morton, F. M. (1975). Assessment of vocal function by air-flow measurements. *Folia Phoniatrica, 27,* 250–262.

Koike, Y., & Hirano, M. (1968). Significance of the vocal velocity index. *Folia Phoniatrica, 20,* 285–296.

Koike, Y., Hirano, M., & von Leden, H. (1967). Vocal initiation: Acoustic and aerodynamic investigations of normal subjects. *Folia Phoniatrica, 19,* 173–182.

McGlone, R. E. (1967). Air flow during vocal fry phonation. *Journal of Speech and Hearing Research, 10,* 299–304.

McGlone, R. E. (1970). Air flow in the upper register. *Folia Phoniatrica, 22,* 231–238.

Rothenberg, M. (1973). A new inverse-filtering technique for deriving the glottal airflow waveform during voicing. *Journal of the Acoustical Society of America, 53,* 1632–1645.

Rothenberg, M. (1977). Measurement of airflow in speech. *Journal of Speech and Hearing Research, 20,* 155–176.

Schneider, P., & Baken, R. J. (1984). Influence of lung volume on the airflow-intensity relationship. *Journal of Speech and Hearing Research, 27,* 430–435.

Stathopoulos, E. T. (1985). Effects of monitoring vocal intensity on oral air flow in children and adults. *Journal of Speech and Hearing Research, 28,* 589–593.

Sullivan, W. J., Peters, G. M., & Enright, P. L. (1984). Pneumotachographs: Theory and clinical application. *Respiratory Care, 29,* 736–749.

Tanaka, S., Hirano, M., & Terasawa, R. (1991). Examination of air usage during phonation: Correlations among test parameters. *Journal of Voice, 5,* 106–112.

Turney, S. Z., & Blumenfeld, W. (1973). Heated Fleisch pneumotachometer: A calibration procedure. *Journal of Applied Physiology, 34,* 117–121.

Yanagihara, N., & Koike, Y. (1967). The regulation of sustained phonation. *Folia Phoniatrica, 19,* 1–18.

Yanagihara, N., Koike, Y., & von Leden, H. (1966). Phonation and respiration: Function study in normal subjects. *Folia Phoniatrica, 19,* 323–340.

Yanagihara, N., & von Leden, H. (1967). Respiration and phonation: The functional examination of laryngeal disease. *Folia Phoniatrica, 19,* 153–166.

Student _____ Date _____

MEAN PHONATORY AIRFLOW USING A PNEUMOTACHOGRAPH

I. SETTING UP AND CALIBRATING THE AIRFLOW SYSTEM

Block Diagram of Your Airflow Instrumentation

Maximum flow: _____ L/s

Chart Calibration: _____ cm vertical height per L/s

(Attach your calibration record to this page.)

Student _____   Date _____

II. MEAN AIRFLOW DURING PHONATION

A. 1. Mean phonatory airflow

Patient *a*: _____ mL/s

Patient *b*: _____ mL/s

2. Normal? _____

_____

_____

_____

Source(s): _____

3. Flow onset/offset: _____

_____

_____

_____

_____

_____

4. Stability: _____

_____

_____

_____

Length: _____

_____

_____

_____

Student _____ Date _____

B. 1. Mean phonatory airflow: _____ mL/s

   2. Normal? _____

_____

_____

      Source(s): _____

   3. Assessment: _____

_____

_____

   4. Expected MPT (show arithmetic):

_____ s

C. Attach all of your labeled data recordings to this page.

   6. Mean phonatory airflow: _____ mL/s

      Normal? _____

_____

_____

      Source(s): _____

   7. Comparison of flow records: _____

_____

_____

_____

_____

Student   Date

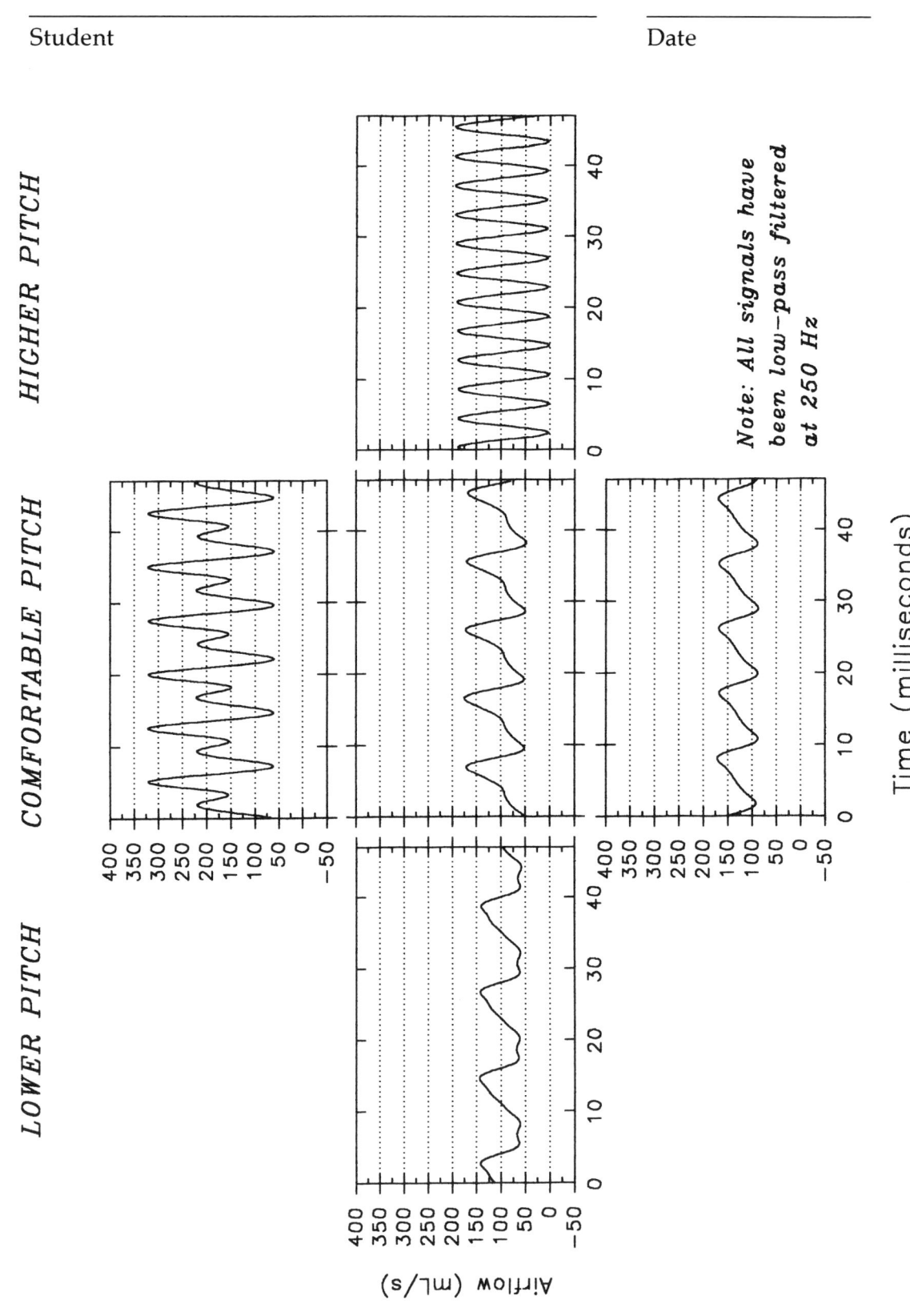

Student _____   Date _____

10. Complete the following table for your patient:

Phonatory Condition	Mean Airflow Rate (mL/s)
Comfortable Pitch, Comfortable Loudness	_____
Low Pitch, Comfortable Loudness	_____
High Pitch, Comfortable Loudness	_____
Soft Phonation, Comfortable Pitch	_____
Loud Phonation, Comfortable Pitch	_____

11. Observed differences in flow rate: _____

_____

_____

_____

_____

_____

12. Patient: _____

Assessment: _____

_____

_____

_____

Student _____ Date _____

_____
_____
_____
_____
_____
_____
_____

UNIT 20

Clinical Application: Airflow During Speech Production

Airflow characteristics associated with the production of consonants are very closely tied to the manner of articulation and voicing. Like measures of intraoral pressure, airflow information can reveal much about articulatory precision, timing, and coordination.

Purpose: In these exercises you will

- Learn to obtain valid measures of peak airflow during consonant production;

- Gain some skill in assessing the validity of the data record; and

- Undertake some basic interpretation of the articulatory behavior based on speech airflow information.

Equipment: A heated pneumotachograph, differential pressure transducer and associated amplifier. A compressed air supply and flow meter (rotameter) will be needed for calibration. In addition, you will need a microphone, audio amplifier, and 2-channel data recording system.

General preparation: Review the general physical principles of airflow and the units of its measurement (Baken, 1987, pp. 277–279). Read about airflow measures obtained during spoken utterances (Baken, 1987, pp. 294–298). In particular, compare measures obtained from children and adults (for example, Stathopoulos and Weismer, 1985) for different classes of speech sounds (for example, Isshiki and

Ringel, 1964; Klatt, Stevens, and Mead, 1968) in different phonetic contexts (for example, Gilbert, 1973).

I. SETTING UP AND CALIBRATING THE AIRFLOW SYSTEM

1. Prepare a block diagram of the airflow instrumentation array that you will use. Be sure to label each of its parts.

2. Indicate the maximum airflow that may be transduced by your system (consult the specifications that accompany your pneumotach). [NOTE: Be sure that your pneumotach system has a linear flow range that extends to at least 1200 mL/s.]

3. Connect the apparatus according to your diagram, and connect the supply tank to the flowmeter as shown in Baken (1987, Fig. 8-12, p. 295) in preparation for calibration of your flow system.

4. Turn on the transducer electronics and the recording system and allow several minutes for them to warm up and stabilize. [NOTE: Be sure that the transducer amplifier and recording systems are set for a "DC response."]

5. Before releasing air from the tank, adjust the trace position on the data recorder. Activate the paper drive of the recorder system and let it run for a few seconds. You will have produced a trace on the chart that represents zero flow. Label the line that you made on the chart "0."

6. Now adjust the tank's regulator valve to release a small but steady stream of air from the tank. Adjust this valve until the flow rate registers 1,000 mL/s (60 L/min) on the flowmeter. Record a couple of seconds at this airflow and mark the new line on your chart "1,000." [NOTE: The lines on your recording should extend over about 2/3 of the available vertical range. If you need to, adjust the sensitivity of your transducer amplifier or data recorder and recalibrate.]

7. Repeat #6 using airflows of 100 mL/s (6 L/min), 200 mL/s (12 L/min), 400 mL/s (24 L/min), and 800 mL/s (48 L/min). Label each line on your chart recording.

8. Disconnect the tank and flowmeter from the input of your airflow system.

9. Measure the vertical distance from the 0 to the 1,000 line on your chart recording as accurately as you can. Use this distance to determine the calibration in terms of "cm height per L/s." Indicate the calibration both on the hand-in sheet and on the chart you have made and include it with the materials you submit to your instructor.

> **WARNING:** Remember that if any of the transducer or recorder amplifier settings are later changed, the calibration will no longer be valid.

II. PEAK AIRFLOW DURING CONSONANT PRODUCTION

1. Firmly attach a clean, cushioned face mask to the pneumotach.

2. Turn on the pneumotach heater and allow several minutes for it to warm up.

3. Place the mask over your patient's nose and mouth. Make sure that your patient maintains a tight seal against the face mask.

4. Have your patient repeat the syllable /pɑ/ at a steady and moderate rate as you gather airflow data with a pen recorder or computer system.

5. Use the calibration data you obtained earlier to scale your data recording. (You may also use the record provided on the hand-in sheet.)

6. Mark and label each flow peak on the data record. Be sure to identify each vowel production as well.

7. Based on your data recording:

    a. Is the frequency response of your system adequate? How do you know? (see Baken, 1987, pp. 295–297).

    b. What is the mean syllable repetition rate?

    c. What is the mean peak airflow associated with the /p/ productions?

    d. How consistent are the peak airflows?[1] Describe your patient's performance.

III. SPEECH AIRFLOW

1. Place the mask over your patient's nose and mouth. Then position a microphone on a stand in front of the patient and orient the microphone toward the pneumotach opening.

2. After making sure that your patient maintains a tight seal against the face mask, begin to record the acoustic and airflow data.

3. Have your patient say the phrase "Today is a sale" using her normal articulation and speech rate. You may wish to record several repetitions of this phrase for comparison. Continue to watch the output to be sure that the data are acceptable.

---

[1] You may wish to report the *SD* or a relative index of variability, such as the coefficient of variation (CV). The CV is defined as the *SD* divided by the mean.

4. Use the calibration data you obtained earlier to scale your record. (A sample record is provided on the hand-in sheet.)

5. Examine your data carefully:

   a. Label the airflow peaks associated with /t/, /d/, /z/, and /s/ on the data record.

   Note that double peaks typify fricative consonants: the first occurring before maximal tract constriction (articulation), and the second following that constriction in transition toward the next articulatory configuration (see Klatt, Stevens, and Mead, 1968).

   b. What evidence in the flow trace signals the presence of voicing?

   c. What flow characteristics are associated with the final /l/ production? How is it distinguished from the preceding vowel? What articulatory behavior accounts for this difference?

   d. Fill in the table to describe the peak airflow associated with each consonant.[2]

   e. Do the data in your table accord with what is known about the airflow relationships of plosives and fricatives? Voiced and unvoiced phones? Why should voicing make a difference in the flow rate?

   f. Based on your airflow trace, what is your best estimate of the mean airflow during the vowel productions? (See Unit 19 "Mean Phonatory Airflow Using a Pneumotachograph.") What might account for the variability in mean phonatory airflow?

6. Repeat your airflow observation with a patient presenting an articulation disorder. (Be sure to use a clean and sterile face mask assembly!) Assess the differences between this patient's record and the normal individual you tested. (You may also use the sample record provided on the next page.)

---

[2] In reporting the peak airflow of fricative consonants, some authors have used the highest peak (see, for example, Klatt et al., 1968), and others have taken the average of the pre- and post-constriction peaks regardless of individual height (see, for instance, Stathopoulos and Weismer, 1985).

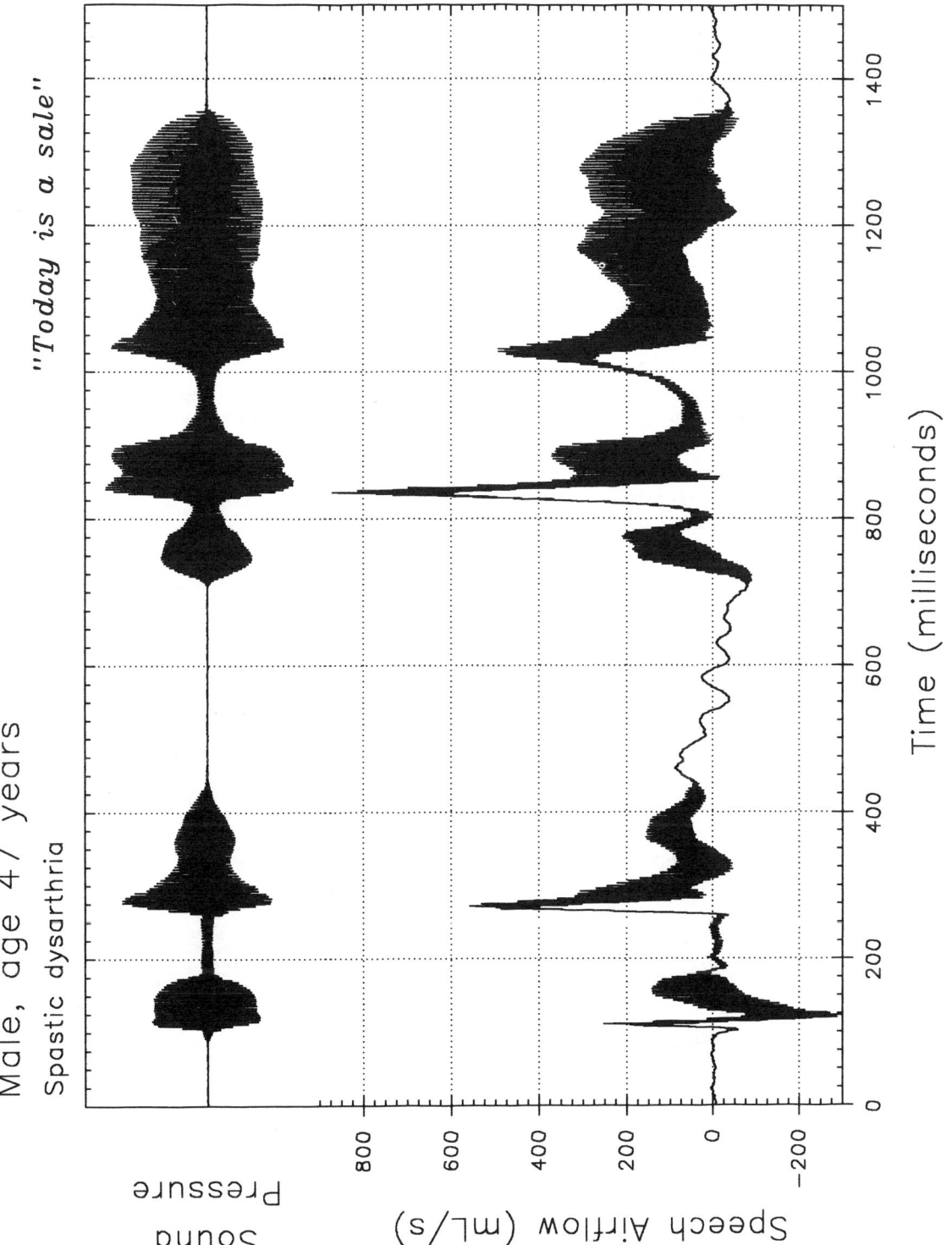

READ MORE ABOUT IT!

Baken, R. J. (1987). *Clinical measurement of speech and voice*. Boston: Little, Brown.

Brown, W. S., Jr., & McGlone, R. E. (1974). Aerodynamic and acoustic study of stress in sentence productions. *Journal of the Acoustical Society of America, 56*, 971–974.

Emanuel, F. W., & Counihan, D. T. (1970). Some characteristics of oral and nasal air flow during plosive consonant production. *Cleft Palate Journal, 7*, 249–260.

Gilbert, H. R. (1973). Oral airflow during stop consonant production. *Folia Phoniatrica, 25*, 288–301.

Isshiki, N., & Ringel, R. (1964). Air flow during the production of selected consonants. *Journal of Speech and Hearing Research, 7*, 233–244.

Klatt, D. H., Stevens, K. N., & Mead, J. (1968). Studies of articulatory activity and airflow during speech. *Annals of the New York Academy of Sciences, 155*, 42–55.

Miller, C. J., & Daniloff, R. (1993). Airflow measurements: Theory and utility of findings. *Journal of Voice, 7*, 38–46.

Netsell, R., Lotz, W. K., & Barlow, S. M. (1989). A speech physiology examination for individuals with dysarthria. In K. M. Yorkston and D. R. Beukelman (Eds.), *Recent advances in clinical dysarthria* (pp. 3–35). San Diego: Singular Publishing Group.

Rothenberg, M. (1977). Measurement of airflow in speech. *Journal of Speech and Hearing Research, 20*, 155–176.

Stathopoulos, E. T. (1985). Effects of monitoring vocal intensity on oral air flow in children and adults. *Journal of Speech and Hearing Research, 28*, 589–593.

Stathopoulos, E. T., & Weismer, G. (1985). Oral airflow and air pressure during speech production: A comparative study of children, youths and adults. *Folia Phoniatrica, 37*, 152–159.

Stevens, K. N. (1971). Airflow and turbulence noise for fricative and stop consonants: Static considerations. *Journal of the Acoustical Society of America, 50*, 1180–1192.

Subtelny, J., Kho, G., McCormack, R. M., & Subtelny, J. D. (1969). Multidimensional analysis of bilabial stop and nasal consonants —Cineradiographic and pressure-flow analysis. *Cleft Palate Journal, 6*, 263–289.

Subtelny, J. D., Worth, J. H., & Sakuda, M. (1966). Intraoral pressure and rate of flow during speech. *Journal of Speech and Hearing Research, 9*, 498–518.

Trullinger, R. W., & Emanuel, F. W. (1983). Airflow characteristics of stop-plosive consonant productions of normal-speaking children. *Journal of Speech and Hearing Research, 26*, 202–208.

van Hattum, R., & Worth, J. H. (1967). Air flow rates in normal speakers. *Cleft Palate Journal, 4*, 137–147.

Warren, D. W. (1976). Aerodynamics of speech production. In N. J. Lass (Ed.), *Contemporary issues in experimental phonetics* (pp. 105–137). New York: Academic Press.

Watson, B. C., & Dembowski, J. (1991). Instrumentation in the evaluation and modification of speech motor control during stuttering therapy. In H. F. M. Peters, W., Hulstijn & C. W. Starkweather (Eds.), *Speech motor control and stuttering* (pp. 503–511). Amsterdam: Elsevier.

Student _____   Date _____

AIRFLOW DURING SPEECH PRODUCTION

I. SETTING UP AND CALIBRATING THE AIRFLOW SYSTEM

Block Diagram of Your Airflow Instrumentation

Maximum flow: _____ L/s

Chart calibration: _____ cm vertical height per L/s

(Attach your calibration record to this page.)

SPEECH AIRFLOW **261**

Student   Date

Attach your labeled data recording to this page.

II. PEAK AIRFLOW DURING CONSONANT PRODUCTION

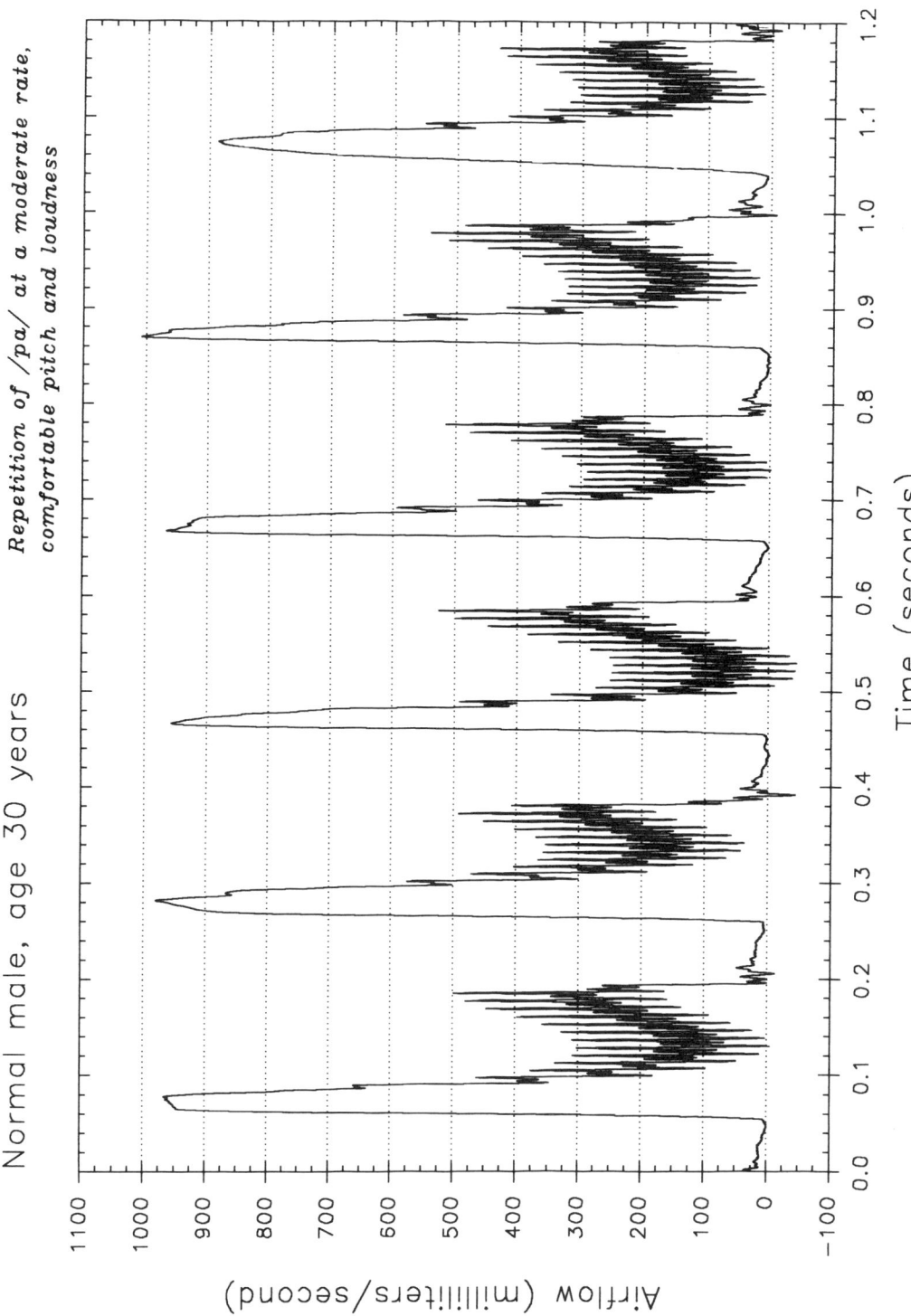

Student _____   Date _____

7. a. Adequacy of frequency response: _____

_____

_____

_____

_____

_____

_____

b. Syllable repetition rate: _____ syllables/s

c. Mean peak airflow rate: _____ mL/s

d. Consistency: _____

_____

_____

_____

_____

_____

_____

Student   Date

III. SPEECH AIRFLOW

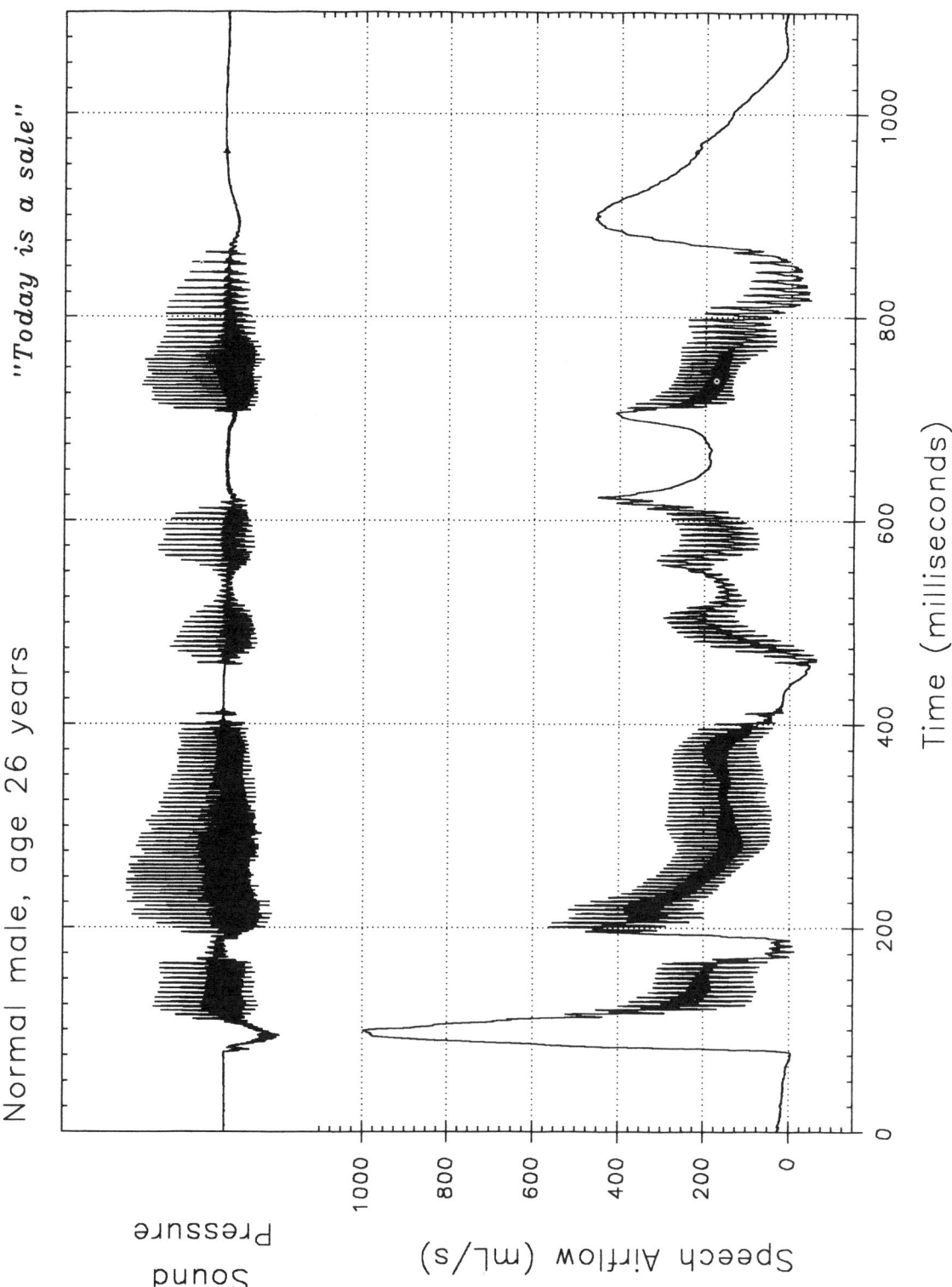

Student _____ Date _____

5. b. Evidence of voicing in the flow record: _____

_____

_____

_____

_____

c. Flow characteristics of /l/ production: _____

_____

_____

_____

_____

_____

d. Complete the following table:

Phone	Peak Flow (mL/s)
[t]	_____
[d]	_____
[z]	_____
[s]	_____

e. Characteristics of consonant classes: _____

_____

_____

_____

_____

Student _____   Date _____

_____
_____

   f. Estimated mean airflow during vowels: _____ mL/s

   Variability: _____

_____
_____
_____
_____

6. Patient: _____

Assessment/comparison of airflow records: _____

_____
_____
_____
_____
_____
_____
_____

UNIT 21

Clinical Application: Estimating Glottal Resistance

The vocal folds vibrate because, when adducted, they represent a significant resistance to the flow of air. In evaluating vocal function, the magnitude of that resistance can often give us important insights concerning the normality of vocal fold adjustment for voicing.

We can measure the glottal resistance (which we will designate R_g) by taking advantage of Ohm's law, which states that resistance is the ratio of pressure to flow. In the context of vocal function, the glottal resistance is the ratio of the pressure drop across the larynx (P_g) to the airflow through the glottis ($Flow_g$). Algebraically,

$$R_g = \frac{P_g}{Flow_g}.$$

You may recall from Unit 18 "Estimating Subglottal Pressure" that, if we are careful, we can estimate the pressure drop across the larynx from the intraoral pressure (P_{io}). Furthermore, it is clear that any airflow from the nose or mouth must have passed through the larynx and that (at least in the case of normal structure!) all of the airflow through the larynx must exit via the nose and mouth. Therefore, measuring glottal airflow involves nothing more than measuring the airflow out of the vocal tract (see Unit 19 "Mean Phonatory Airflow Using a Pneumotachograph"). So our algebraic statement becomes:

$$R_g = \frac{P_{io}}{Flow}.$$

The unit of pressure is cm H$_2$O, and the unit of flow is liters per second (abbreviated L/s or LPS). Therefore, the unit of resistance is "cm H$_2$O/LPS," read "cm H$_2$O per liter per second." (It is sometimes written "cm H$_2$O/L/s.")

Smitheran and Hixon (1981) have proposed a method for using these facts to estimate the phonatory glottal resistance that we will apply in these exercises.

Purpose: In these exercises you will learn to estimate the mean glottal resistance to airflow during phonation and to interpret the results of your measurements in clinical terms.

Equipment: Instrumentation for the measurement of intraoral pressure (see Unit 17 "Intraoral Pressure During Consonant Production") and vocal tract airflow (see Unit 19 "Mean Phonatory Airflow Using a Pneumotachograph") and a way of obtaining a permanent record of the instrument output.

General preparation: Review, if necessary, the general physics of airflow and pressure as well as the means of their transduction and quantification (Baken, 1987, pp. 241–254, 277–294). Also, study the original proposal for the method we will use (Smitheran & Hixon, 1981) and the discussions concerning its validity (Rothenberg, 1982; Hixon & Smitheran, 1982).

Background: Beyond ensuring accurate measurement of P_{io} and flow, two important conditions must be satisfied for this method to be valid:

1. The vocal folds must represent the only significant resistance in the vocal tract at the time R_g is determined; and

2. Vocal intensity and frequency must be well controlled. This is particularly important in evaluating changes in R_g over time.

The first condition poses a problem whose solution dictates the method to be used and the compromise that must be accepted in using it. Specifically, we can use repeated /pi/ syllables to estimate P_s, but there is labial closure for /p/ at the instant we take the pressure measure. Hence, we can't get a flow measure at the same instant that we get a pressure reading. We can measure the flow during /i/ (when the larynx is the only significant resistance in the vocal tract), but we can't use P_{io} to estimate P_s during the vowel. The required solution is to make the assumption that the P_s during /i/ is the same as the peak P_{io} during the /p/'s that immediately precede and follow it.

I. ESTIMATING GLOTTAL RESISTANCE

1. Set up and carefully calibrate the instrumentation for measuring airflow (using a face mask) and intraoral pressure (using an intraoral pressure probe tube). Prepare a block diagram of your instrumentation array.

2. Estimating R_g requires that P_{io} and flow be measured together. This means that the probe tube and face mask must both be appropriately positioned at the same time. Remember that, when in the patient's mouth, the opening of the probe tube must be perpendicular to the airflow. Also, the face mask must make a tight seal so that air does not escape around it. Practice fitting the tube and the mask to achieve correct positioning. [NOTE: You can test for air escape around the mask by suddenly closing off the mask outlet with your hand while your patient phonates. High pressure should build up inside the mask. Don't forget to remove your hand!]

3. Once you have mastered the required positioning, record P_{io} and flow while your subject repeats /pi/ (using a comfortable pitch and loudness) at a rate of about 1.5 syllables per second.

4. Examine your data record. It should be similar to that of the figure on the hand-in sheet. Put your record aside for the moment. We will use the sample record to learn the details of the measurement method.

5. The peaks in the pressure record show P_{io} during the closure phase of /p/, while the troughs show P_{io} during /i/.

    a. Mark the sample figure to show a pressure peak associated with labial closure and a pressure trough during the following vowel production.

    b. Note any evidence of voicing on the figure.

6. Now look at the airflow record. The peaks represent the burst of air at the release of /p/. Each peak is followed by a plateau that represents airflow during /i/. (Note that the data have been low-pass filtered to smooth the trace somewhat.)

7. Mark a vertical line to demonstrate the time relationship between the duration of lip closure for /p/ and airflow and the release of lip closure and airflow. Write a brief description of these relationships on the figure.

8. Two important characteristics should be noted. First, the peak P_{io} for /p/ varies slightly from repetition to repetition; This suggests that the P_s is changing relatively slowly. Secondly, the vowel occurs between two pressure peaks. Clearly, the P_s during the vowel must be somewhere between the pressure of the two peaks that surround it. We can estimate P_s during the vowel by doing the following (as indicated for one of the vowels on the sample figure):

    a. Draw a line from one pressure peak to the next;

    b. Find the midpoint of that line; and

    c. Determine the pressure at that midpoint.

The pressure at the midpoint of the connecting line is the best estimate of the P_s during the vowel. In the example provided, the pressure is 7.05 cm H_2O.

9. Now draw a vertical line from the midpoint of the pressure line down through the flow trace.

The vertical line crosses the pressure trace during the vowel. The pressure at this point is an estimate of the *pharyngeal pressure* (P_p, sometimes called the supraglottal pressure) during the vowel. In the example, the pressure trace is a thick band, so we take the pressure at half the width of the trace. The P_p in the example is 0.83 cm H_2O.

10. The vowel airflow is measured at the point where the vertical line intersects the flow trace. This is the flow value we will use to estimate R_g.

    In the example, the flow is 0.15 LPS.

11. We can now derive R_g:

$$R_g = \frac{(\text{estimated } P_s - P_p)}{\text{Flow}}$$

$$= \frac{(7.05 - 0.83)}{0.15}$$

$$= \frac{6.22}{0.15}$$

$$= 41.5 \text{ cm } H_2O/LPS$$

12. Fill in the table on the hand-in sheet for the other repetitions of /pi/ in the sample figure. To avoid start-up and termination effects, ignore the first and last two repetitions in the record.

13. Mark the data record you have produced to show the peak pressures and the vowel flows. Then fill in the data on the second table on the hand-in sheet. Attach your data record and turn in your work to your instructor.

II. EFFECT OF VOCAL FREQUENCY AND INTENSITY ON GLOTTAL RESISTANCE

1. Use the Smitheran and Hixon method to evaluate R_g under the following conditions:

   a. Lower-than-comfortable pitch at a comfortable loudness;

   b. Comfortable pitch at a comfortable loudness;

   c. Higher-than-comfortable pitch at a comfortable loudness;

   d. Greater-than-comfortable loudness at a comfortable pitch;

   e. Comfortable loudness at a comfortable pitch; and

   f. Less-than-comfortable loudness at a comfortable pitch.

2. Fill in the tables on the hand-in sheet, and attach your marked and labeled data records.

3. What conclusions can you derive concerning the effect of vocal fold adjustments for regulating fundamental frequency and intensity on the glottal resistance? Are your observations consistent with published research findings?

READ MORE ABOUT IT!

Baken, R. J. (1987). *Clinical measurement of speech and voice*. Boston: Little, Brown.

Hillman, R. E., Holmberg, E. G., Perkell, J. S., Walsh, M., & Vaughan, C. (1989). Objective assessment of vocal hyperfunction: An experimental framework and initial results. *Journal of Speech and Hearing Research, 32*, 373–392.

Hixon, T. J., & Smitheran, J. R. (1982). A reply to Rothenberg. *Journal of Speech and Hearing Disorders, 47*, 220–223.

Hoit, J. D., & Hixon, T. J. (1992). Age and laryngeal airway resistance during vowel production in women. *Journal of Speech and Hearing Research, 35*, 309–313.

Isshiki, N. (1964). Regulatory mechanism of voice intensity variation. *Journal of Speech and Hearing Disorders, 7*, 17–29.

Isshiki, N. (1969). Remarks on mechanism for vocal intensity variation. *Journal of Speech and Hearing Disorders, 12*, 665–672.

Kitajima, K., & Fujita, F. (1990). Estimation of subglottal pressure with intraoral pressure. *Acta Otolaryngologica, 109*, 473–478.

Leeper, H. A., Jr., & Graves, K. K. (1984). Consistency of laryngeal airway resistance in adult women. *Journal of Communication Disorders, 17*, 153–163.

McGlone, R. E., & Shipp, T. (1971). Some physiologic correlates of vocal-fry phonation. *Journal of Speech and Hearing Research, 14*, 769–775.

Melcon, M. C., Hoit, J. D., & Hixon, T. J. (1989). Age and laryngeal airway resistance during vowel production. *Journal of Speech and Hearing Disorders, 54*, 282–286.

Netsell, R., Lotz, W., & Shaughnessy, A. O. (1984). Laryngeal aerodyanmics associated with selected voice disorders. *American Journal of Otolaryngology, 5*, 397–403.

Rothenberg, M. (1982). Interpolating subglottal pressure from oral pressure. *Journal of Speech and Hearing Disorders, 47*, 219–220.

Shipp, T. (1973). Intraoral air pressure and lip occlusion in midvocalic stop consonant production. *Journal of Phonetics, 1*, 167–170.

Smitheran, J. R., & Hixon, T. J. (1981). A clinical method for estimating laryngeal airway resistance during vowel production. *Journal of Speech and Hearing Disorders, 46*, 138–146.

Warren, D. W. (1976). Aerodynamics of speech production. In N. J. Lass (Ed.), *Contemporary issues in experimental phonetics* (pp. 105–137). New York: Academic Press.

Student _____ Date _____

GLOTTAL RESISTANCE

I. ESTIMATING GLOTTAL RESISTANCE

Block Diagram of Your Instrumentation Array

Maximum pressure: _____ cm H_2O

Chart calibration: _____ cm vertical height per cm H_2O

Maximum flow: _____ L/s

Chart calibration: _____ cm vertical height per L/s

(Attach your calibration record to this page.)

Student Date

SAMPLE DATA RECORD

Normal male, age 48. Repeated /pi/

Intraoral probe tube with Statham pressure transducer. Face mask and Fleisch #0 pneumotach with Validyne pressure transducer.

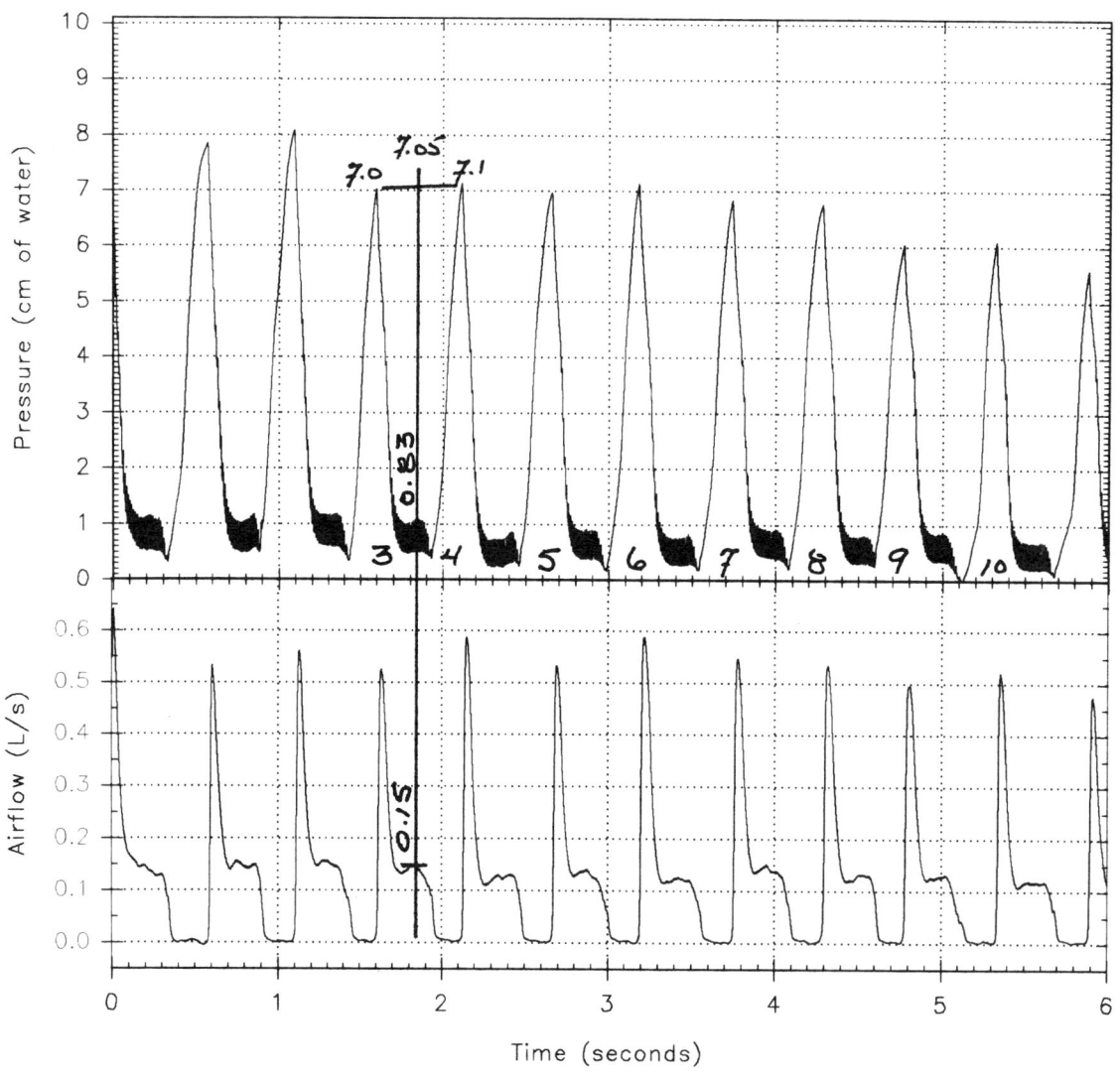

Student _____ Date _____

7. Relationship between duration of lip closure and airflow:

_____
_____
_____
_____
_____

12. Complete the following table for the *sample* figure:

Syllable Number	Peak P_{io} during /p/ (cm H_2O)	Estimated P_s at vowel (cm H_2O)	P_p at vowel midpoint (cm H_2O)	Flow (LPS)	Estimated R_g (cm H_2O/LPS)
3	7.0	7.05	0.83	0.15	41.5
4	7.1				
5	___	___	___	___	___
6	___	___	___	___	___
7	___	___	___	___	___
8	___	___	___	___	___
9	___	___	___	___	___
MEAN					___
SD					___

Student _____ Date _____

13. Patient: _____ sex: _____ age: _____

Phonatory conditions: _____

Complete the following table for your patient's aerodynamic records:

Syllable Number	Peak P_{io} during /p/ (cm H_2O)	Estimated P_s at vowel (cm H_2O)	P_p at vowel midpoint (cm H_2O)	Flow (LPS)	Estimated R_g (cm H_2O/LPS)
3	_____				
4	_____	_____	_____	_____	_____
5	_____	_____	_____	_____	_____
6	_____	_____	_____	_____	_____
7	_____	_____	_____	_____	_____
8	_____	_____	_____	_____	_____
9	_____	_____	_____	_____	_____
10	_____	_____	_____	_____	_____
11	_____	_____	_____	_____	_____
12	_____	_____	_____	_____	_____
MEAN					_____
SD					_____

(Attach your data record to this page.)

Student   Date

II. EFFECT OF VOCAL FREQUENCY AND INTENSITY ON GLOTTAL RESISTANCE

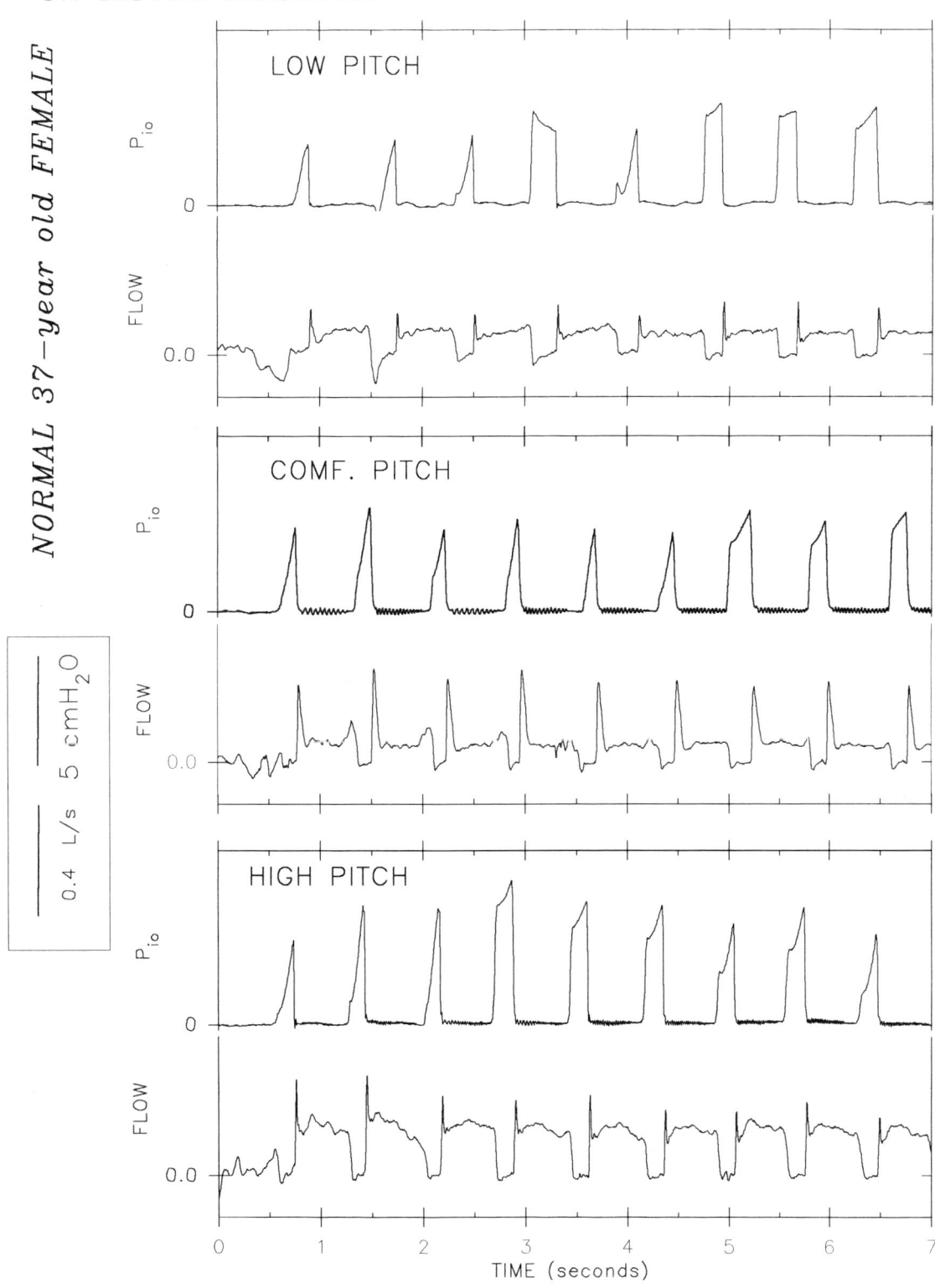

Student   Date

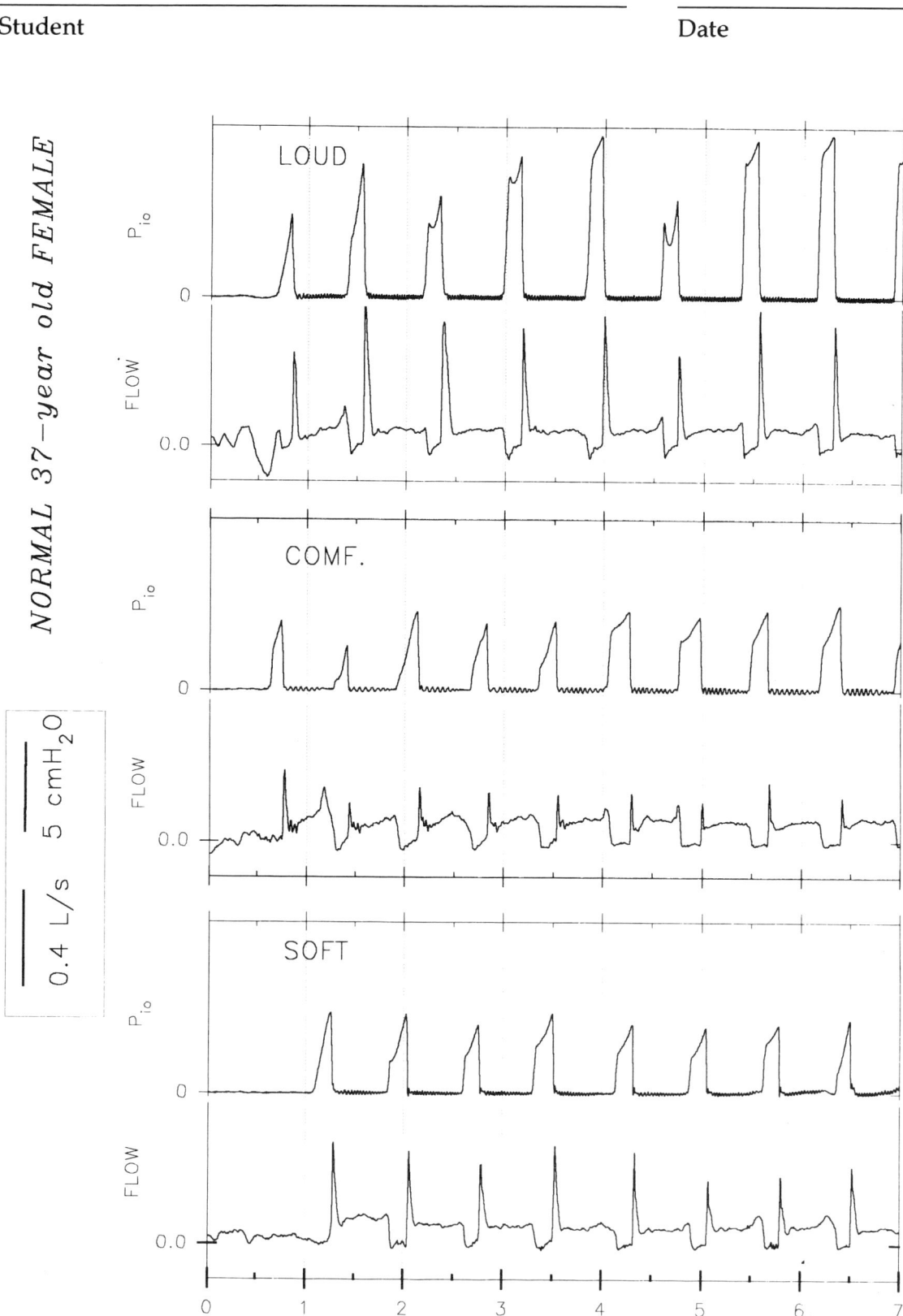

Student _____   Date _____

2. Fill in the following tables from your data:

Patient: _____ sex: _____ age: _____

Phonatory conditions: __Low pitch, comfortable loudness__

Complete the following table for your patient's aerodynamic record:

Syllable Number	Peak P_{io} during /p/ (cm H_2O)	Estimated P_s at vowel (cm H_2O)	P_p at vowel midpoint (cm H_2O)	Flow (LPS)	Estimated R_g (cm H_2O/LPS)
3	_____				
4	_____	_____	_____	_____	_____
5	_____	_____	_____	_____	_____
6	_____	_____	_____	_____	_____
7	_____	_____	_____	_____	_____
8	_____	_____	_____	_____	_____
9	_____	_____	_____	_____	_____
10	_____	_____	_____	_____	_____
11	_____	_____	_____	_____	_____
12	_____	_____	_____	_____	_____
MEAN					_____
SD					_____

(Attach your data record to this page.)

Student _____   Date _____

Patient: _____ sex: _____ age: _____

Phonatory conditions: _Comfortable pitch, comfortable loudness_

Complete the following table for your patient's aerodynamic record:

Syllable Number	Peak P_{io} during /p/ (cm H_2O)	Estimated P_s at vowel (cm H_2O)	P_p at vowel midpoint (cm H_2O)	Flow (LPS)	Estimated R_g (cm H_2O/LPS)
3	_____				
4	_____	_____	_____	_____	_____
5	_____	_____	_____	_____	_____
6	_____	_____	_____	_____	_____
7	_____	_____	_____	_____	_____
8	_____	_____	_____	_____	_____
9	_____	_____	_____	_____	_____
10	_____	_____	_____	_____	_____
11	_____	_____	_____	_____	_____
12	_____	_____	_____	_____	_____
MEAN					_____
SD					_____

(Attach your data record to this page.)

Student _____   Date _____

Patient: _____ sex: _____ age: _____

Phonatory conditions: __High pitch, comfortable loudness__

Complete the following table for your patient's aerodynamic record:

Syllable Number	Peak P_{io} during /p/ (cm H_2O)	Estimated P_s at vowel (cm H_2O)	P_p at vowel midpoint (cm H_2O)	Flow (LPS)	Estimated R_g (cm H_2O/LPS)
3	_____				
4	_____	_____	_____	_____	_____
5	_____	_____	_____	_____	_____
6	_____	_____	_____	_____	_____
7	_____	_____	_____	_____	_____
8	_____	_____	_____	_____	_____
9	_____	_____	_____	_____	_____
10	_____	_____	_____	_____	_____
11	_____	_____	_____	_____	_____
12	_____	_____	_____	_____	_____
MEAN					_____
SD					_____

(Attach your data record to this page.)

Student _____   Date _____

Patient: _____ sex: _____ age: _____

Phonatory conditions: <u>Relatively loud, comfortable pitch</u>

Complete the following table for your patient's aerodynamic record:

Syllable Number	Peak P_{io} during /p/ (cm H_2O)	Estimated P_s at vowel (cm H_2O)	P_p at vowel midpoint (cm H_2O)	Flow (LPS)	Estimated R_g (cm H_2O/LPS)
3	_____				
4	_____	_____	_____	_____	_____
5	_____	_____	_____	_____	_____
6	_____	_____	_____	_____	_____
7	_____	_____	_____	_____	_____
8	_____	_____	_____	_____	_____
9	_____	_____	_____	_____	_____
10	_____	_____	_____	_____	_____
11	_____	_____	_____	_____	_____
12	_____	_____	_____	_____	_____
MEAN					_____
SD					_____

(Attach your data record to this page.)

Student _____   Date _____

Patient: _____ sex: _____ age: _____

Phonatory conditions: __Comfortable loudness, comfortable pitch__

Complete the following table for your patient's aerodynamic record:

Syllable Number	Peak P_{io} during /p/ (cm H_2O)	Estimated P_s at vowel (cm H_2O)	P_p at vowel midpoint (cm H_2O)	Flow (LPS)	Estimated R_g (cm H_2O/LPS)
3	_____				
4	_____	_____	_____	_____	_____
5	_____	_____	_____	_____	_____
6	_____	_____	_____	_____	_____
7	_____	_____	_____	_____	_____
8	_____	_____	_____	_____	_____
9	_____	_____	_____	_____	_____
10	_____	_____	_____	_____	_____
11	_____	_____	_____	_____	_____
12	_____	_____	_____	_____	_____
MEAN					_____
SD					_____

(Attach your data record to this page.)

Student _____ Date _____

Patient: _____ sex: _____ age: _____

Phonatory conditions: <u>Relatively soft, comfortable pitch</u>

Complete the following table for your patient's aerodynamic record:

Syllable Number	Peak P_{io} during /p/ (cm H_2O)	Estimated P_s at vowel (cm H_2O)	P_p at vowel midpoint (cm H_2O)	Flow (LPS)	Estimated R_g (cm H_2O/LPS)
3	_____				
4	_____	_____	_____	_____	_____
5	_____	_____	_____	_____	_____
6	_____	_____	_____	_____	_____
7	_____	_____	_____	_____	_____
8	_____	_____	_____	_____	_____
9	_____	_____	_____	_____	_____
10	_____	_____	_____	_____	_____
11	_____	_____	_____	_____	_____
12	_____	_____	_____	_____	_____
MEAN					_____
SD					_____

(Attach your data record to this page.)

Student _____   Date _____

3. How is increased vocal frequency reflected in R_g? _____

_____

_____

_____

_____

_____

_____

What is the effect of increasing vocal intensity on R_g? _____

_____

_____

_____

_____

_____

_____

Previous findings in the literature: _____

_____

_____

_____

_____

_____

_____

_____

_____

Source(s): _____

UNIT 22

Clinical Application: Determining Lung Volume Change and Mean Phonatory Airflow from Spirometric Records

The efficient management of an adequate air supply is a basic requisite of normal speech. Spirometry is a time-honored way of evaluating lung volume management. It finds considerable use in clinical assessment of speech problems.

Purpose: In these exercises you will learn to use a spirometer to

- Measure a patient's forced vital capacity (FVC) and assess its normality;
- Evaluate maximum phonation volume;
- Derive estimates of mean airflow from a volume record;
- Estimate the lung volume (in absolute terms and as a percentage of the FVC) used for each breath group during reading of a standard passage.

Equipment: A recording spirometer and face mask assembly. A meter stick will also be needed for measuring the patient's height.

General preparation: Familiarize yourself with the several common methods of measuring lung volume and the relationship between air volume and flow (see, for example, Baken, 1987, pp. 279–284, 302–311). Then examine the spirometer you will be using and read its manual carefully. Determine the maximum volume of air that it can contain, and be sure that you understand how it produces a data record. Identify its critical parts, including the spirometer "bell," the pen linkage (on chart-writing instruments), and the paper drive system. If your spirometer produces an electrical output, identify the function of its output connections (there may be more than one!) and be sure you understand how you will convert that output into a written record.

Examine the face mask, paying particular attention to the cushion that will be in contact with the patient's face. Make sure you understand how the mask is connected to the spirometer.

Prepare a block diagram of how your equipment will be set up. Show the spirometer bell, associated linkage to the pen assembly, and any associated electronics. On your block diagram indicate: (1) The maximal capacity of the spirometer; (2) Whether an upward movement of the recording pen indicates increasing or decreasing lung volume; and (3) Whether time proceeds from right-to-left or left-to-right on the printed record.

Now connect the hose and face mask assembly to the spirometer. Adjust the position of the spirometer bell so it is filled with air to a convenient volume (perhaps 5 liters or about half of its capacity). We will refer to this as the "baseline volume." Note exactly what your baseline volume is, because you will have to reset the spirometer to it several times during the exercises that follow.

I. FORCED VITAL CAPACITY

Forced vital capacity (FVC) is defined as the maximum volume of air that can be expired after a maximal inspiration. As such, it represents the total amount of air that (in some theoretical sense) is available for "use."

To measure the FVC, you must get your patient to fill her lungs as fully as possible and then to exhale all the air she can possibly "squeeze out." The expiration should be fairly rapid. Because it is absolutely critical that the patient put in a *maximal* effort, your interaction with the patient is critical to obtaining a good measurement of the FVC. Your instructions must make it clear that you want the patient first to inhale absolutely to the "bursting point," and then to exhale rapidly, "squeezing out every last drop of air." During the test, you should keep encouraging your patient to inhale more and more, and then to exhale just another bit — always more, MORE, **MORE!**

1. Measure your patient's height.

2. Seat your patient comfortably, and allow her to breathe quietly for a while. Have her practice exhaling to her resting expiratory level (REL) and then holding her breath. Then instruct the patient about the task to be performed.

3. Set the spirometer to its baseline volume (about half its capacity).

4. With the patient holding her breath at her REL, press the mask snugly against the patient's face. It should be held tightly enough to prevent any leakage.

5. Instruct the patient to inhale maximally and then to exhale maximally while the spirometer records lung volume change. You will obtain a graphic tracing the height of which represents the patient's FVC. Label this "Trial 1."

6. Remove the face mask and give the patient a minute or so rest period, during which you should empty the spirometer bell and reset it to the baseline volume.

7. Repeat steps 3 through 6 two more times to obtain three traces (or *spirograms*) in all. Label the traces "Trial 2" and "Trial 3," respectively. Record each of the volumes on the hand-in sheet.

8. The patient's FVC is the largest volume represented in the three tracings. Write the FVC on this record and be sure to save it for later use.

9. Determine your patient's *expected* forced vital capacity using the regression equation (provided in Appendix G) appropriate for your patient's sex, age, and height. Write this expected FVC near the patient's name on the chart recording. Is your patient's FVC normal?

II. PHONATION VOLUME AND ESTIMATED MEAN FLOW RATE

The *phonation volume* (PV) is defined as "the maximum amount of air that is available for a maximally sustained phonation" (Yanagihara & Koike, 1967).

1. Empty the spirometer bell and reset it to the baseline volume.

2. If available, attach an event marker to the spirometer's recording system to mark where phonation begins and ends.

3. Instruct your patient that, once the face mask is in place, he is to breathe normally. When told to begin, he is to fill his lungs to their maximal volume and then to hold the vowel /ɑ/ at a comfortable pitch and loudness until it cannot be sustained any longer. (You may want to rephrase these instructions to suit your patient's level of sophistication!) Encourage your patient to produce /ɑ/ until it becomes absolutely impossible to continue. (*Voice*, not *voice quality*, is of importance here.)

4. Instruct your patient to exhale to REL. Fit the mask snugly against his face, start the spirometer's recording system, and have him accomplish the task. Activate the event marker (if you have one) when phonation starts, and deactivate it when phonation ends. (A sample record is provided on the hand-in sheet.)

5. On the basis of the record you have obtained,

   a. What was your patient's maximum phonation time (MPT)? (Provide this information on the hand-in sheet and under the section of the spirogram where phonation occurs.)

   b. What volume of air was used to produce /ɑ/? If your test was valid, this is the phonation volume. (Provide this datum on the hand-in sheet and to the left of that part of the record that represents the phonatory event.)

   c. Is your patient's PV normal? How do you know?

   d. In what kinds of pathology might the PV be abnormal? Name some specific disorders.

6. The PV divided by the duration of phonation (the MPT) provides an estimate of the mean phonatory airflow. Based on this estimate:

   a. What is your patient's estimated mean flow rate?

   b. Is it normal?

   c. Why is this way of evaluating phonatory airflow not as good as methods that measure flow more directly (see Unit 19 "Mean Phonatory Airflow using a Pneumotachograph")?

III. VOLUME OF BREATH GROUPS IN READING

Spirometric assessment of lung volume change during a speaking task lets us see how a patient manages air for speech purposes. In this exercise, you will examine the duration and relative volume (that is, the amount of air expressed as a percentage of the patient's FVC) of each breath group, and you will get some idea of how the chest wall is used by comparing the volumes to the REL.

1. Empty the spirometer bell and reset it to the baseline volume.

2. Provide your patient with a copy of the Rainbow Passage (Appendix D) and allow her to practice reading it.

3. Instruct your patient that, after the face mask is in place, she is to breathe normally and then, at your signal, she is to read the Rainbow Passage as normally as possible until you tell her to stop.

4. Have your patient exhale to her REL and hold her breath until the mask is in place. Fit the mask snugly to the patient's face.

5. Activate the spirometer's recording system. After about a minute of quiet breathing, instruct the patient to begin reading.

Analysis:

6. Line up the FVC recording to the left of the recording of speech breathing you have just obtained. Align the two records so that the baseline volume is at the same horizontal position, and tape the two records together. (A sample composite spirogram is provided on the hand-in sheet.)

7. Examine the record of quiet breathing that precedes reading of the Rainbow Passage. Locate the resting expiratory level, and extend a heavy line across the entire record to represent REL.

8. Divide the full height of the FVC trace into ten equal segments. Each interval now represents 10% of the vital capacity. Draw horizontal lines across the entire record, thereby establishing a "percent vital capacity" scale for the speech breathing record. Label the vertical axis on the right side of your combined record as "Percent VC" and mark the percentage represented by each horizontal line across the recording.

9. Now mark off and number each breath group. Fill in the table on the hand-in sheet with the data from your recording. Attach it to your data record for submission to your instructor.

10. Write a brief evaluation of your patient's performance. Suggest reasons for any abnormality you might detect. Attach it to your data record. Consider not only the durations and size of breath groups, but also the relationship of the breath groups to REL.

READ MORE ABOUT IT!

Baken, R. J. (1987). *Clinical measurement of speech and voice.* Boston: Little, Brown.

Beckett, R. L. (1971). The respirometer as a diagnostic and clinical tool in the speech clinic. *Journal of Speech and Hearing Disorders, 36,* 235–241.

Beckett, R. L., Thoelke, W., & Cowan, L. (1971). A normative study of airflow in children. *British Journal of Disorders of Communication, 6,* 13–16.

Horii, Y., & Cooke, P. A. (1978). Some airflow, volume, and duration characteristics of oral reading. *Journal of Speech and Hearing Research, 21,* 470–481.

Itoh, M., & Horii, Y. (1985). Airflow, volume, and durational characteristics of oral reading by the hearing-impaired. *Journal of Communication Disorders, 18,* 393–407.

Loudon, R. G., Lee, L., & Holcomb, B. J. (1988). Volumes and breathing patterns during speech in healthy and asthmatic subjects. *Journal of Speech and Hearing Research, 31,* 219–227.

Painter, C. (1979). *An introduction to instrumental phonetics* (pp. 55–59). Baltimore: University Park Press.

Snidecor, J. C., & Isshiki, N. (1965). Air volume and air flow relationships of six male esophageal speakers. *Journal of Speech and Hearing Disorders, 30,* 205–215.

Yanagihara, N., & Koike, Y. (1967). The regulation of sustained phonation. *Folia Phoniatrica, 19,* 1–18.

Yanagihara, N., Koike, Y., & von Leden, H. (1966). Phonation and respiration: Function study in normal subjects. *Folia Phoniatrica, 18,* 323–340.

Yanagihara, N., & von Leden, H. (1967). Respiration and phonation: The functional examination of laryngeal disease. *Folia Phoniatrica, 19,* 153–166.

Student _____   Date _____

DETERMINING LUNG VOLUME CHANGE AND MEAN PHONATORY AIRFLOW FROM SPIROMETRIC RECORDS

Block Diagram of Your Instrumentation

Spirometer capacity: _____ Liters

Increasing lung volume will be: upward   downward

Time advances from: right-to-left   left-to-right

Student _____   Date _____

I. FORCED VITAL CAPACITY

Patient: _____ Sex: _____ Age: _____

Height: _____ cm

7. Forced vital capacity measurements:

Trial 1: _____ liters

Trial 2: _____ liters

Trial 3: _____ liters

9. Expected forced vital capacity: _____ liters

Assessment of patient's FVC: _____

_____

_____

_____

_____

Student _____   Date _____

II. PHONATION VOLUME AND ESTIMATED MEAN FLOW RATE

Patient: _____ Sex: _____ Age: _____

Height: _____ cm

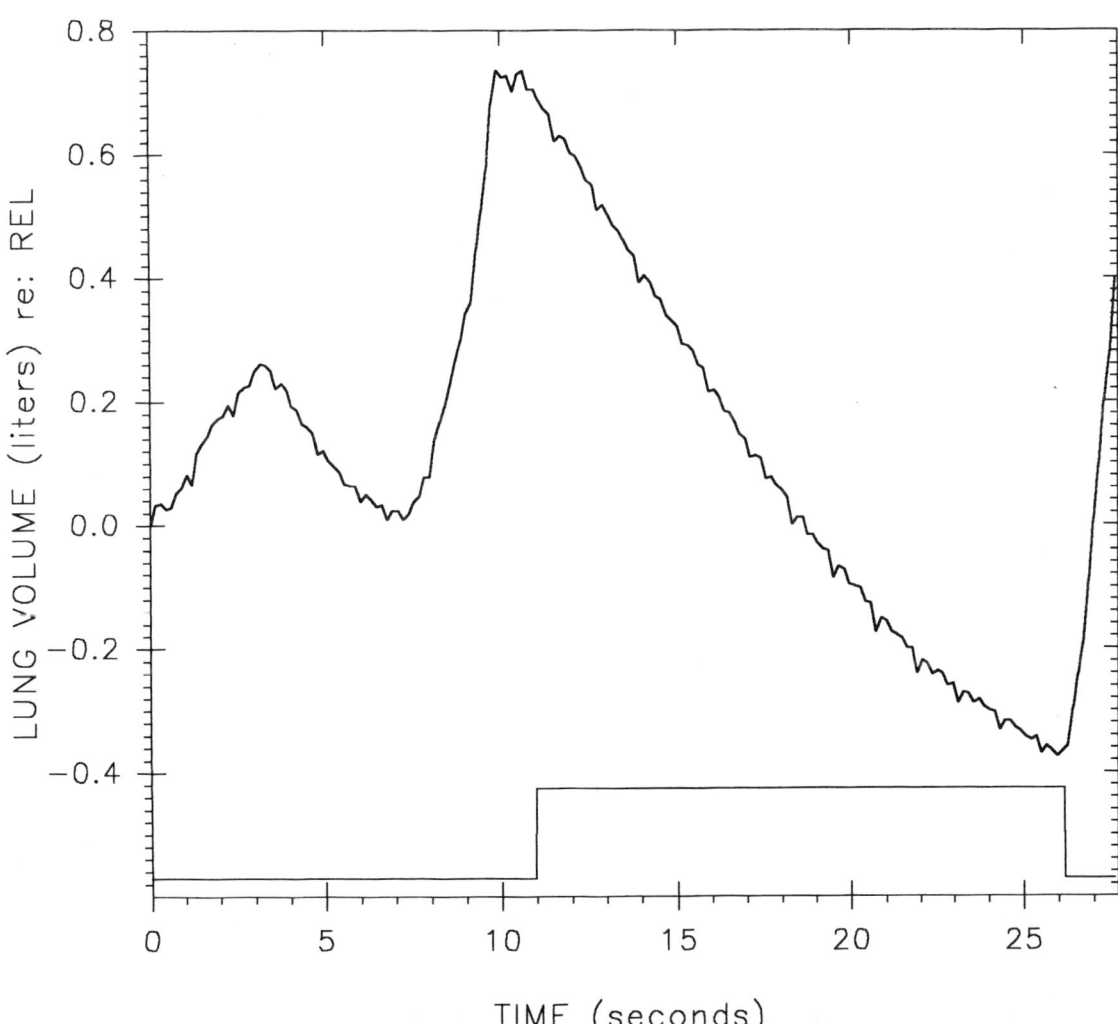

Sustained /a/, comfortable pitch and loudness.

(Attach your labeled data recording to this page.)

DETERMINING LUNG VOLUME CHANGE

Student _____   Date _____

5. a. Maximum phonation time: _____ seconds

  b. Phonation volume: _____ liters

  c. Assessment: _____
  _____
  _____
  _____
  _____

    Source(s): _____

  d. Pathologies in which PV might be abnormal include: _____
  _____
  _____

6. a. Estimated mean phonatory airflow (show your arithmetic):
  _____

  b. Assessment: _____
  _____
  _____
  _____
  _____

    Source(s): _____

  c. Why might other airflow measurement methods be better?
  _____
  _____
  _____

Student   Date

II. VOLUME OF BREATH GROUPS IN READING

Patient: _____ Sex: _____ Age: _____

FVC: _____ liters

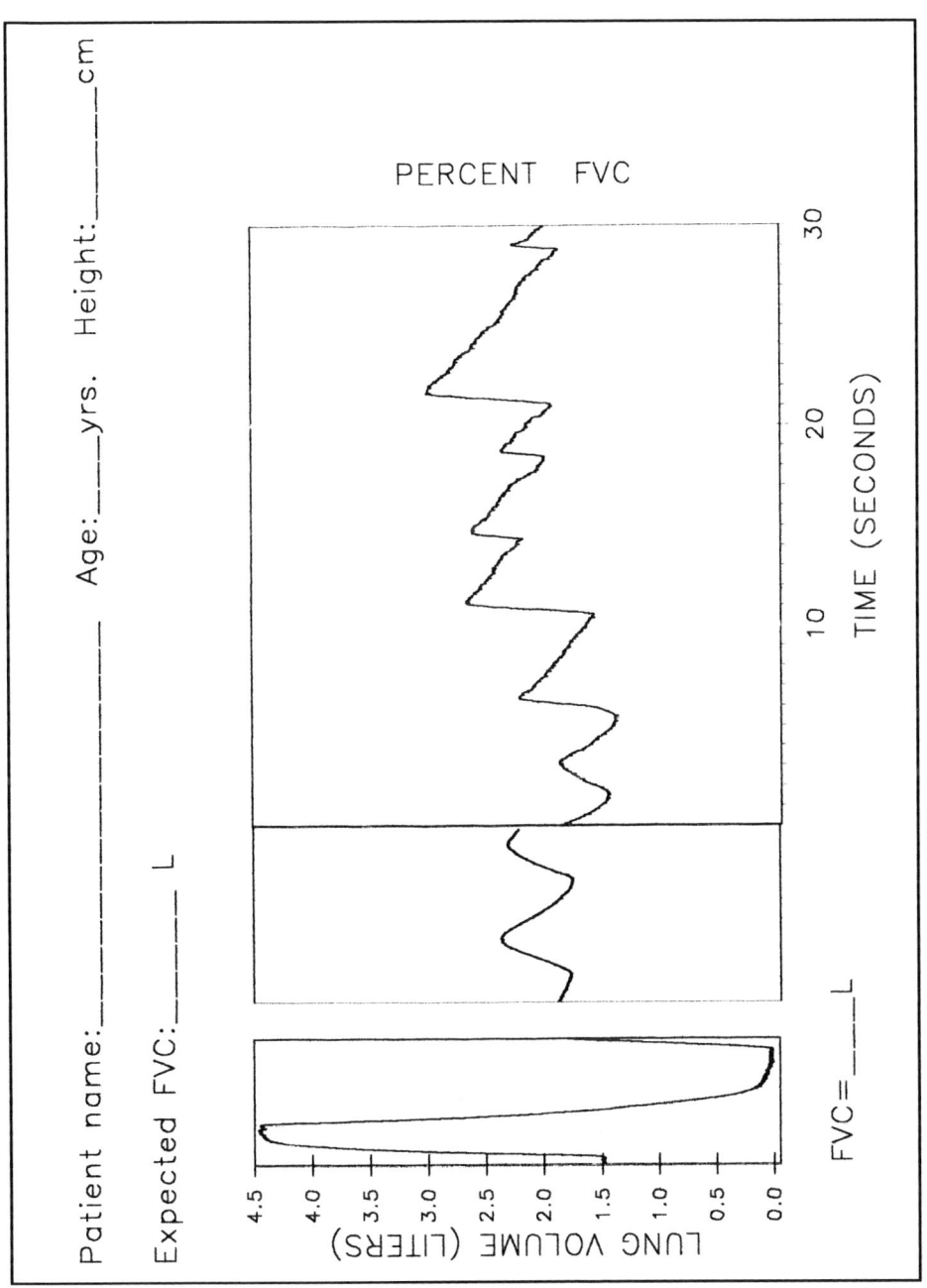

(Attach your labeled data recording to this page.)

DETERMINING LUNG VOLUME CHANGE

Student _____   Date _____

9. Complete the following table based on your patient's spirometric data:

Breath Group Number	Duration (in s)	Volume (in liters)	Volume (in % FVC)
1	_____	_____	_____
2	_____	_____	_____
3	_____	_____	_____
4	_____	_____	_____
5	_____	_____	_____
6	_____	_____	_____
7	_____	_____	_____
8	_____	_____	_____
9	_____	_____	_____
10	_____	_____	_____
MEAN	_____	_____	_____
SD	_____	_____	_____

10. Evaluation: _____

_____

_____

_____

_____

UNIT 23

Clinical Application: Estimating Mean Speech Airflow From Spirometric Records

Mean airflow data may be of value when attempting to assess more general characteristics of ventilatory, laryngeal, and/or articulatory function. The mean speech airflow may be derived by dividing the volume of air a speaker uses over the course of an utterance by the time taken to produce the utterance. Such volume records can be obtained by a recording spirometer (Baken, 1987, pp. 277–311, see also Unit 20 "Airflow During Speech Production").

Purpose: In these laboratory exercises you will use a recording spirometer to measure a patient's mean airflow during spoken utterances.

Equipment: A recording spirometer with a non-rebreathing valve and face mask assembly (see Baken, 1987, p. 298).

General preparation: Familiarize yourself with the relationship between air volume and flow. Review the nature of breath groups and lung volume change during speech (see Unit 22 "Determining Lung Volume Change and Mean Air Flow From Spirometric Records"). Also familiarize yourself with the instruction manual accompanying the spirometer you will be using. Be sure you understand how it produces a data record. Prepare a block diagram of how your equipment will be set up — identifying all critical components. On your block diagram, indicate:

   a. The maximal capacity of the spirometer;
   b. Whether an upward movement of the recording pen indicates increasing or decreasing lung volume; and

c. Whether time proceeds from right-to-left or left-to-right.

Equipment setup: Connect the face mask and non-rebreathing valve to the spirometer intake hosing. (This valve will allow the patient to inhale room air, but all expired air will be passed to the spirometer.) Empty the spirometer and adjust the position of the spirometer's bell so that it is filled with air to a convenient "baseline" volume (about 5 liters).

I. MEAN FLOW DURING THE RAINBOW PASSAGE

1. Seat your patient comfortably. Provide him with a copy of the Rainbow Passage (Appendix D), and allow him to practice reading it.

2. Set the spirometer to an appropriate "baseline volume."

3. Instruct your patient that, once the face mask is in place, he is breathe normally. Then, when told, he is to begin to reading the Rainbow Passage at a comfortable rate and loudness until told to stop.

4. Press the mask snugly against the patient's face.[1] (Be sure that there are no air leaks!)

5. After a few moments, instruct your patient to begin reading. Continue to watch the output to be sure that the data are acceptable.

6. Tell your patient to stop and remove the mask before his expiratory volume fills the spirometer.

7. Mark your spirogram to indicate when speech began and when it ended. From your record determine:

    a. The "baseline" volume when your patient began speaking;

    b. The spirometer volume when your patient finished; and

    c. The total volume of air used by your patient while speaking.

8. Identify each speech expiration (breath group) on the data record. Mark and number each of these expirations. [NOTE: Because of the non-rebreathing valve, inspirations appear as "plateaus" on the record.]

An example of a marked spirogram is provided on the next page. Here a normal male speaker read the first paragraph of the Rainbow Passage while his expiratory volume was collected using a 9-liter Collins spirometer.

---

[1] The face mask may be held by you or by the patient, if capable. Alternatively, it may be firmly attached with an adjustable harness available with many mask assemblies.

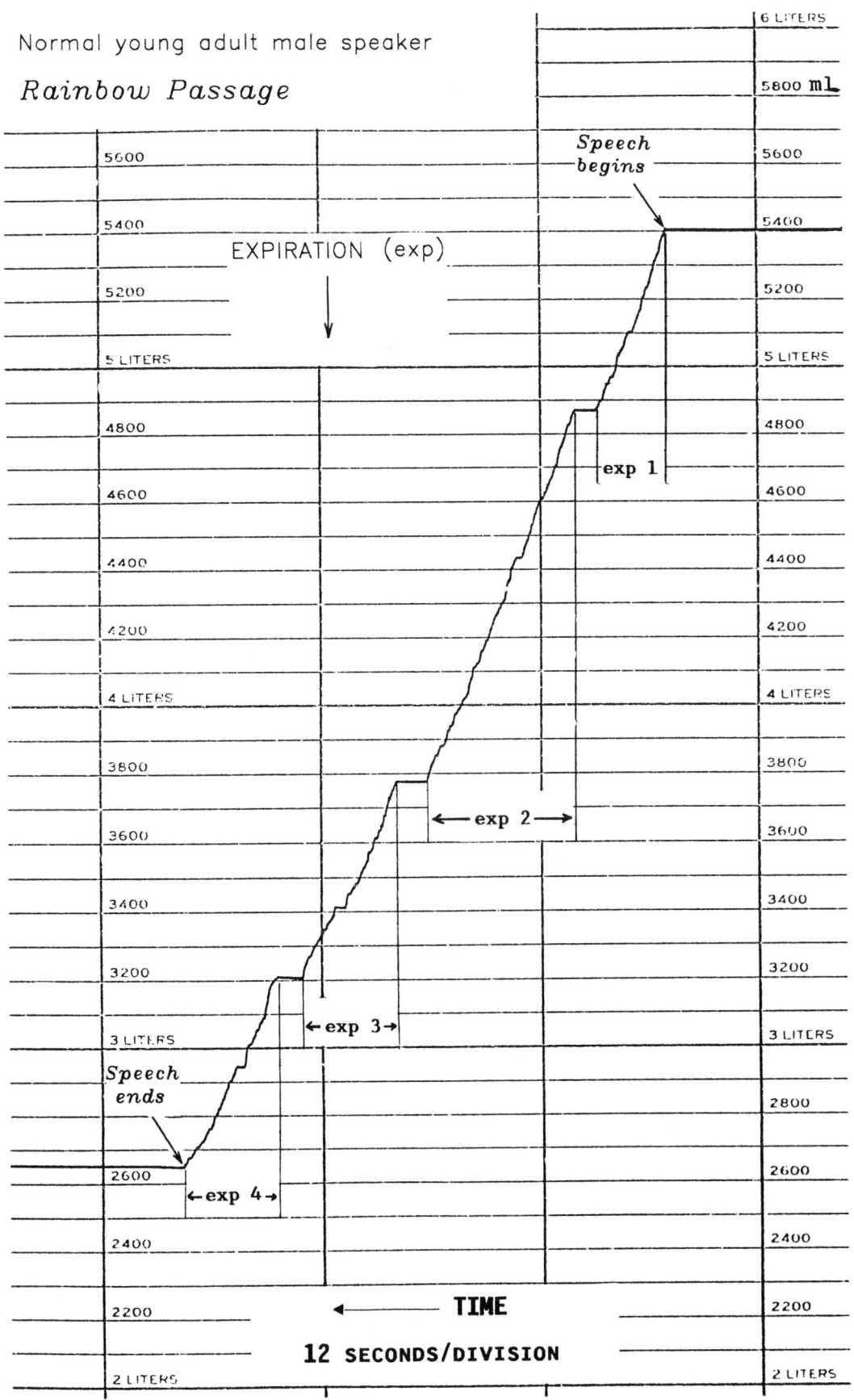

MEAN SPEECH AIRFLOW 301

9. For each breath group, determine the volume of air expired and the duration of each expiration. As you do so, fill in the table provided on the hand-in sheet.

10. Add all of the speech volumes and expiratory durations for your sample and divide the total volume by the total expiratory time. What is the estimated mean speech airflow?

11. Write a brief evaluation of your patient's performance. Suggest reasons for any abnormality you might detect. Attach your marked and labeled spirogram to your evaluation and turn them in to your instructor.

CLINICAL NOTE: Although the spirometer does not have the frequency response to provide detailed information about airflow for isolated speech sounds, any gross irregularities in the record may reflect pathology, especially those of structural or neurologic origin.

II. MEAN FLOW DURING "LOW-FLOW" AND "HIGH-FLOW" READING PASSAGES

Average speech airflow will be strongly influenced by the nature of the spoken material. Under some circumstances, it may be desirable to evaluate speech airflow while the patient recites a passage loaded with low-flow sounds (such as voiced phones) or with high-flow sounds (such as voiceless plosives and fricatives). Passages of these sorts are provided in Appendices H and I, respectively. (Sample volume records for each passage are provided on the hand-in sheet.) Repeat the procedure you used to record and evaluate the Rainbow Passage using these passages, or construct ones of your own. If you use your own passages be sure to include them with your lab report.

READ MORE ABOUT IT!

Baken, R. J. (1987). *Clinical measurement of speech and voice* (pp. 296–298). Boston: Little, Brown.

Horii, Y., & Cooke, P. A. (1978). Some airflow, volume, and duration characteristics of oral reading. *Journal of Speech and Hearing Research, 21,* 470–481.

Itoh, M., & Horii, Y. (1985). Airflow, volume, and durational characteristics of oral reading by the hearing-impaired. *Journal of Communication Disorders, 18,* 393–407.

Klatt, K. H., Stevens, K. N., & Mead, J. (1968). Studies of articulatory activity and airflow during speech. *Annals of the New York Academy of Sciences, 155,* 42–54.

Rothenberg, M. (1977). Measurement of airflow in speech. *Journal of Speech and Hearing Research, 20,* 155–176.

Snidecor, J. C., & Isshiki, N. (1965). Air volume and air flow relationships of six male esophageal speakers. *Journal of Speech and Hearing Disorders, 30,* 205–215.

Stathopoulos, E. T. (1985). Effects of monitoring vocal intensity on oral air flow in children and adults. *Journal of Speech and Hearing Research, 28,* 589–593.

Subtelny, J. D., Worth, H. H., & Sakuta, M. (1966). Intraoral pressure and rate of flow during speech. *Journal of Speech and Hearing Research, 9,* 498–518.

Van Hattum, R. J., & Worth, J. H. (1967). Air flow rates in normal speakers. *Cleft Palate Journal, 4,* 137–147.

Student _____   Date _____

MEAN SPEECH AIRFLOW

Block Diagram of Your Instrumentation

a. Spirometer capacity: _____ liters

b. Increasing lung volume is: upward   downward

c. Time advances from: right-to-left   left-to-right

Student _____   Date _____

Attach your labeled data recordings to this page.

I. MEAN FLOW DURING THE RAINBOW PASSAGE

7. a. Approximate baseline volume: _____ mL

   b. Approximate end volume: _____ mL

   c. Approximate speech volume: _____ mL

9. Complete the following table:

Expiration Number	Speech Volume (in mL)	Expiratory Duration (in seconds)
1	_____	_____
2	_____	_____
3	_____	_____
4	_____	_____
5	_____	_____
6	_____	_____
Sum	_____	_____

10. Estimated mean airflow rate: _____ mL/s

Student _____   Date _____

11. Evaluation: _____

_____

_____

_____

_____

_____

_____

_____

_____

Source(s) of normative data: _____

_____

Student   Date

II. "LOW-FLOW" AND "HIGH-FLOW" READING PASSAGES

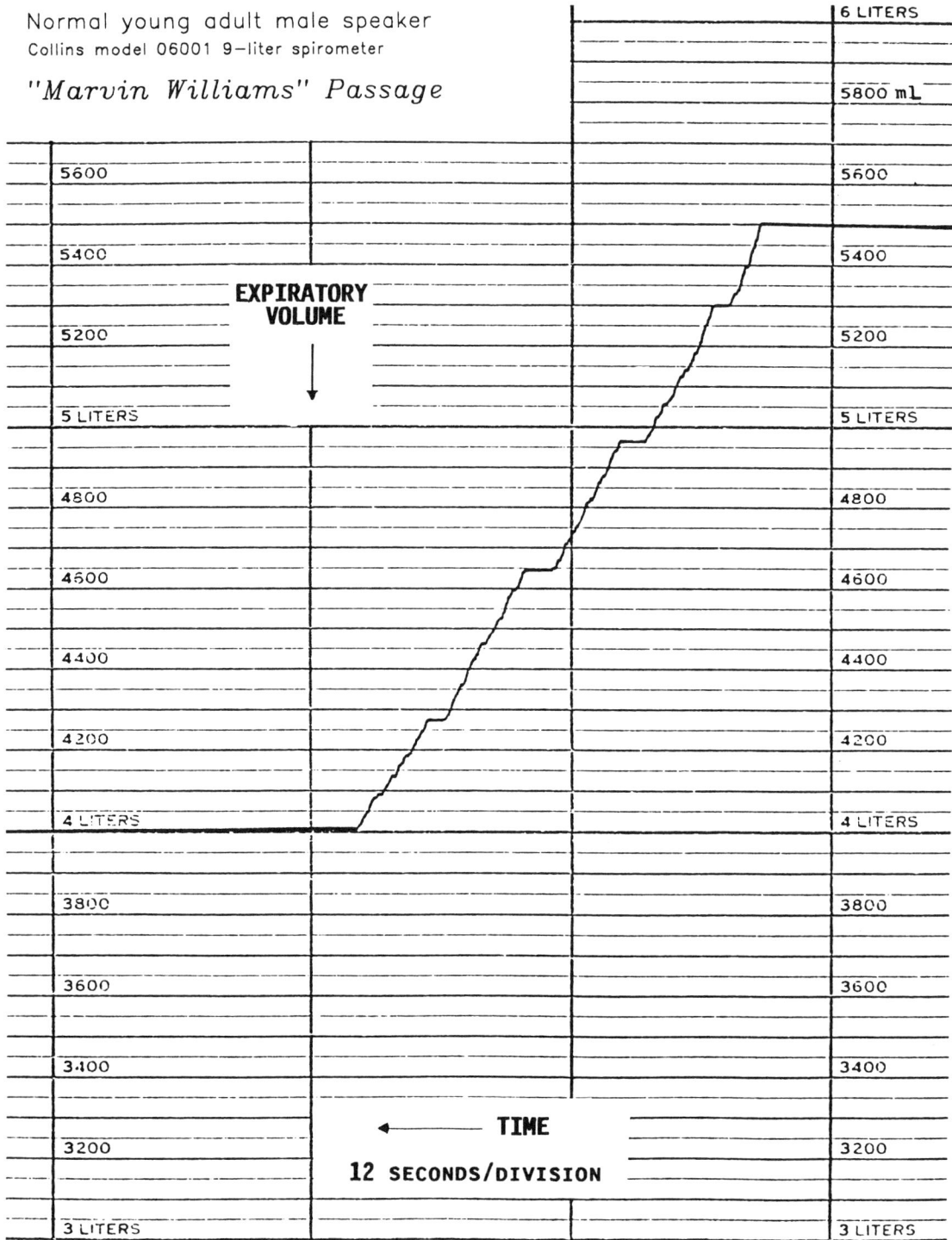

Student _____ Date _____

Low-Flow passage used: _____

Approximate baseline volume: _____ mL

Approximate end volume: _____ mL

Approximate speech volume: _____ mL

Complete the following table:

Expiration Number	Speech Volume (in mL)	Expiratory Duration (in seconds)
1	_____	_____
2	_____	_____
3	_____	_____
4	_____	_____
5	_____	_____
6	_____	_____
Sum	_____	_____

Estimated mean airflow rate: _____ mL/s

Evaluation: _____
_____
_____
_____
_____
_____

Student _____   Date _____

Normal young adult male speaker
Collins model 06001 9-liter spirometer

"Harrison Cook" Passage

EXPIRATORY VOLUME ↓

6 LITERS
5800 mL

← TIME
12 SECONDS/DIVISION

310 CLINICAL SPEECH AND VOICE MEASUREMENT

Student _____   Date _____

High-Flow passage used: _____

Approximate baseline volume: _____ mL

Approximate end volume: _____ mL

Approximate speech volume: _____ mL

Complete the following table:

Expiration Number	Speech Volume (in mL)	Expiratory Duration (in seconds)
1	_____	_____
2	_____	_____
3	_____	_____
4	_____	_____
5	_____	_____
6	_____	_____
Sum	_____	_____

Estimated mean airflow rate: _____ mL/s

Evaluation: _____

_____

_____

_____

_____

_____

NASALIZATION

UNIT 24

Clinical Application: Nasalance

Nasality (more properly *hypernasality*) is a speech symptom commonly associated with many structurally and neurologically based communication disorders. Perceived nasality is tied, in quite complex ways, to an inappropriate coupling of the nasal cavity to the vocal tract that disrupts normal speech resonance. This physical *nasalization* is associated with varied and variable spectral features that may, for instance, be assessed via spectrographic means (see Baken, 1987, pp. 393–401). To derive an acoustic index of perceived nasality, Fletcher (1970) developed an electronic system, *The Oral Nasal Acoustic Ratio* (TONAR). Kay Elemetrics presently markets an instrument, the Nasometer™, which uses the TONAR system.[1] This device uses two directional microphones mounted on either side of a sound-separating plate to transduce oral and nasal sound pressure signals individually. After each is identically bandpass filtered and conditioned, the ratio of these two signals (nasal sound pressure/oral sound pressure) is termed nasalance (see Baken, 1987, pp. 403–404). The nasalance measure appears to be moderately correlated with nasality; that is, as nasalance increases from 0 to 100%, perceived nasality tends to increase. There appears to be a better correlation when data are averaged over speech sounds using sets of sentences or short reading passages.

Purpose: In these exercises you will become familiar with the instrumentation and procedures required to measure nasalance.

Equipment: Computer-based Nasometer™ or other nasalance (TONAR) system with a printer.

---

[1] The Kay Elemetrics™, model 6200, uses dual nasal/oral filters centered at 500 Hz with a 300-Hz bandwidth, as does the TONAR II on which it is based.

General preparation: Review thoroughly the instruction manual for your nasalance system. Clean and calibrate the instrument according to the manufacturer's instructions. Carefully adjust the headpiece and microphones for your patient. Make sure that the headpiece is securely fitted and that the sound separation plate is perpendicular to the patient's face and rests securely between his nose and mouth.

I. VOCALIZATION

1. From a time history or bar display, record the mean nasalance for your patient as he comfortably sustains the consonant /m/.

    a. Is this value appropriate for a normal speaker?

    b. What condition(s) might result in an inappropriately low nasalance?

2. Record the mean nasalance for your patient sustaining the vowel /ɑ/ at a comfortable pitch and loudness.

    a. Is this value appropriate for a normal speaker?

    b. What condition(s) might result in an inappropriately high nasalance?

3. Below are bar displays of nasalance obtained while a normal adult male speaker comfortably sustained /m/ and /ɑ/.

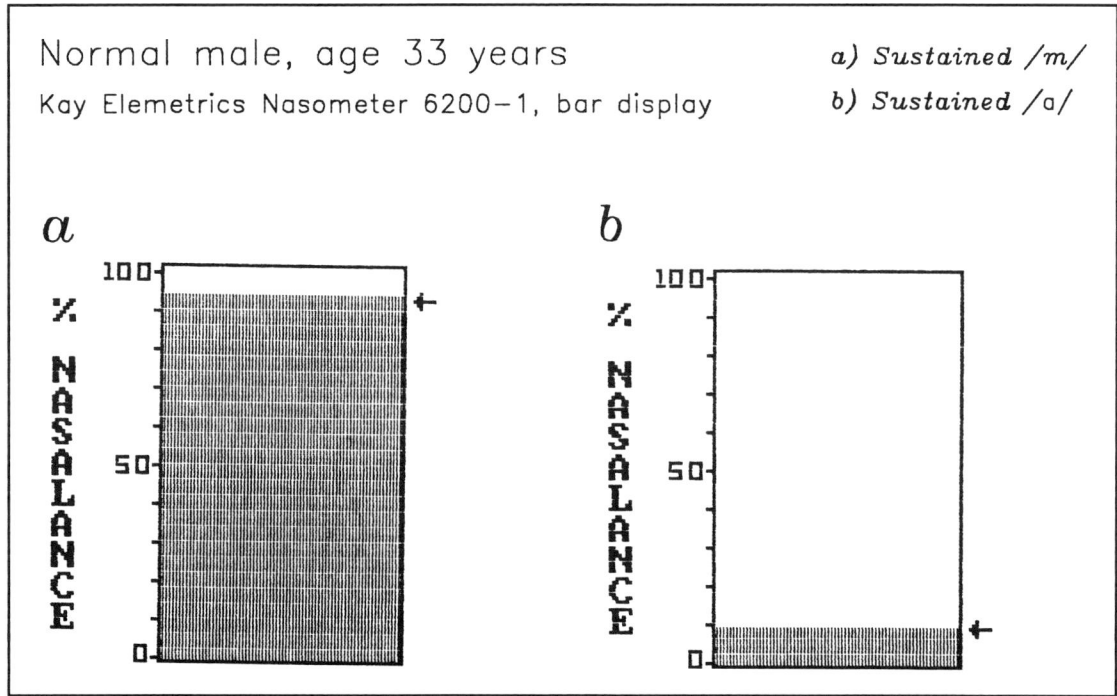

a. Record the mean nasalance for each production; and

b. Compare this speaker's performance to that of your patient.

4. From a bar or time history display, describe differences in mean nasalance you observe for the vowels /æ/, /i/, and /u/ sustained at a comfortable pitch and loudness. Why might mean nasalance differ by vowel type?

II. SPEECH

1. Have your patient repeat the syllable /mɑ/ at a moderate rate using his normal articulation and resonance. (You may also use the normal record provided on the hand-in sheet.)

   a. Mark the display, identifying and delineating the consonant and vowel productions.

   b. Record the mean and standard deviation of the nasalance for the entire production.

   c. Record the mean nasalance associated with the consonant and with the vowel. How do they compare to the nasalance of the isolated productions of each examined earlier?

2. Record a patient with a resonance disorder while he or she repeats the syllable /mɑ/ at a comfortable rate. (You may also use the record provided.) Assess the differences between the record of this patient and the speaker you tested previously. As before:

   a. Mark the display, identifying and delineating the consonant and vowel productions;

   b. Record the mean and standard deviation of the nasalance for the entire production; and

   c. Record the mean nasalance associated with the consonant and with the vowel. How do they compare with the nasalance values of the previous speaker? Be sure to describe the consistency (or variability) of each speaker's nasalance record.

3. Compare previous findings with those obtained from a normal speaker repeating the syllable /bɑ/ at a comfortable rate.

   a. Mark the display, identifying and delineating each consonant and vowel.

   b. Record the mean and standard deviation of the nasalance for the entire production.

c. Record the mean nasalance associated with the consonant and with the vowel. Explain why you might expect different vowel nasalance than you had observed during repetition of /mɑ/.

4. Record from one or more normal speakers the reported mean nasalance and standard deviation for the sentences:

a. "Mama made some lemon jam"; and

b. "Please put the five cupcakes back."

(Several examples are provided on the following pages.)

Normal speakers

a "Mama made some lemon jam"

1) Male, age 33 years

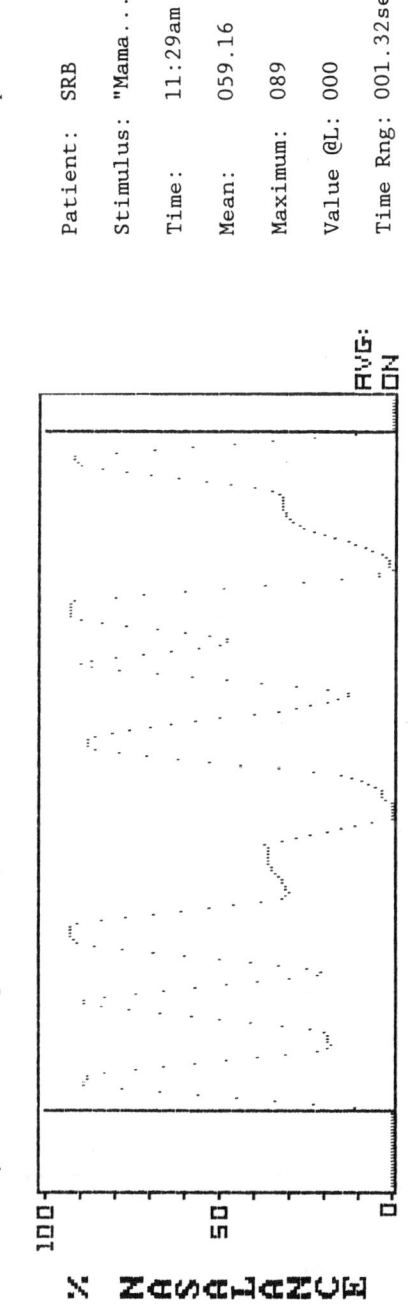

2) Male, age 5 years

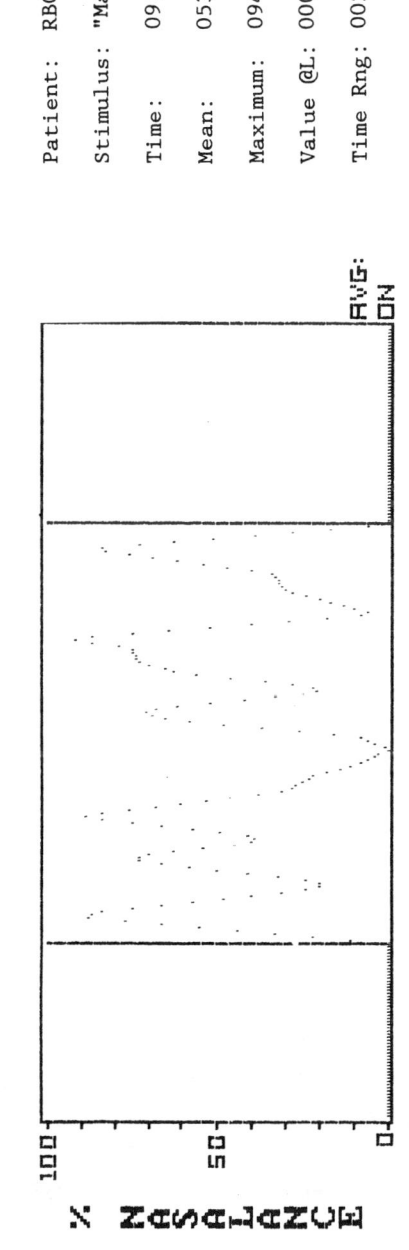

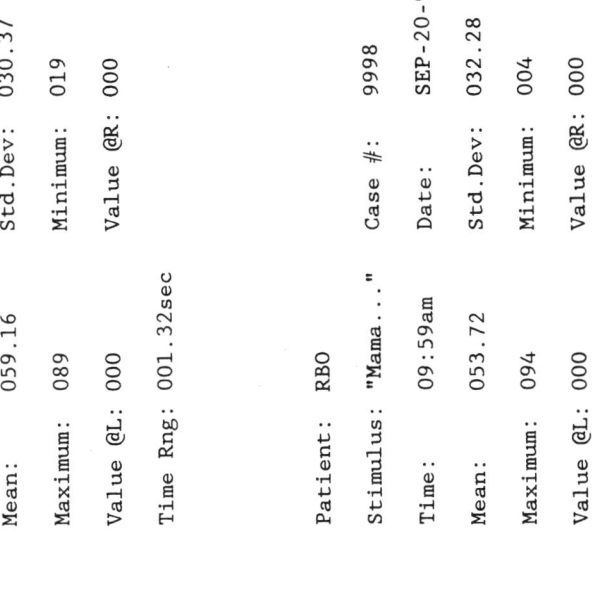

```
              Statistics
          Memphis State University

Patient:    SRB
Stimulus:   "Mama..."      Case #:      9999
Time:       11:29am        Date:        OCT-16-92
Mean:       059.16         Std.Dev:     030.37
Maximum:    089            Minimum:     019
Value @L:   000            Value @R:    000
Time Rng:   001.32sec


Patient:    RBO
Stimulus:   "Mama..."      Case #:      9998
Time:       09:59am        Date:        SEP-20-92
Mean:       053.72         Std.Dev:     032.28
Maximum:    094            Minimum:     004
Value @L:   000            Value @R:    000
Time Rng:   002.17sec
```

b "Please put the five cupcakes back"

1) Female, age 24 years

```
Patient:    CAF
Stimulus:   "Please..."   Case #:    9997
Time:       02:36pm       Date:      OCT-12-92
Mean:       006.82        Std.Dev:   004.72
Maximum:    020           Minimum:   001
Value @L:   000           Value @R:  000
Time Rng:   001.71sec
```

2) Male, age 5 years

```
Patient:    RBO
Stimulus:   "Please..."   Case #:    9998
Time:       10:02am       Date:      SEP-20-92
Mean:       006.20        Std.Dev:   004.64
Maximum:    026           Minimum:   002
Value @L:   000           Value @R:  000
Time Rng:   002.12sec
```

5. Using the same two sentences, repeat your nasalance observation with a patient presenting with a resonance disorder. (You may also use the records provided on page 322). Assess the differences between the patient's record and the normal individual you tested.

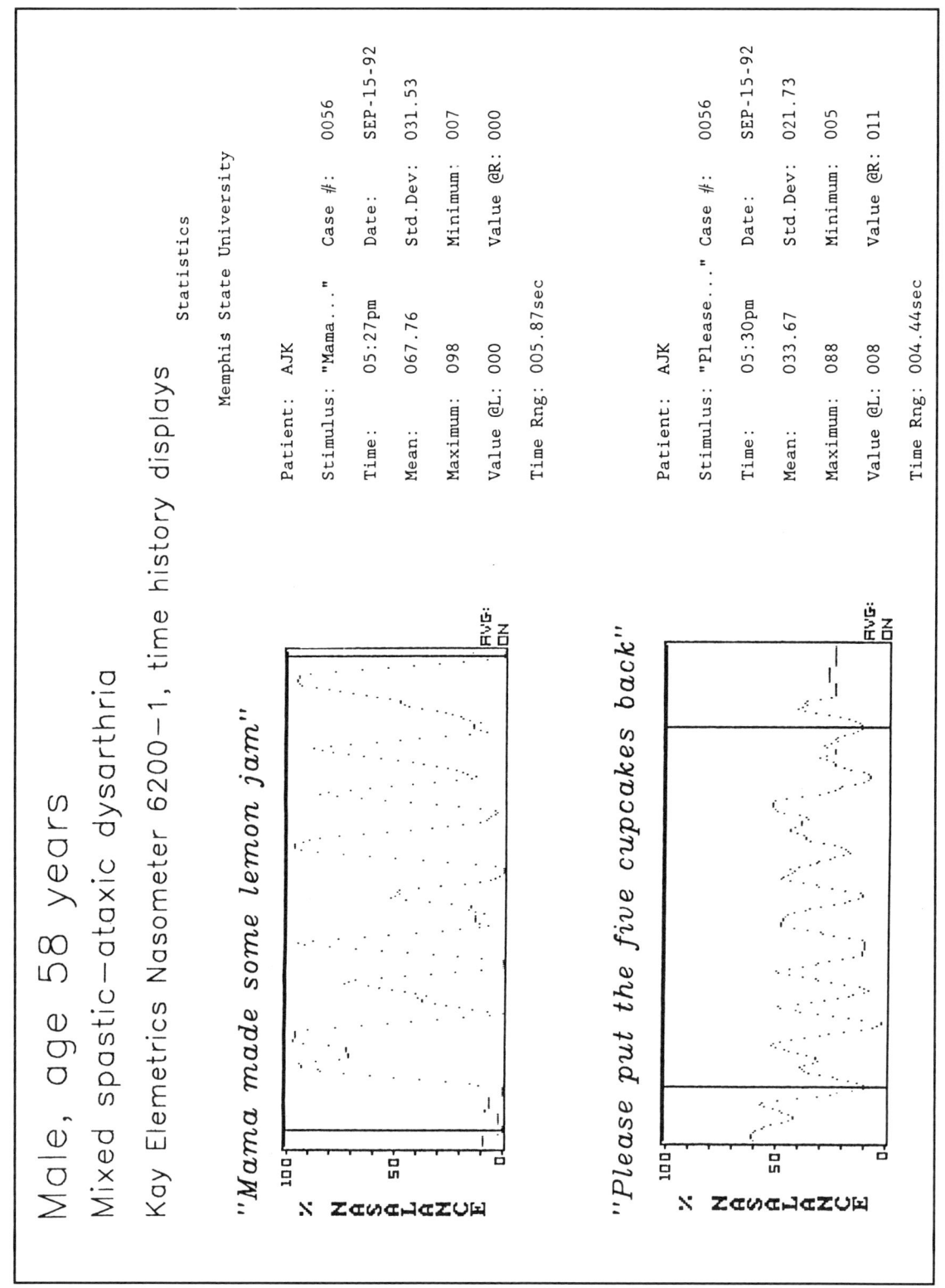

READ MORE ABOUT IT!

Baken, R. J. (1987). *Clinical measurement of speech and voice* (pp. 393–407). Boston: Little, Brown.

Clarke, W. M. (1975). The measurement of oral and nasal sound pressure levels of speech. *Journal of Phonetics, 3,* 257–262.

Clarke,, W. M. (1978). The relationship between subjective measures of nasality and measures of the oral and nasal sound pressure ratio. *Language and Speech, 21,* 69–75.

Colyar, T. C., & Christensen, J. M. (1980). Nasalance patterns in esophageal speech. *Journal of Communication Disorders, 13,* 43–48.

Dalston, R. M., & Warren, D. W. (1986). Comparison of Tonar II, pressure-flow, and listener judgments of hypernasality in the assessment of velopharyngeal function. *Cleft Palate Journal, 23,* 108–115.

Dalston, R. M., Warren, D. W., & Dalston, E. T. (1991). A preliminary investigation concerning the use of nasometry in identifying patients with hyponasality and/or nasal airway impairment. *Journal of Speech and Hearing Research, 34,* 11–18.

Fletcher, S. G. (1970). Theory and instrumentation for quantitative measurement of nasality. *Cleft Palate Journal, 7,* 601–609.

Fletcher, S. G. (1976). 'Nasalance' vs. listener judgements of nasality. *Cleft Palate Journal, 13,* 31–44.

Fletcher, S. G., & Daly, D. A. (1976). Nasalance in utterances of hearing-impaired speakers. *Journal of Communication Disorders, 9,* 63–73.

Horii, Y. (1983). An accelerometric measure as a physical correlate of perceived hypernasality in speech. *Journal of Speech and Hearing Research, 26,* 476–480.

Kuehn, D. P. (1982). Assessment of resonance disorders. In N. J. Lass, L. V. McReynolds, J. L. Northern, & D. E. Yoder (Eds.), *Speech, language, and hearing* (Vol. 2, pp. 499–525). Philadelphia: W. B. Saunders.

Netsell, R. (1969). Evaluation of velopharyngeal function in dysarthria. *Journal of Speech and Hearing Disorders, 34,* 113–122.

Seaver, E. J., Dalston, R. M., Leeper, H. A., & Adams, L. E. (1991). A study of nasometric values for normal nasal resonance. *Journal of Speech and Hearing Research, 34,* 715–721.

Shelton, R. L., Jr., Knox, A. W., Arndt, W. B., Jr., & Elbert, M. (1967). The relationship between nasality score values and oral and nasal sound pressure level. *Journal of Speech and Hearing Research, 10,* 549–557.

Warren, D. W. (1975). The determination of velopharyngeal incompetence by aerodynamic and acoustical techniques. *Clinics in Plastic Surgery, 2,* 299–304.

Student _____ Date _____

NASALANCE

I. VOCALIZATION

1. Nasalance for sustained /m/: _____ %

   a. Appropriate? _____

       Source(s): _____

   b. Low nasalance: _____

2. Nasalance for sustained /ɑ/: _____ %

   a. Appropriate? _____

       Source(s): _____

   b. High nasalance: _____

3. a. Nasalance for sustained /m/: _____ %

     Nasalance for sustained /ɑ/: _____ %

Student _____   Date _____

b. Comparison: _____
_____
_____

4. Nasalance and vowel type: _____
_____
_____

II. SPEECH

1. Use the display below or attach your record to this page.

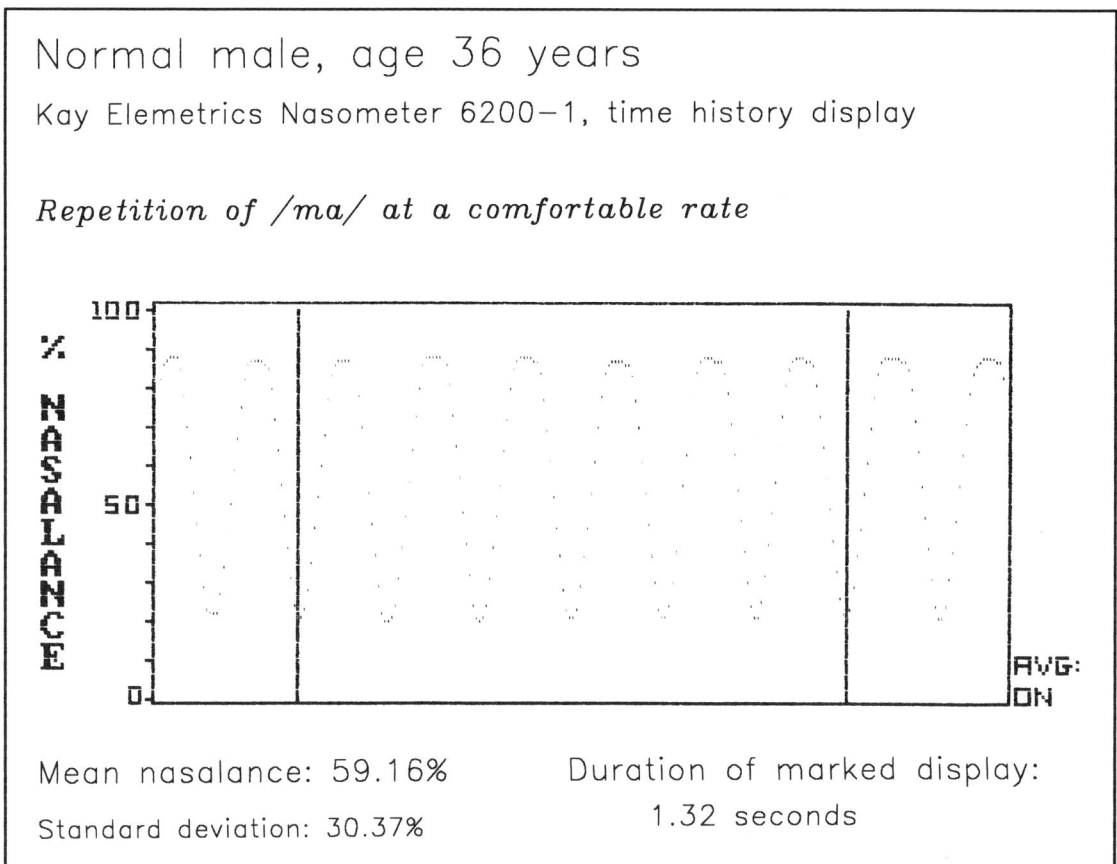

Student _____   Date _____

Patient: _____

b. Nasalance for /ma/ repetitions: _____ %

Mean nasalance: _____ %

Standard deviation: _____ %

c. Typical nasalance for /m/: _____ %

Typical nasalance for /ɑ/: _____ %

Comparison: _____

_____

_____

_____

2. Use the display below or attach your patient's record to this page.

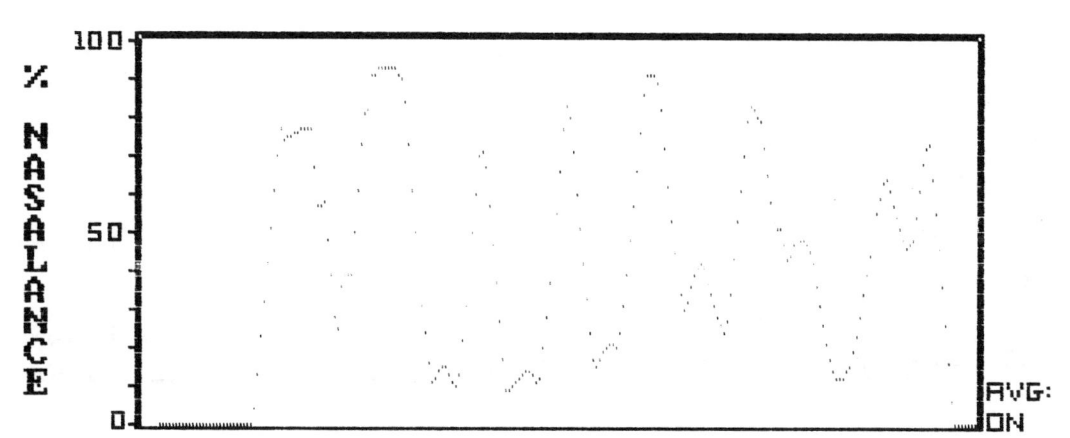

Male, age 58 years
Mixed spastic–ataxic dysarthria
Kay Elemetrics Nasometer 6200–1, time history display

Repetition of /ma/ at a comfortable rate

Mean nasalance: 51.27%   Duration of display: 6.12 seconds
Standard deviation: 32.08%

Student _____   Date _____

Patient: _____

b. Nasalance for /mɑ/ repetitions: _____ %

Mean nasalance: _____ %

Standard deviation: _____ %

c. Typical nasalance for /m/: _____ %

Typical nasalance for /ɑ/: _____ %

Comparison: _____

_____

_____

_____

3. Use the display below or attach your patient's record to this page.

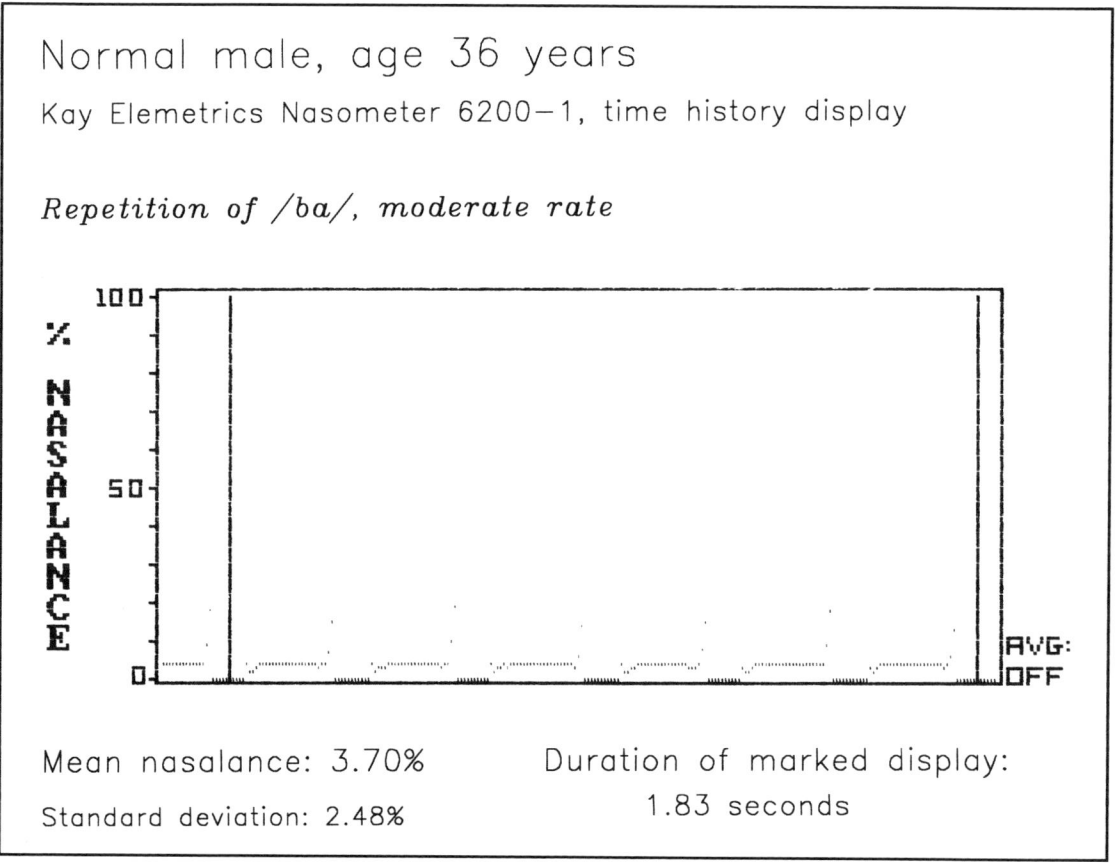

Student _____ Date _____

Patient: _____

b. Nasalance for /bɑ/ repetitions:

Mean nasalance: _____ %

Standard deviation: _____ %

c. Typical nasalance for /b/: _____ %

Typical nasalance for /ɑ/: _____ %

Vowel difference: _____

_____

_____

_____

_____

4. If you are using records other than those provided, attach them to this page and indicate speaker information below.

Patient: _____

"Mama made some lemon jam"

Mean nasalance: _____ %

Standard deviation: _____ %

Patient: _____

"Please put the five cupcakes back"

Mean nasalance: _____ %

Standard deviation: _____ %

Student _____   Date _____

5. Attach your records to this page and indicate your patient below.

   Patient: _____

   "Mama made some lemon jam"

       Mean nasalance: _____ %

       Standard deviation: _____ %

   Patient: _____

   "Please put the five cupcakes back"

       Mean nasalance: _____ %

       Standard deviation: _____ %

   Nasalance assessment: _____

   _____

   _____

   _____

   _____

   _____

   _____

   _____

   _____

   _____

   _____

UNIT 25

Clinical Application: Nasalization

Hypernasality and hyponasality are prevalent symptoms of many disorders of speech. Nasality, however, is a perceptual attribute that cannot be directly measured (although its degree can be scaled by listeners). Nasality generally has its roots in *nasalization,* which is the coupling of the nasal cavity to the lower pharynx. Nasalization can be observed and evaluated fairly easily using standard laboratory methods.

If the velopharyngeal port is open (or if there is some other open channel between the oral and nasal regions) a rise in pressure in the oropharynx will result in a flow of air through the nose. Therefore, observing the intraoral pressure and nasal flow provides information about the extent and, equally important, the timing, of nasalization.

Purpose: This exercise will provide you with practice in the simultaneous measurement of intraoral pressure and nasal airflow and will introduce you to the basic considerations needed to interpret the resulting data records.

Equipment: Instrumentation (including probe tube) for transducing and recording intraoral pressure and airflow. You will need some means of collecting only *nasal* airflow, such as a nose mask or nasal olives. You will also require a microphone and amplifier for capturing the speech signal.

General preparation: Review the basic principles of nasalization and of testing velopharyngeal function (Baken, 1987, pp. 393–396), paying particular attention to aerodynamic methods (Baken, 1987, pp. 407–421; Netsell, 1969). Also, review methods of measuring intraoral pressure (see Unit 17 "Intraoral Pressure During Consonant Production") and vocal tract airflow (see Unit 20 "Airflow During Speech Production").

I. SETTING UP AND CALIBRATING THE PRESSURE-FLOW SYSTEM

1. Normal speakers rarely generate intraoral pressures (P_{io}) greater than 15 cm H_2O. Choose a pressure transduction system that is suitable for this maximum, set it up, and calibrate it (see Unit 11 "Calibration" and Unit 17 "Intraoral Pressure During Consonant Production").

2. Airflow can be very high for short periods of time (such as at the release of a plosive), but generally flow is moderate. It is unlikely that nasal airflow will exceed 500 mL/s. Select a flow transducer suitable for this range, connect it to its support electronics, and calibrate it (see Unit 11 "Calibration" and Unit 20 "Airflow During Speech Production").

3. Shape an intraoral pressure probe for you patient and couple it to the pressure transducer (see Unit 17 "Intraoral Pressure During Consonant Production" for details).

4. You will need to measure only the air that is emitted via the nose. Therefore, you will need some means of capturing nasal airflow. Your instructor will provide you with a nose mask, nasal olives, or other apparatus for this. Couple it to the flow transducer.

5. Place the intraoral pressure probe in your patient's mouth and allow her to become accustomed to speaking as normally as possible with it in place. At the same time, you should practice your ability to clear the probe of saliva (using the syringe/stopcock system). Observe the data traces you obtain during this "warm up" period and, if they are either too small or too large, adjust the gain on the transducer system. [Remember: If you change the settings you will have to recalibrate! But you could do so after you have gathered your data.]

6. Remove the probe tube from your patient's mouth when you are satisfied that you will be able to get good pressure recordings.

7. Similarly, practice getting measurements of nasal airflow. It is vitally important that all of the air that leaves the nose goes through the flow transducer. Therefore, whatever means you are using to collect nasal air must fit tightly to the patient — with *no leaks*. Have your patient slowly repeat /imi/ as you observe the output of the flow measurement system. If the data trace is either too small or too large, adjust the gain of the transduction system. [NOTE: As with your pressure transduction system, if you change the settings, you will have to recalibrate your flow system — but, again, you could do so after you have gathered your data.]

8. Remove the nasal mask (or olives) from your patient's nose when you are satisfied that you will be able to get good flow data.

9. Place a microphone in front of your patient and have her say a few words at her customary loudness while you adjust the amplifier gain to a suitable level.

10. Sketch a block diagram of your instrumentation array on the hand-in sheet.

II. RECORDING ORAL PRESSURE AND NASAL FLOW

1. With all of the instrumentation (pressure, flow, and audio transducers) in place, have your patient repeat the sentence "I tied the bale" (which has no nasalized phonemes) at a moderate rate while you obtain recordings of her nasal flow, P_{io}, and speech signal. (A sample recording from a normal adult male speaker is provided on the hand-in sheet.)

2. Examine all three traces on your data record and mark it to show:

  a. The location of each phone; and

  b. The regions of nasal flow.

  Attach your data recording to the hand-in sheet.

3. Fill in the table on the hand-in sheet to show the approximate magnitude of nasal flow during each of the phones.

4. Is there a relationship between P_{io} and nasal flow? What can you conclude about the tightness of velopharyngeal closure in this patient?

5. Now obtain data while your patient repeats the sentence "I tend the mail" (which, of course, *does* have nasal phonemes). (Again, a sample recording from a normal adult male speaker is provided on the hand-in sheet.)

6. Mark the resulting record as you did the first one, showing each phone and regions of significant nasal airflow. Attach this record to the hand-in sheet.

7. Measure nasal flow and P_{io} during each phone of this production and enter the data on the hand-in sheet.

8. Look at the data for "I tend the mail." Is nasalization limited to the nasal phones [n] and [m]? What accounts for this "hypernasality" (even in this normal speaker)?

III. VELOPHARYNGEAL TIMING

Perceived nasality can result not only from an abnormal degree of velopharyngeal opening, but also from *inappropriately timed* nasal coupling. This is often clearly demonstrated in patients with problems of speech motor control.

The figure on the facing page is the record of P_{io}, nasal flow, and (integrated) sound pressure during the production of /tʌdʌ/ by a 6-year-old dyspraxic boy. He is perceptually hypernasal, and was referred by a surgeon for evaluation of his "incomplete velopharyngeal closure."

1. Examine this record carefully, paying particular attention to the relationship between P_{io} and nasal flow and the timing of velopharyngeal movements as they might be evidenced in the nasal flow trace. Write a brief description of this child's velopharyngeal function and draw any conclusions you feel are warranted on the basis of these data.

2. Obtain a similar record from a hypernasal patient presenting with a known dysarthria. Write a brief description of your patient's velopharyngeal function and draw any conclusions you feel are warranted on the basis of these data. Compare your patient's performance with that of the dyspraxic child above.

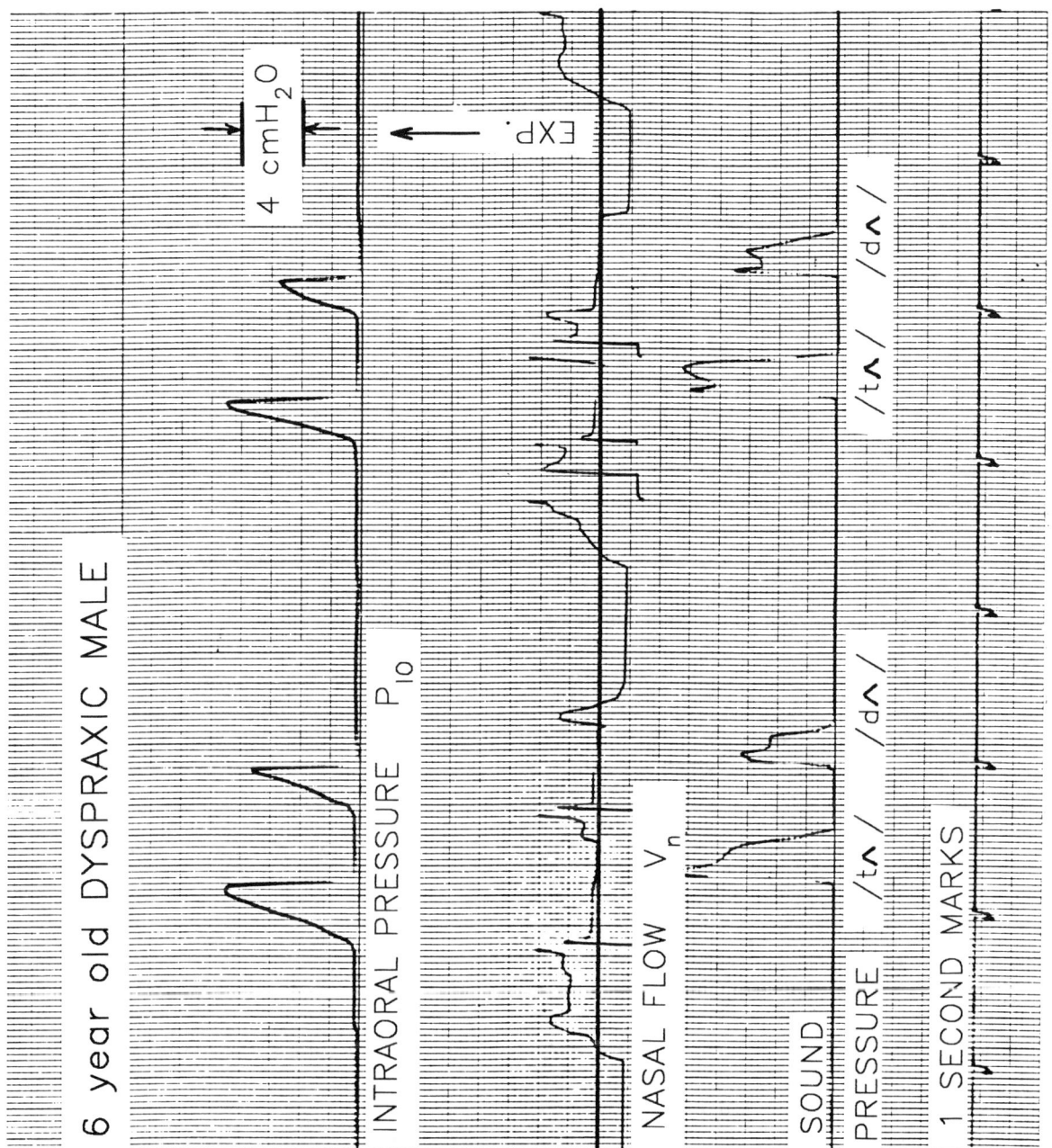

READ MORE ABOUT IT!

Andreassen, M. L., Smith, B. E., & Guyette, T. W. (1991). Pressure-flow measurements for selected oral and nasal sound segments produced by normal adults. *Cleft Palate-Craniofacial Journal, 28,* 398-407.

Baken, R. J. (1987). *Clinical measurement of speech and voice.* Boston: Little, Brown.

Chase, R. A. (1960). An objective evaluation of palatopharyngeal competence. *Plastic and Reconstructive Surgery, 26,* 23-29.

Dalston, R. M., & Warren, D. W. (1986). Comparison of Tonar II, pressure-flow, and listener judgments of hypernasality in the assessment of velopharyngeal function. *Cleft Palate Journal, 23,* 108-115.

Fletcher, S. G. (1970). Theory and instrumentation for quantitative measurement of nasality. *Cleft Palate Journal, 7,* 601-609.

Gilbert, H. R., & Ferrand, C. T. (1987). A respirometric technique to evaluate velopharyngeal function in speakers with cleft palate, with and without prostheses. *Journal of Speech and Hearing Research, 30,* 268-275.

Gilbert, H. R., & Hoodin, R. B. (1984). Effect of speaking rate on nasal airflows in hearing-impaired speakers. *Folia Phoniatrica, 36,* 183-189.

Hardy, J. C. (1961). Intraoral breath pressure in cerebral palsy. *Journal of Speech and Hearing Disorders, 26,* 309-319.

Hardy, J. C., Netsell, R., Schweiger, J. W., & Morris, H. L. (1969). Management of velopharyngeal function in cerebral palsy. *Journal of Speech and Hearing Disorders, 34,* 123-137.

Hattori, S., Yamamoto, K., & Fujimura, O. (1958). Nasalization of vowels in relation to nasals. *Journal of the Acoustical Society of America, 30,* 267-274.

Hoodin, R. B., & Gilbert, H. R. (1989). Parkinsonian dysarthria: An aerodynamic and perceptual description of velopharyngeal closure for speech. *Folia Phoniatrica, 41,* 249-258.

Hyde, S. R. (1968). Nose trumpet: Apparatus for separating the oral and nasal outputs in speech. *Nature, 219,* 763-765.

Kuehn, D. P. (1982). Assessment of resonance disorders. In N. J. Lass, L. V. McReynolds, J. L. Northern, & D. E. Yoder (Eds.), *Speech, language, and hearing* (Vol. 2, pp. 499-525). Philadelphia: W. B. Saunders.

Laine, T., Warren, D. W., Dalston, R. M., Hairfield, W. M., & Morr, K. E. (1988). Intraoral pressure, nasal pressure, and airflow rate in cleft palate speech. *Journal of Speech and Hearing Research, 31,* 432-437.

Lubker, J. F. (1970). Aerodynamic and ultrasonic assessment techniques in speech-dentofacial research. *ASHA Reports, 5,* 207-223.

Lubker, J. F., Schweiger, J. W., & Morris, H. L. (1970). Nasal airflow characteristics during speech in prosthetically managed cleft palate speakers. *Journal of Speech and Hearing Research, 13,* 326-338.

Moll, K. L. (1964). 'Objective' measures of nasality. *Cleft Palate Journal, 1,* 371-374.

Morr, K. E., Warren, D. W., Dalston, R. M., Smith, L. R., Seaton, D., & Hairfield, W. M. (1988). Intraoral speech pressures after experimental loss of velar resistance. *Folia Phoniatrica, 40,* 284-289.

Netsell, R. (1969). Evaluation of velopharyngeal function in dysarthria. *Journal of Speech and Hearing Disorders, 34,* 113-122.

Netsell, R., & Daniel, B. (1979). Dysarthria in adults: Physiologic approach to rehabilitation. *Archives of Physical Medicine and Rehabilitation, 60,* 502-508.

Peterson-Falzone, S. J., & Graham, M. S. (1990). Phoneme-specific nasal emission in children with and without physical anomalies of the velopharyngeal mechanism. *Journal of Speech and Hearing Disorders, 55,* 132-139.

Ruscello, D. M., Shuster, L. I., & Sandwisch, A. (1991). Modification of context-specific nasal emission. *Journal of Speech and Hearing Research, 34,* 27-32.

Shelton, R. L., Jr., & Blank, J. L. (1984). Oronasal fistulas, intraoral air pressure, and nasal air flow during speech. *Cleft Palate Journal, 21,* 91-99.

Thompson, A. E., & Hixon, T. J. (1979). Nasal air flow during normal speech production. *Cleft Palate Journal, 16,* 412-420.

Warren, D. W. (1964). Velopharyngeal orifice size and upper pharyngeal pressure-flow patterns in normal speech. *Plastic and Reconstructive Surgery, 33,* 148-162.

Warren, D. W. (1964). Velopharyngeal orifice size and upper pharyngeal pressure-flow patterns in cleft palate speech: A preliminary study. *Plastic and Reconstructive Surgery, 34,* 15-26.

Warren, D. W. (1967). Nasal emission of air and velopharyngeal function. *Cleft Palate Journal, 4,* 148-156.

Warren, D. W. (1975). The determination of

velopharyngeal incompetence by aerodynamic and acoustical techniques. *Clinics in Plastic Surgery, 2,* 299–304.

Warren, D. W., & DuBois, A. B. (1964). A pressure-flow technique for measuring velopharyngeal orifice area during continuous speech. *Cleft Palate Journal, 1,* 52–71.

Warren, D. W., Duany, L. F., & Fischer, N. D. (1969). Nasal pathway resistance in normal and cleft lip and palate subjects. *Cleft Palate Journal, 6,* 134–140.

Warren, D. W., Hinton, V. A., Pillsbury, H. C., & Hairfield, W. M. (1987). Effects of size of the nasal airway on nasal airflow rate. *Archives of Otolaryngology, 113,* 405–408.

Student _____ Date _____

NASALIZATION

I. SETTING UP AND CALIBRATING THE PRESSURE-FLOW SYSTEM

Block Diagram of Your Instrumentation Array

Maximum pressure: _____ cm H$_2$O

Chart calibration: _____ cm vertical height per cm H$_2$O

Maximum airflow: _____ L/s

Chart calibration: _____ cm vertical height per L/s

(Attach your calibration records to this page.)

Student _____ Date _____

II. RECORDING ORAL PRESSURE AND NASAL FLOW

Attach your patient's labeled data record to this page.

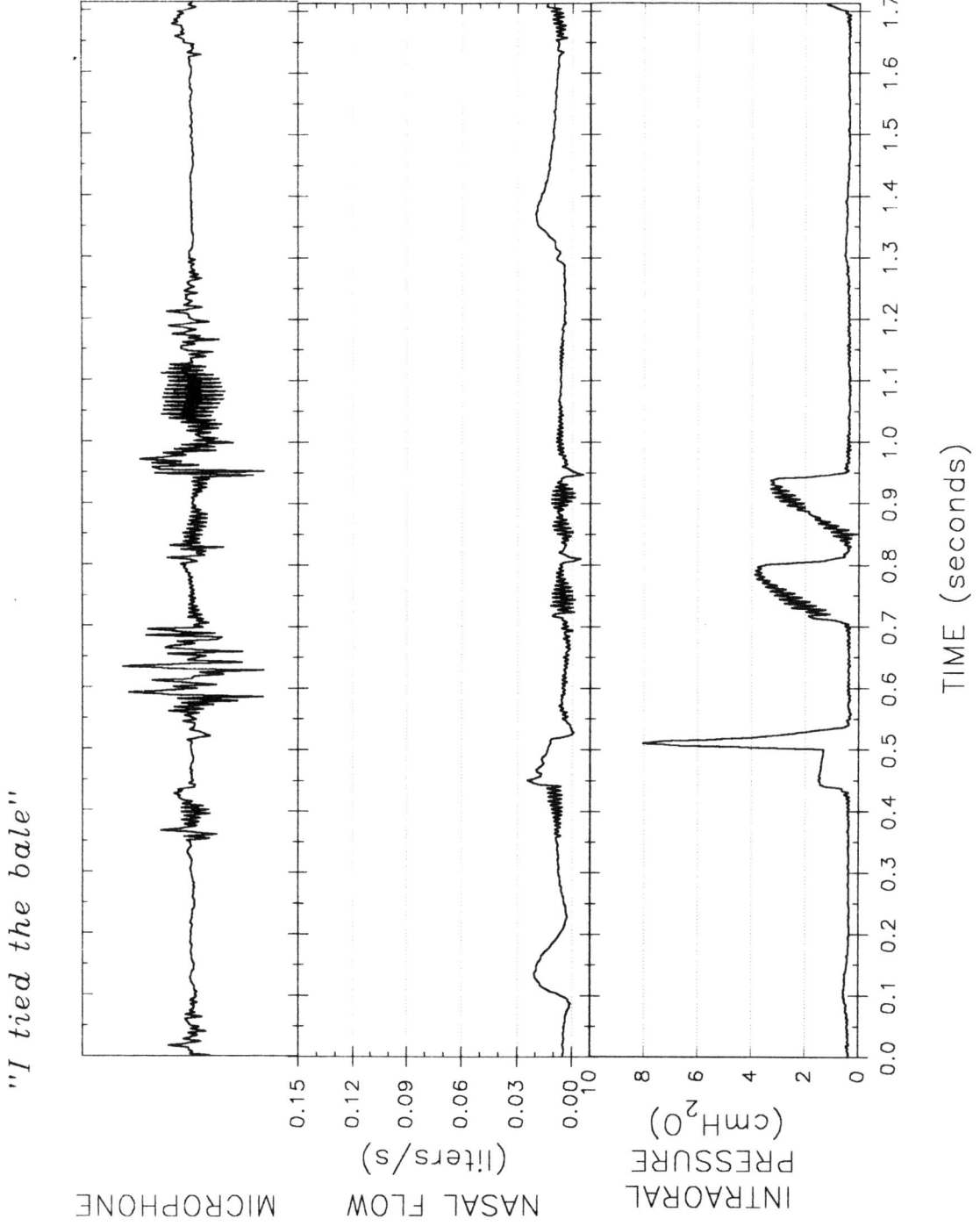

Student   Date

3. Complete the following table based on your patient's aerodynamic data for the phrase: "I tied the bale"

Phone	Intraoral Pressure (cm H$_2$O)	Nasal Airflow (L/s)
[aɪ]	_____	_____
[t]	_____	_____
[aɪ]	_____	_____
[dð]	_____	_____
[ə]	_____	_____
[b]	_____	_____
[eɪ]	_____	_____
[l]	_____	_____

4. Relationship between P$_{io}$ and nasal flow: _____

_____

_____

_____

_____

Velopharyngeal closure (in a normal speaker): _____

_____

_____

_____

_____

Student   Date

Attach your patient's labeled data record to this page.

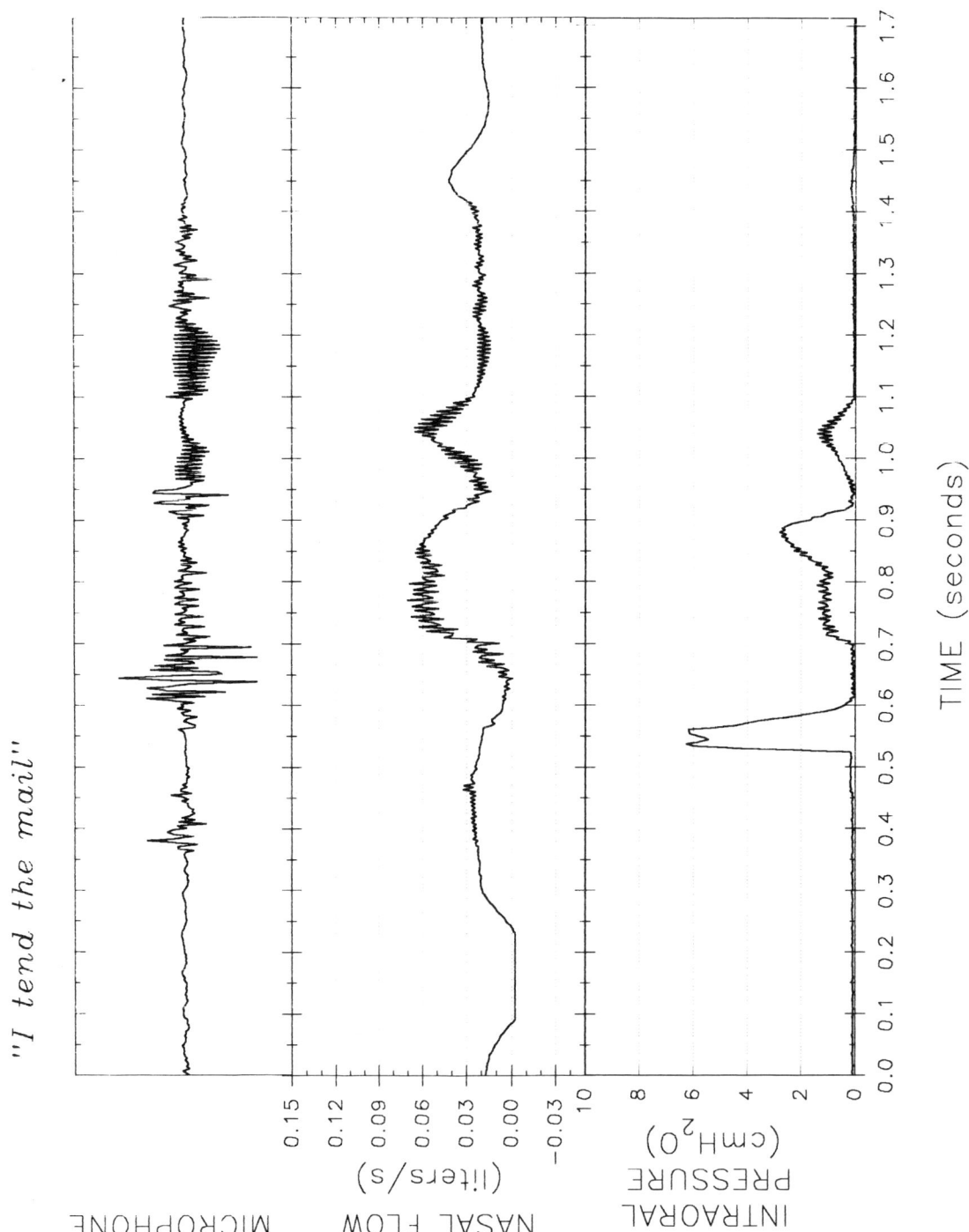

Student _____   Date _____

7. Complete the following table based on your patient's aerodynamic data for the phrase: "I tend the mail"

Phone	Intraoral Pressure (cm H$_2$O)	Nasal Airflow (L/s)
[aɪ]	_____	_____
[t]	_____	_____
[ɛ]	_____	_____
[n]	_____	_____
[dð]	_____	_____
[ə]	_____	_____
[m]	_____	_____
[eɪ]	_____	_____
[l]	_____	_____

8. Nasalization during "I tend the mail": _____

_____

_____

_____

_____

Increased nasalization: _____

_____

_____

_____

_____

_____

Student _____ Date _____

III. VELOPHARYNGEAL TIMING

1. Patient: _6-year-old dyspraxic male_

Assessment: _____

Student _____ Date _____

6. Patient: _____

Assessment: _____

_____
_____
_____
_____
_____
_____
_____
_____
_____
_____
_____
_____
_____
_____
_____
_____
_____
_____
_____
_____

(Attach you patient's labeled data recording to this page.)

ELECTROGLOTTOGRAPHY

UNIT 26

Basic Skills: Electroglottography

Electroglottography demonstrates vocal fold contact area. It is a useful technique in drawing inferences about certain aspects of vocal fold vibration and therefore is very helpful in assessing laryngeal function.

Purpose: In this laboratory exercise you will learn to set up the electroglottograph (EGG), to position the electrodes correctly, and to do some elementary interpretation of the EGG record.

Equipment: An electroglottograph and a means of generating a printed output (such as an oscilloscope and camera, computer system, oscillograph).

General preparation: Review the general principles underlying electroglottography and the interpretation of the electroglottographic waveform (Baken, 1987, pp. 216–227; Baken, 1992; Childers & Krishnamurthy, 1985; Titze, 1990). If necessary, review the physiology of vocal fold vibration. Read the instruction manual for your EGG instrument and answer the following questions:

1. Is the EGG powered by batteries or is it powered from the electrical mains?

2. If battery-powered, how can you tell if the batteries need to be charged?

3. Do you need to use electrode paste (conductive cream) on the electrodes?

4. Does the manufacturer recommend any special procedures or precautions that you should take?

I. EGG SETUP AND ELECTRODE PLACEMENT

The electroglottograph senses changes in the electrical resistance of the neck in the region of the larynx. Changes associated with vibration of the vocal folds are fast (they have the same frequency as the vocal F_0), but there are other, much slower changes caused by neck movement, arterial pulses, breathing, and the like. In the most common manner of using the EGG, these slow (low-frequency) changes are removed from the output, leaving a "high-pass filtered" signal often referred to as "Lx." It is this output with which we will be concerned.

1. Connect the electrodes to the EGG and connect the EGG output to the recording device. (If your EGG unit has more than one output, choose the one labeled "glottal vibrations," "Lx," or "filtered.") On the hand-in sheet, draw a block diagram of your instrumentation setup. Make sure that you label each block clearly, including the model numbers where appropriate.

2. If your instrument requires it, apply paste to the electrodes before turning the instrument on; rub the electrodes together to distribute the paste evenly over their surfaces.

3. Turn on the EGG and the output device. Allow both a few minutes to stabilize.

4. Seat your patient in the examination chair. If the chair has a headrest, use it to comfortably stabilize the patient's head in an upright position. Using gentle palpation, locate the following landmarks on your patient's neck: the hyoid bone, thyroid notch, cricothyroid space, and thyroid alae (see Unit 3 "Physical Examination").

5. Apply the electrodes on either side of your patient's neck, directly over the thyroid alae. Strap the electrodes in place so firmly that they will not slip, but not so tightly that your patient is uncomfortable.

6. If your EGG unit requires that the system be balanced, rotate the balance control until the meter indicator is centered. (You may have to change the coarse balance setting — see your EGG instruction manual for details.)

7. Have your patient sustain the vowel /i/ at a comfortable pitch and loudness while you adjust the sensitivity (gain) of the instrument until the signal is about 2/3 as large as the largest signal that your display device can show.

8. Now obtain a recording of another production of /i/ sustained at a comfortable pitch and loudness. Label this record with the date, the patient's initials, and the electrode position ("thyroid alae") and save it. [NOTE: Do not readjust any settings on the electroglottograph for the rest of this exercise!]

9. Relocate the electrodes so that they are positioned just below the hyoid bone and the same distance apart as they were in step #5 above. (You should re-

move any electrode paste from your patient's neck and, if necessary, apply more paste to the electrodes before reattaching them.) Rebalance the EGG if necessary, but do NOT change the sensitivity or gain control.

10. Now obtain another recording of your patient's comfortable /i/. Label it with the date, the patient's initials, and location ("subhyoid") and save it.

11. Finally, reposition the electrodes at the level of the cricoid cartilage, with the same separation as in step #5. As before, you may need to rebalance the EGG, but be certain not to adjust the EGG gain control. Label this new recording with the date, the patient's initials, and the electrode location ("cricoid") and save it.

12. Examine the three recordings you have made. How do the recordings differ with respect to signal size and/or to signal noisiness? What conclusions can you draw?

13. Write a summary of your conclusions about the effect(s) of electrode placement. Include your three recordings with your lab report. (Sample electroglottograms are provided on the hand-in sheet.)

II. THE Lx WAVE

1. Apply the electrodes on either side of your patient's neck, directly over the thyroid alae. Strap the electrodes in place so firmly that they will not slip, but not so tightly that your patient is uncomfortable.

2. Instruct your patient to produce several comfortable vowel prolongations while you adjust the sensitivity and "time base" of your recording system. Set your recording system to clearly display the details of the EGG waveshape. (On an oscillograph, for instance, choose a fast paper speed.) Be sure that your data printout has a time calibration; your instructor will help you set this up if necessary. Once you have completed the setup and verified its adequacy, do not change any settings for the rest of this exercise.

3. Prepare EGG records (Lx electroglottograms) of /ɑ/ sustained at:

    a. A comfortable pitch and loudness;

    b. A somewhat lower pitch at the same loudness;

    c. A somewhat higher pitch at the same loudness;

    d. A comfortable pitch at a softer than comfortable loudness; and at

    e. A comfortable pitch at a greater than comfortable loudness.

    (Sample records are provided on the hand-in sheet.)

4. Examine the Lx record of the vowel sustained at a comfortable pitch and loudness. Mark it to show what is happening during each phase of the Lx wave. [NOTE: Be cautious in using terms: Can we really speak of "glottal opening" or "closing"? Why not?]

5. Determine the fundamental frequency (F_0) of each of the productions and mark it on the data record (see Unit 10 "Reading Oscillograms" or Unit 12 "Vocal Fundamental Frequency").

6. Compare the records for higher and lower pitch and for louder and softer phonations. What conclusions can you draw about the Lx wave as phonatory conditions change? Can you explain the changes you see in terms of what we know about how the vocal folds are adjusted for frequency and intensity?

III. Lx AND VOCAL REGISTERS

Vocal physiologists generally recognize three vocal registers: modal, falsetto (or loft), and pulse (Hollien, 1974).

1. Obtain a good recording of /ɑ/ sustained in modal register. Adjust your equipment sensitivity for a signal that is about 2/3 of the largest your system can display. Do not change any settings after this recording.

2. Now obtain a recording of the same vowel sustained in pulse register (glottal fry).

3. Finally, record /ɑ/ produced in falsetto register. (Sample Lx records at each register are supplied on the hand-in sheet.)

4. Mark your data records to indicate the mean F_0 of each sample.

5. What are the salient Lx characteristics that identify each register?

IV. Lx AND VOCAL DISORDER

1. Obtain an EGG Lx recording of a sustained vowel by a patient with known vocal pathology. (Again, a sample data record is provided on the hand-in sheet.)

2. Mark your data record to show the F_0 of the sample, and indicate any peculiarities of the Lx wave.

3. What inferences concerning this patient's vocal fold behavior can you draw?

READ MORE ABOUT IT!

Baken, R. J. (1987). *Clinical measurement of speech and voice.* Boston: Little, Brown.

Baken, R. J. (1992). Electroglottography. *Journal of Voice, 6,* 98–110.

Borden, G. J., Baer, T., & Kenney, M. K. (1985). Onset of voicing in stuttered and fluent utterances. *Journal of Speech and Hearing Research, 28,* 363–372.

Childers, D. G., Alsaka, Y. A., Hicks, D. M., & Moore, G. P. (1987). Vocal fold vibrations: An EGG model. In T.Baer, C. Sasaki, & K. S. Harris (Eds.), *Laryngeal function in phonation and respiration* (pp. 181–202). Boston: Little, Brown.

Childers, D. G., & Krishnamurthy, A. K. (1985). A critical review of electroglottography. *CRC Critical Reviews in Biomedical Engineering, 12,* 131–161.

Colton, R. H., & Conture, E. G. (1990). Problems and pitfalls of electroglottography. *Journal of Voice, 4,* 10–24.

Fourcin, A. J. (1981). Laryngographic assessment of phonatory function. *ASHA Reports, 11,* 116–127.

Fourcin, A. J. (1982). Electrolaryngographic assessment of vocal fold function. *Journal of Phonetics, 14,* 435–442.

Hollien, H. (1974). On vocal registers. *Journal of Phonetics, 2,* 125–143.

Kitzing, P. (1982). Photo- and electroglottographic recording of the laryngeal vibratory pattern during different registers. *Folia Phoniatrica, 34,* 234–241.

Motta, G., Cesari, U., Iengo, M., & Motta, G., Jr. (1990). Clinical application of electroglottography. *Folia Phoniatrica, 42,* 111–117.

Orlikoff, R. F. (1991). Assessment of the dynamics of vocal fold contract from the electroglottogram: Data from normal male subjects. *Journal of Speech and Hearing Research, 34,* 1066–1072.

Painter, C. (1988). Electroglottogram waveform types. *Archives of Oto-Rhino-Laryngology, 245,* 116–121.

Reinsch, M., & Gobsch, H. (1972). Zur quantitativen Auswertung elektroglottographischer Kurven bei Normal personen [On the quantitative evaluation of electroglottographic curves from normal people]. *Folia Phoniatrica, 24,* 1–6.

Rothenberg, M., & Mahshie, J. J. (1988). Monitoring vocal fold abduction through vocal fold contact area. *Journal of Speech and Hearing Research, 31,* 338–351.

Titze, I. R. (1990). Interpretation of the electroglottographic signal. *Journal of Voice, 4,* 1–9.

Unger, E., Unger, H., & Tietze, G. (1981). Stimmuntersuchungen mittels der elektroglottographischen Einzelkurven [Voice studies by means of electroglottographic curves]. *Folia Phoniatrica, 33,* 168–180.

Watson, B. C., & Alfonso, P. J. (1991). Noninvasive instrumentation in the treatment of stuttering. In D. Vogel & M. P. Cannito (Eds.), *Treating disordered speech motor control* (pp. 319–340). Austin, TX: PRO-ED.

Watson, B. C., & Dembowski, J. (1991). Instrumentation in the evaluation and modification of speech motor control during stuttering therapy. In H. F. M. Peters, W. Hulstijn, & C. W. Starkweather (Eds.), *Speech motor control and stuttering* (pp. 503–511). Amsterdam: Elsevier.

Student _____   Date _____

ELECTROGLOTTOGRAPHY

Block Diagram of Your Instrumentation Array

1. _____
2. _____
3. _____
4. _____

Student   Date

I. EGG SET UP AND ELECTRODE PLACEMENT

(Attach your labeled data recordings to this page.)

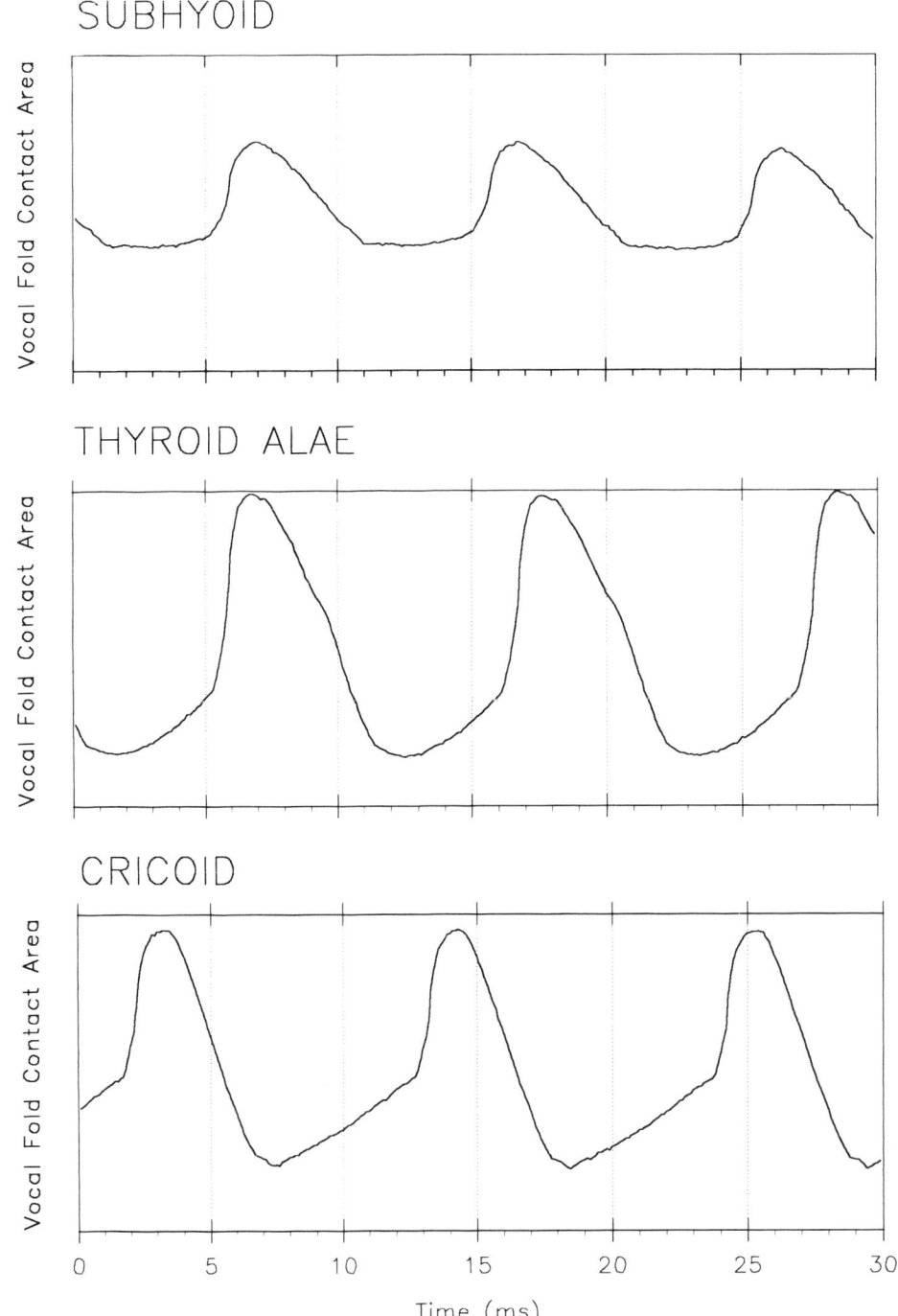

Normal 40-year-old male, sustained /a/

Student _____ Date _____

12. Effect(s) of electrode placement: _____

_____

_____

_____

_____

_____

_____

13. Conclusions: _____

_____

_____

_____

_____

_____

_____

_____

_____

Student _____   Date _____

II. THE Lx WAVE

(Attach your labeled data recordings to this page.)

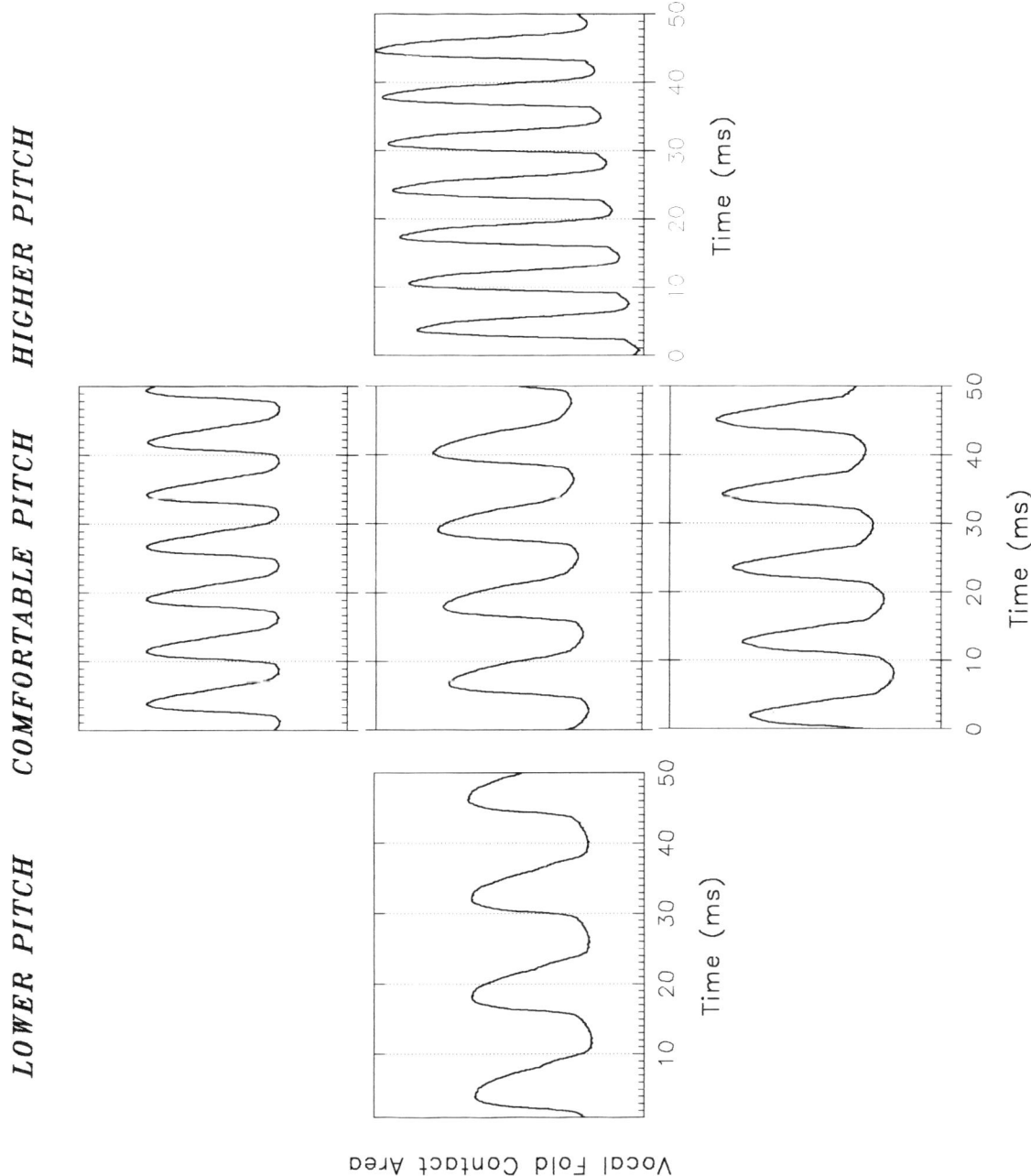

Student _____   Date _____

4. Why are the terms "opening," "closing," and the like not technically appropriate?

_____

_____

_____

_____

_____

6. How does the Lx record change with changes in vocal F_0 and intensity?

_____

_____

_____

_____

_____

_____

_____

_____

_____

Student   Date

III. Lx AND VOCAL REGISTERS

(Attach your labeled data recordings to this page.)

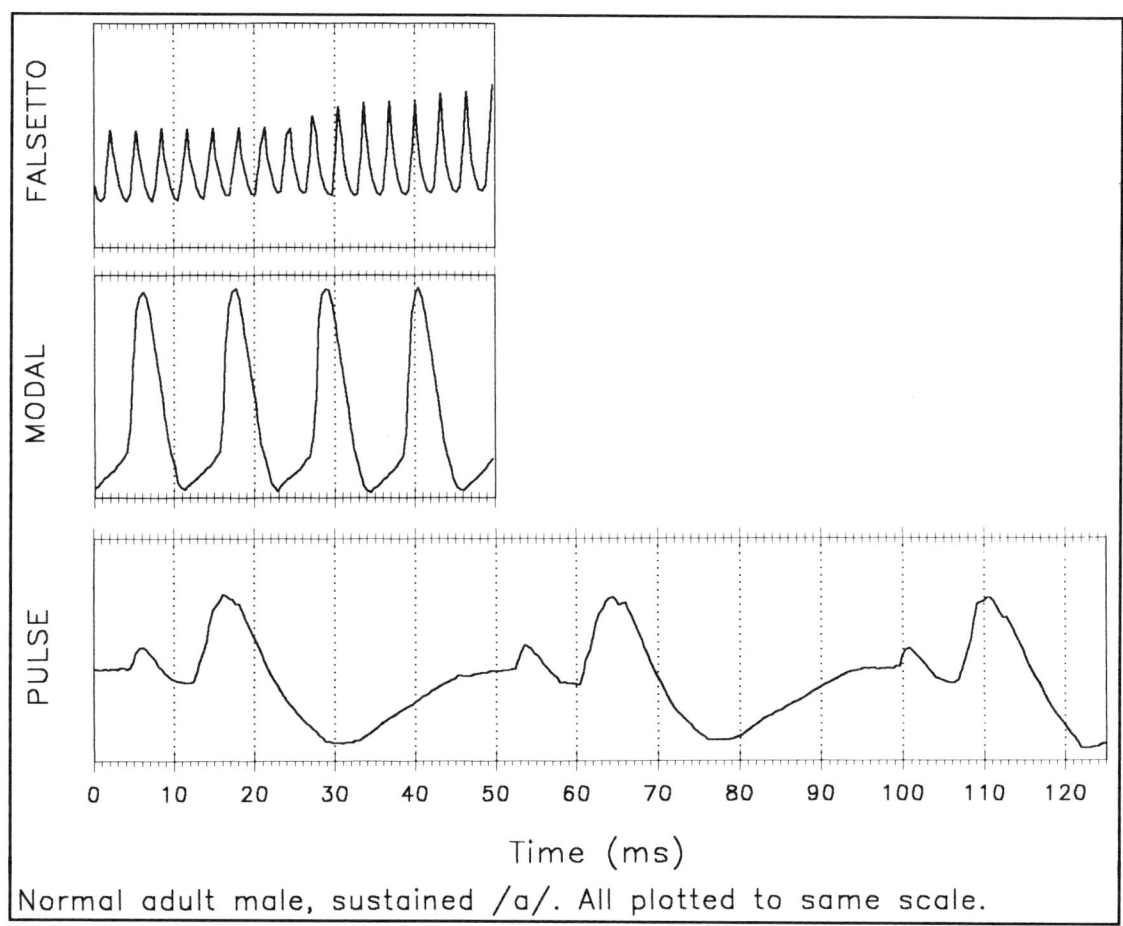
Normal adult male, sustained /a/. All plotted to same scale.

Student _____   Date _____

6. How does the Lx record change with changes in vocal register? _____

Student   Date

V. Lx AND VOCAL DISORDER

(Attach your labeled data recording to this page.)

1. Patient: _____

Medical diagnosis: _____

Lx record, sustained /a/, comfortable pitch and loudness

Female, age 21, vocal nodes of 3 years duration.

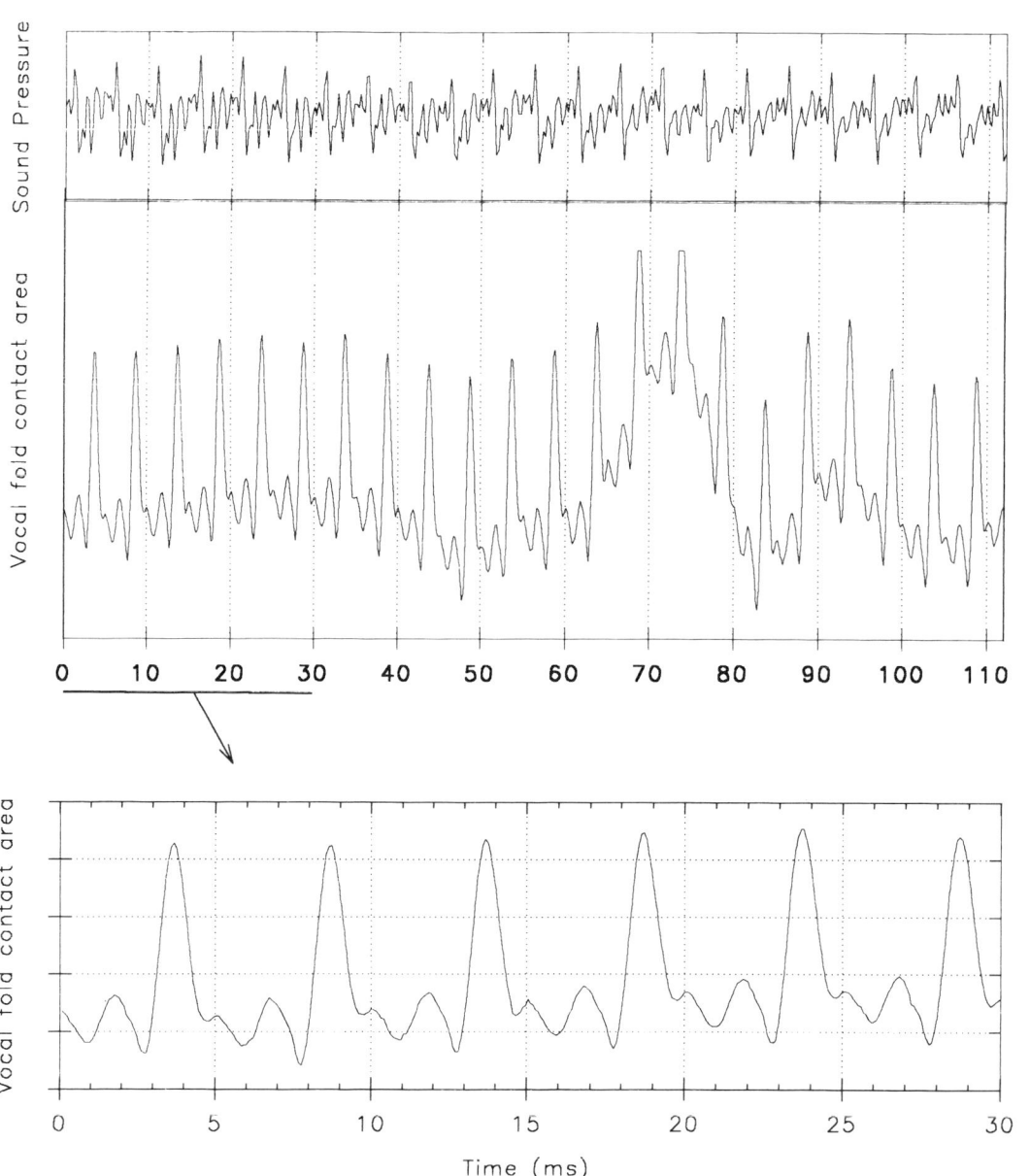

Student   Date

3. Inferences concerning your patient's vocal fold behavior:

SOUND SPECTROGRAPHY

UNIT 27

Basic Skills: Sound Spectrography I — Getting Acquainted

The *sound spectrograph* is the instrument of choice for analyzing the acoustic components of the speech signal, their interrelationships, and the way in which they change over time. With careful and conservative application of basic principles of acoustics and speech physiology, the *sound spectrogram,* the printed spectrographic output, can provide important insights into the processes underlying speech production. Sound spectrography is, therefore, one of the most important analytic techniques available to the speech-language pathologist.

A number of factors — not the least of which is the enormous complexity of the speech signal — conspire to make sound spectrography a more complicated undertaking than many other evaluative procedures. Good sound spectrograms require that the examiner make several important decisions about how a given analysis is to be performed and about how the results are to be displayed. Inappropriate decisions will result in spectrograms that are at best marginally useful and at worst misleading. So, before anything else, it is important that the examiner understand the basis for the several decisions that must be made and the consequences of those decisions in terms of the display that is achieved.

Previously, sound spectrography was almost always conducted with electromechanical instruments that subjected a recording on a magnetic surface to repeated analysis by an ever-changing electronic filter network. (Most commonly the instrument was a Kay Elemetrics "Sonagraph," many continuing in active and reliable service.) But such devices have been superseded by faster and much more versatile computer-based digital instruments.

Purpose: These exercises will be your first introduction to the techniques of digital sound spectrography. You will learn about choosing sampling rates and selecting filter bandwidths appropriate for the types of evaluations you might wish to perform.

Equipment: A computer-based digital sound spectrograph, microphone and speaker system. (The specific techniques in our exercise are intended for the Kay Elemetrics Computerized Speech Lab [CSL™]. Your instructor will provide you with alternative instructions if you have different instrumentation.)

General preparation: More than most other analytic methods, interpretation of sound spectrograms depends on a thorough understanding of basic science. Therefore, it is very important that you review the general principles of speech acoustics and the bases of speech sound spectrography. Recommended review materials include Kent and Read (1992, pp. 41–50 and 70–75) and Baken (1987, pp. 315–345). Also, carefully study the operating manual for the sound spectrographic system you will be using.

I. RECORDING THE SAMPLE: SAMPLING RATE

The first step in making a sound spectrogram is recording the signal to be analyzed. The digital sound spectrograph is a computer system that can only operate on discrete numbers. But the speech signal (after microphone transduction) is in the form of an electrical voltage that continuously varies. Before anything else can be done, this continuous (analog) microphone signal has to be converted to numerical (digital) form. This is accomplished by the *analog-to-digital converter* (commonly referred to as an "A-to-D" or "A/D") that is built into the spectrograph.

What the A-to-D does is to "look" at the microphone signal repeatedly and convert its magnitude at each "glance" into a number that gets saved in the computer's memory. The result is a long series of numbers representing the "size" of the microphone signal each time it was observed. The A-to-D "looks at" (or *samples*) the input at regular intervals, so the numbers it generates could be plotted on graph paper with uniform spacing to reconstruct the original microphone signal. The frequency at which the A-to-D measures the signal is called the *sampling rate*. The sampling rate must be high enough to ensure the accuracy of the numerical representation of the signal.

In this first exercise you will examine the effect of sampling rate to enable you to choose an adequate rate for a given spectrographic analysis.

1. The manual for your sound spectrograph will show you how to change the sampling rate and sample duration. Follow the instructions and set the sampling rate of the sound spectrograph to 20,000 samples/second. Set the sample duration for as short a time as possible.

2. Record a sustained /ɑ/ at this sampling rate. Adjust the input gain to prevent the signal from overloading the amplifier. (On the Kay Elemetrics CSL™, for example, the red indicator light should not go on.)

3. Display just 5 or 6 cycles of the sound waveform of this sample on the screen. (You can use the spectrograph's cursor controls and display options to do this.)

4. Now change the sampling rate to about 5,000 samples/s. Record another /ɑ/ and display a few cycles of it below the first displayed recording.

5. Finally, change the sampling rate to about 2,500 samples/s. Record one more /ɑ/ and display a few cycles of it below the other two.

6. Prepare a printout of the computer screen (a sample CSL display is provided on the hand-in sheet). Label each waveform display with its sampling rate and attach the printout to the hand-in sheet. DO NOT ERASE THE SCREEN YET!

7. Compare the three oscillograms you have produced. What happens to the appearance of the waveform of /ɑ/ as the sampling rate drops?

Any complex waveform is composed of a large number of frequencies. (Specifying *which* frequencies is one of the objectives of spectrography!) The distortion of the waveform at lower sampling rates occurs because the higher frequencies have not been "captured."

There is a definite relationship between the sampling rate and the highest frequency that can be captured. It is stated by the *Nyquist sampling theorem,* which says that the highest frequency that can be represented in a digital record is the frequency equal to half of the sampling rate. So, if you wish to analyze a speech sample and show its spectrum from 0 to 8000 Hz, you would have to set the A-to-D sampling rate to *at least* 16,000 samples/s. (In practice, you would leave yourself a little "head room" and sample at a somewhat higher rate, perhaps 20,000 samples/s.)

8. Prepare sound spectrograms of the three samples of /ɑ/ you have recorded at different sampling rates. (Do the spectrograms using the narrowest filter bandwidth available.) Print the spectrograms and attach them to the hand-in sheet (examples are also provided). What is the highest frequency that each spectrogram shows? How do you explain this?

II. FILTER BANDWIDTH

1. Set up the sound spectrograph so that you will be able to do a spectrographic analysis of a speech signal lasting about 2 seconds. You will want to see all frequency components from 0 to 8 kHz (8000 Hz).

2. Now record the statement "I am tall," spoken as naturally as possible.

3. Set the spectrograph's filter bandwidth to about twice your normal vocal F_0. (You can probably set the filter bandwidth to 200 Hz or so if you're an average male, or to about 400 Hz if you're an average female.)

4. Produce a spectrogram of your sample. Print it and label it "Wide-band filter."

5. Change the filter bandwidth to no more than half your usual F_0 (about 50 Hz for a typical male or about 100 Hz for a typical female). Do a new spectrogram, print it, and label it "Narrow-band filter." (Samples of both filter bandwidths are shown on the hand-in sheet.)

6. Examine the spectrograms. You should be able to identify the following features on one or the other (or both):

    a. harmonic lines;

    b. formant bands;

    c. vertical striations; and

    d. an acoustic indication of release of air pressure for [t].

   Mark your spectrograms to show at least one example of each feature. Attach both spectrograms to the hand-in sheet.

7. Being able to see distinct harmonic lines requires that the spectrogram have relatively good *frequency resolution*. That is, the display can show the frequency difference even when two frequencies are close to each other. Which spectrogram (wide- or narrow-band) has better frequency resolution? Enter your opinion in the table provided on the hand-in sheet.

8. Formant bands are regions on the frequency axis in which harmonics are emphasized. It is easier to see the formant bands if we are not distracted by having to look at the individual harmonics that lie within them. Which spectrogram (wide- or narrow-band) makes the formant bands easier to see? Enter your choice in the table.

9. The vertical striations represent the sounds created each time the glottis closes. Voiced sounds, as you can see from the spectrogram, are actually composed of a

series of such short pulses of sound. Being able to see the very brief glottal pulses requires good *time resolution*. That is, the spectrogram must be able to show the separation between two events that are close together in time. Which spectrogram (wide- or narrow-band) has better time resolution? Mark your answer in the table.

10. Look over your conclusions about time and frequency resolution. What is the relationship between filter bandwidth and resolution?

11. Now set up the spectrograph to analyze frequencies from 0 to 4 kHz.

12. Prepare both wide-band and narrow-band spectrograms of each of the following (underscored words are to be emphasized when spoken):

    a. I am tall.

    b. I am tall.

    c. I am tall.

    d. I am tall?

13. Which spectrograms show the intonation contour ("melody pattern") of the statements? Print out and label one spectrogram that provides a clear indication of the intonation contour (an example is provided on the hand-in sheet). Label it to show which statement it represents and with what filter it was analyzed. Draw a line on this spectrogram tracing the intonation contour you find. Attach it to the hand-in sheet.

14. On the hand-in sheet, summarize what you have learned by indicating whether you would choose a wide- or narrow-band analyzing filter for evaluating each of the following:

    a. The regularity of vocal fold vibration;

    b. The normality of vowel pronunciation;

    c. Vowel duration;

    d. The intonation contour;

    e. Syllable diadochokinesis; and

    f. Hypernasality.

READ MORE ABOUT IT!

Baken, R. J. (1987). *Clinical measurement of speech and voice.* Boston: Little, Brown.

Borden, G. J., & Harris, K. S. (1984). *Speech science primer: Physiology, acoustics, and perception of speech* (2nd ed.) Baltimore: Williams and Wilkins.

Davis, R. O. (1986). Digital signal processing in studies of animal acoustical communication, including human speech. *Computer Methods and Programs in Biomedicine, 23,* 171–196.

Decker, T. N. (1990). *Instrumentation: An introduction for students in the speech and hearing sciences* (pp. 99–118). New York: Longman.

Denes, P. B., & Pinson, E. N. (1993). *The speech chain: The physics and biology of spoken language* (2nd ed., pp. 139–151). New York: W. H. Freeman.

Farmer, A. (1984). Spectrography. In C. Code & M. Ball (Eds.), *Instrumentation in speech-language pathology* (pp. 21–40). San Diego: College-Hill Press.

*Huggins, A. W. (1980). Better spectrograms from children's speech: A research note. *Journal of Speech and Hearing Research, 23,* 19–27.

Kent, R. D., & Read, C. (1992). *The acoustic analysis of speech.* San Diego: Singular Publishing Group.

*Koenig, W., Dunn, H. K., & Lacy, L. Y. (1946). The sound spectrograph. *Journal of the Acoustical Society of America, 18,* 19–49.

Painter, C. (1979). *An introduction to instrumental phonetics* (pp. 11–25). Baltimore: University Park Press.

*Peterson, G. E. (1952). Parameter relationships in the portrayal of signals with sound spectrography techniques. *Journal of Speech and Hearing Disorders, 17,* 427–432.

Pickett, J. M. (1980). *The sounds of speech communication.* Austin, TX: Pro-Ed.

Weismer, G. (1984). Acoustic descriptions of dysarthric speech: Perceptual correlates and physiological inferences. *Seminars in Speech and Language, 5,* 293–313.

Weismer, G., & Liss, J. M. (1991). Acoustic/perceptual taxonomies of speech production deficits in motor speech disorders. In C. A. Moore, K. M. Yorkston, & D. R. Beukelman (Eds.), *Dysarthria and apraxia of speech: Perspectives on management* (pp. 245–270). Baltimore: Paul H. Brookes.

---

*Reprinted in: Baken, R. J., & Daniloff, R. G. (1991). *Readings in clinical spectrography of speech.* San Diego: Singular Publishing Group and Kay Elemetrics Corp.

Student _____   Date _____

SOUND SPECTROGRAPHY I — GETTING ACQUAINTED

I. RECORDING THE SAMPLE: SAMPLING RATE

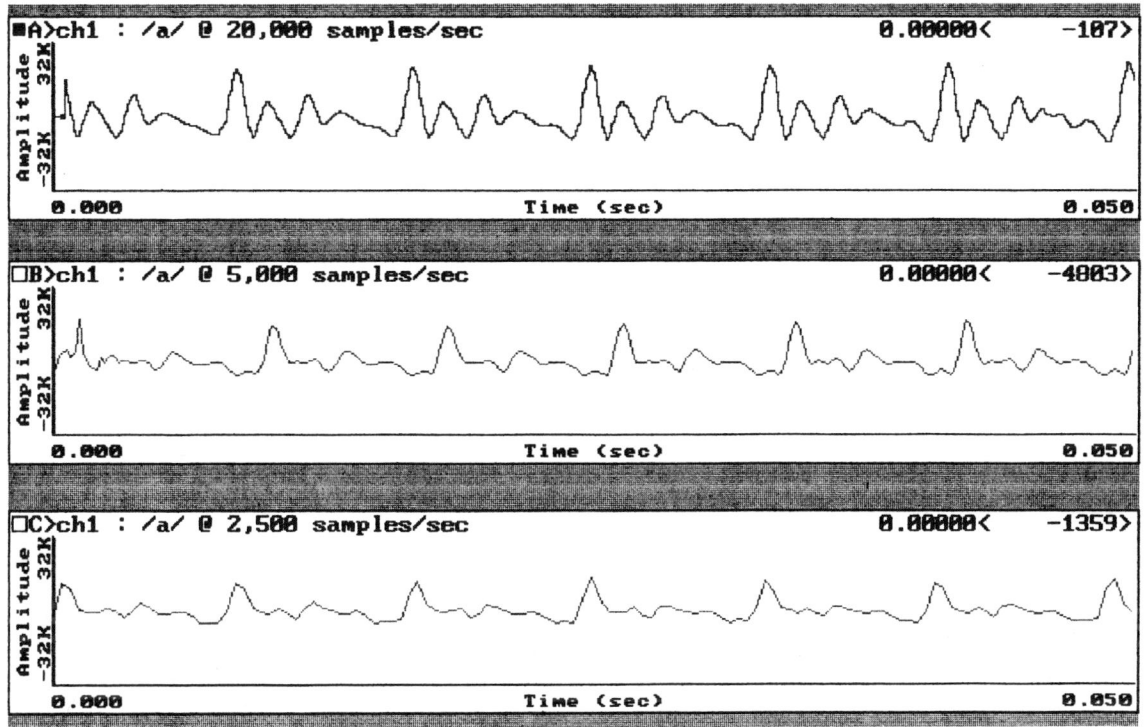

Attach your labeled oscillograms to this page.

Student _____   Date _____

7. Describe how the appearance of the waveform changes as the sampling rate drops: _____

_____

_____

_____

_____

_____

_____

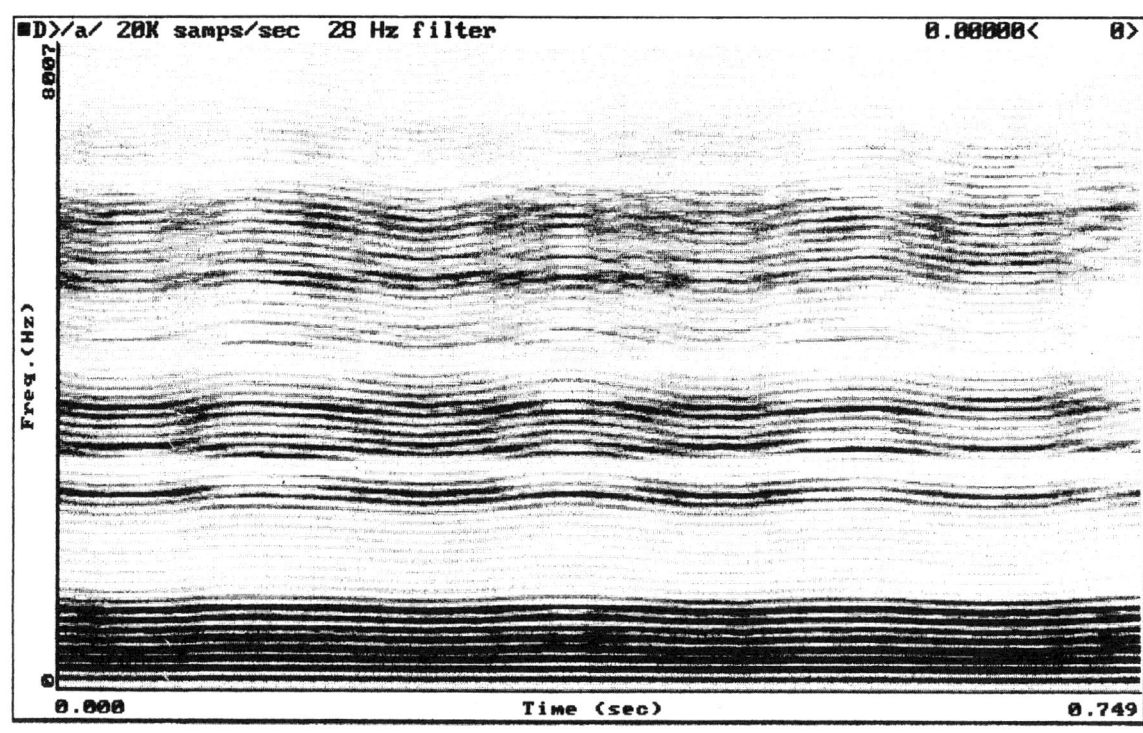

Student   Date

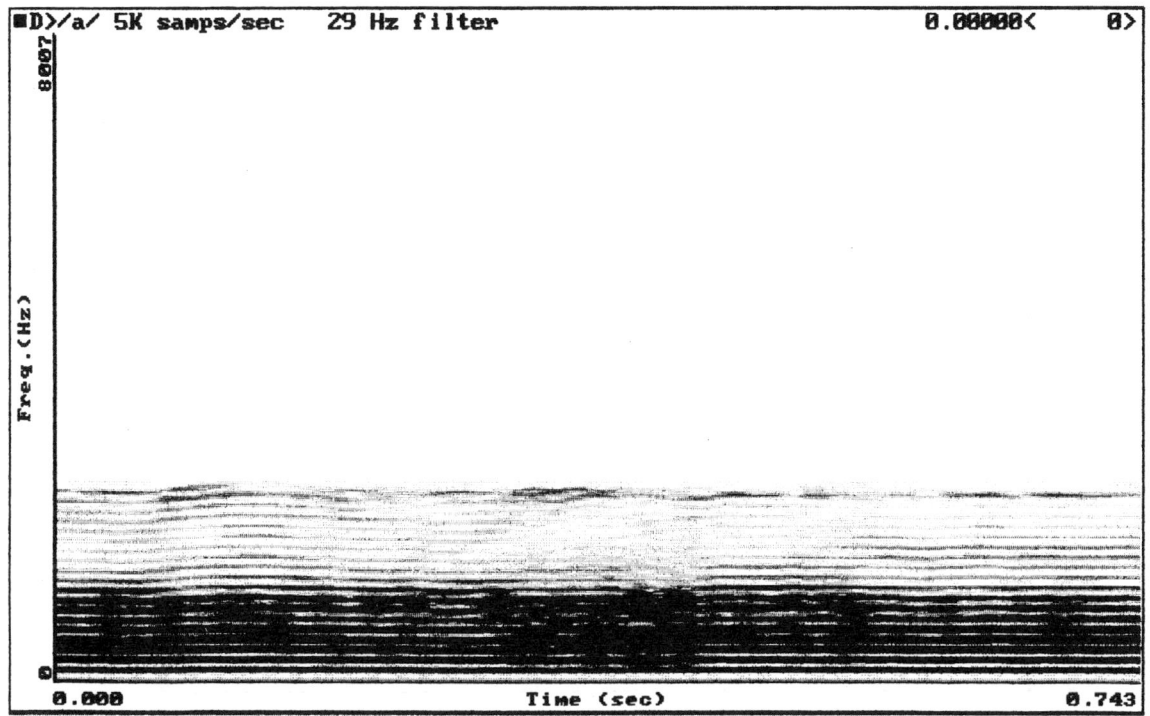

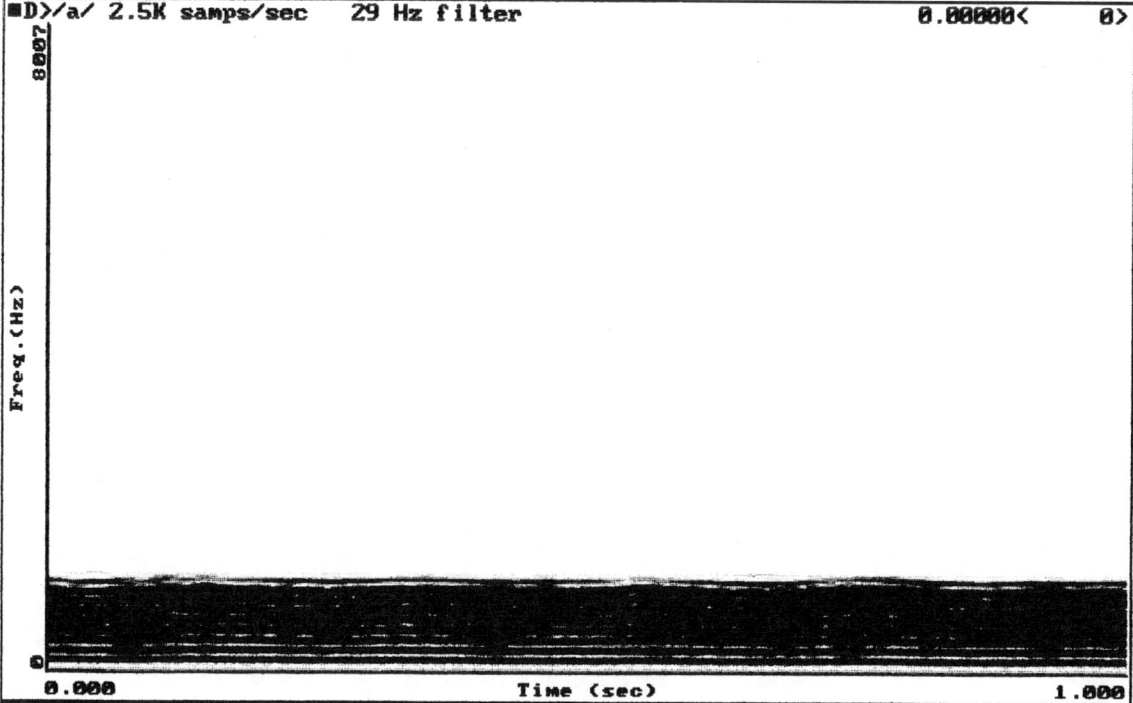

Attach your labeled spectrograms to this page.

Student _____   Date _____

8. SAMPLING RATE: HIGHEST FREQUENCY IN SPECTROGRAM:

20,000 samples/s   _____ Hz

5,000 samples/s   _____ Hz

2,500 samples/s   _____ Hz

Explain: _____

_____

_____

_____

_____

_____

_____

_____

Student   Date

II. FILTER BANDWIDTH

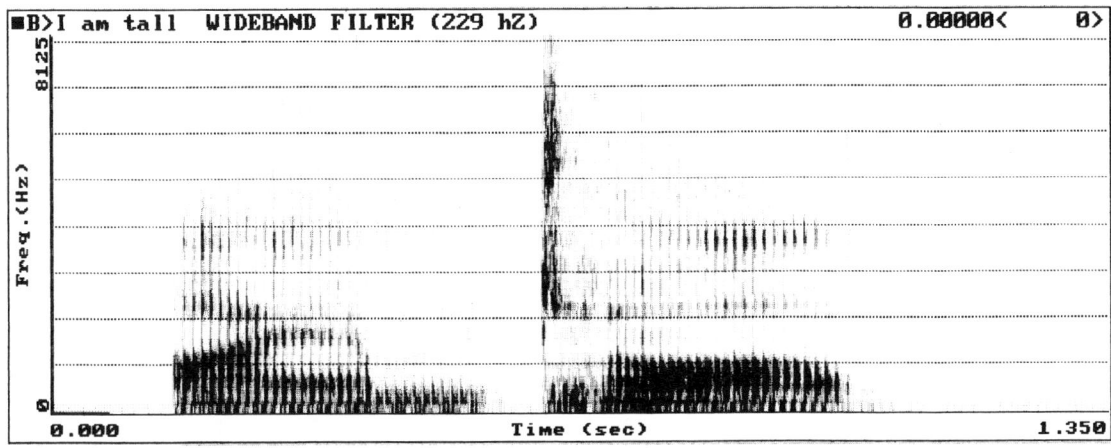

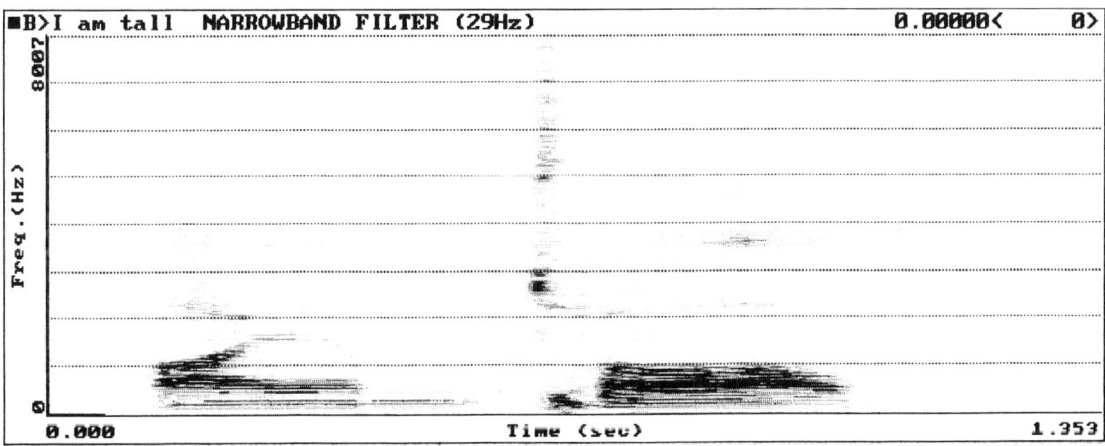

Attach your labeled spectrograms to this page.

Student _____   Date _____

Which spectrogram has better (circle your choice):

7. Frequency resolution: Wide-band   Narrow-band

8. Formant visibility: Wide-band   Narrow-band

9. Time resolution: Wide-band   Narrow-band

10. Relationship between time and frequency resolution: _____

_____
_____
_____
_____
_____
_____
_____

Student _____ Date _____

13. "I am tall   " (Underline the stressed word or add a question mark.)

Filter bandwidth used: _____

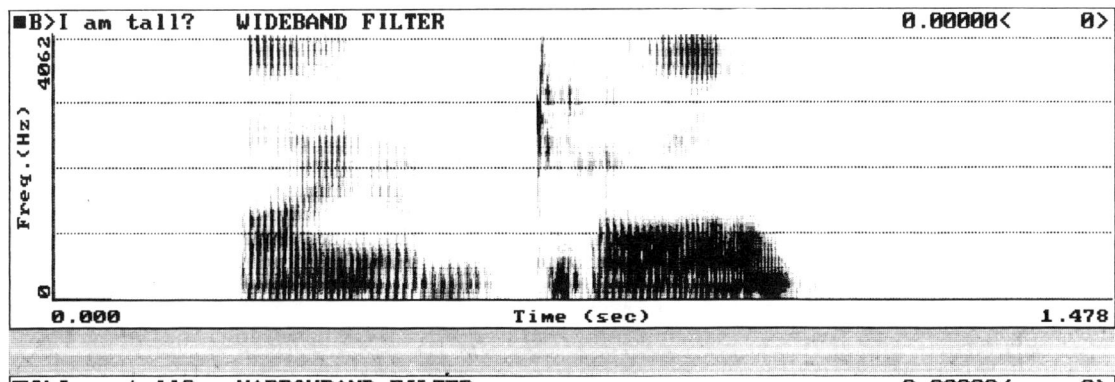

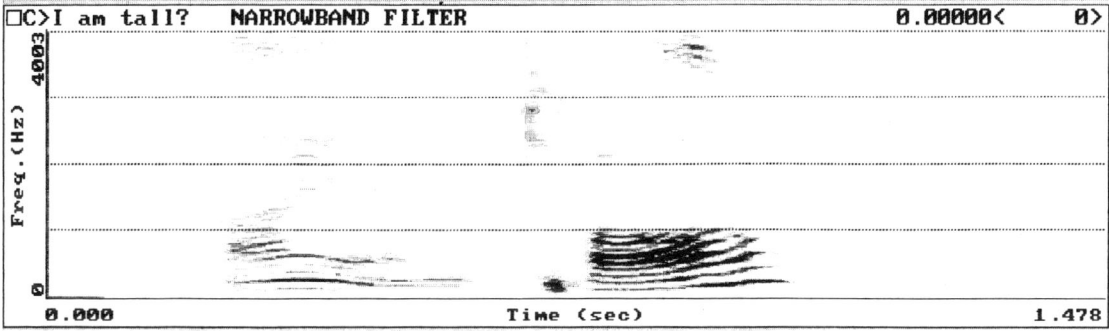

Attach your spectrogram to this page.

Student _____   Date _____

14. EVALUATION OBJECTIVE: FILTER BANDWIDTH OF CHOICE:

    a. Regularity of vocal fold
       vibration   _____

    b. Vowel normality   _____

    c. Vowel duration   _____

    d. Intonation contour   _____

    e. Syllable diadochokinesis   _____

    f. Hypernasality   _____

UNIT 28

Basic Skills: Sound Spectrography II — Identifying "Source" and "Filter" Contributions to the Speech Signal

The "source-filter" theory holds that the acoustic characteristics of vowels are created by the actions of the resonant properties of the vocal tract (referred to as the "filter") interacting with and modifying the acoustic content of a (quasi)periodic tone produced by the larynx (called the "source signal"). Sound spectrography provides a means of evaluating both the source and filter aspects of a vowel production, thereby allowing us to make judgments about where a problem lies.

Purpose: These exercises will help you learn to observe the contributions of the vocal source and vocal tract filter to the acoustic signal of a vowel. You will gain skill in evaluating harmonics and in seeing formant structure.

Equipment: A sound spectrograph and microphone and speaker system.

General preparation: Review the general principles of the acoustics of speech and of the source-filter model of vowel production. (Good sources include Baken, 1987; Borden & Harris, 1984; and Kent & Read, 1992.) Be sure that you understand the concepts of harmonic and formant frequencies.

I. CHANGING THE FILTER

1. Practice saying /i:u:i:/ as one continuous utterance with no change of pitch. Your production should have a duration between one and two seconds. Record your production on the spectrograph. [NOTE: It is VERY important that you produce the vowel combination with no intonation; Your production should sound flat and mechanical.]

2. Prepare two sound spectrograms of your vowel sample. (If you are using a Kay Elemetrics CSL™ system or similar instrument, use the cursors to expand your sample so that it fills the entire width of your spectrograms.) The **first** spectrogram should be done with an analyzing filter with a bandwidth that is about twice your estimated fundamental frequency (F_0). The **second** spectrogram should be done with an analyzing filter with a bandwidth that is no more than half your F_0. Adjust the spectrograph so that:

   a. The harmonic lines are visible across the entire length of the speech sample in the narrow-band spectrogram; and

   b. The formant bands are clear and optimally distinct from each other in the wide-band spectrogram.

   (Examples I-A and I-B are shown on the hand-in sheet.)

3. Mark the filter bandwidth on each spectrogram. Label each to show the region of each vowel.

4. Examine both spectrograms. Identify and label the spectrographic representation of the voice harmonics, formant frequencies, and glottal pulses. Attach your spectrograms to the hand-in sheet.

Harmonics

5. Which spectrogram (narrow- or wide-band filtered) better shows the harmonics?

6. What is the relationship between the spacing of the harmonic lines and the vocal F_0?

7. How does the strength of the harmonics (represented by their darkness) change as their frequency increases?

8. What changes as the signal moves from vowel to vowel — the harmonics or the formants?

9. Do the harmonic lines "move" to create the formant bands or do the formants simply reflect increasing "emphasis" of different harmonics?

Formants

10. Which spectrogram shows the formants more clearly?

11. What are the formant frequencies of the two vowels?

12. Do the harmonics change significantly as the formants shift?

13. Can you detect any relationship between the formant frequencies and the harmonic frequencies?

14. What do the formants *do* to the harmonics?

II. CHANGING THE SOURCE

1. Practice sustained the vowel /i/ using a low-pitch, high-pitch, low-pitch pattern. That is, the "melody" of your production should be ⌐⌐. Do not let the vowel change as you alter your pitch, and be sure that you produce one *continuous* utterance, not three separate vowels.

2. As you did in Exercise I, record your production on the sound spectrograph and prepare two sound spectrograms of your vowel sample. (Again, the first should be done with an analyzing filter with a bandwidth that is 1½ to 2 times your estimated fundamental frequency, and the second should be done with an analyzing filter with a bandwidth that is no more than 50% of your F_0. Adjust the spectrograph so that the harmonic lines are visible across the entire length of the speech sample and that the formant bands are clear and optimally distinct from each other.) Mark the filter bandwidth on each spectrogram. (Examples II-A and II-B are shown on the hand-in sheet.)

3. Examine your spectrograms. Identify and label the spectrographic representation of the voice harmonics, formant frequencies, and glottal pulses.

4. Label the spectrograms to show the regions of high and low pitch. Attach your spectrograms to the hand-in sheet.

5. What is the relationship between harmonic spacing and vocal F_0?

6. Do the formants change significantly as F_0 changes?

III. SUMMARY

The following spectrogram was produced using a Kay Elemetrics model 7800 spectrograph.[1] Here, a normal 25-year-old male speaker has prolonged a vocalization. The frequency scale extends from 0 to 7000 Hz (the thin horizontal lines are frequency marks, spaced every 1000 Hz)

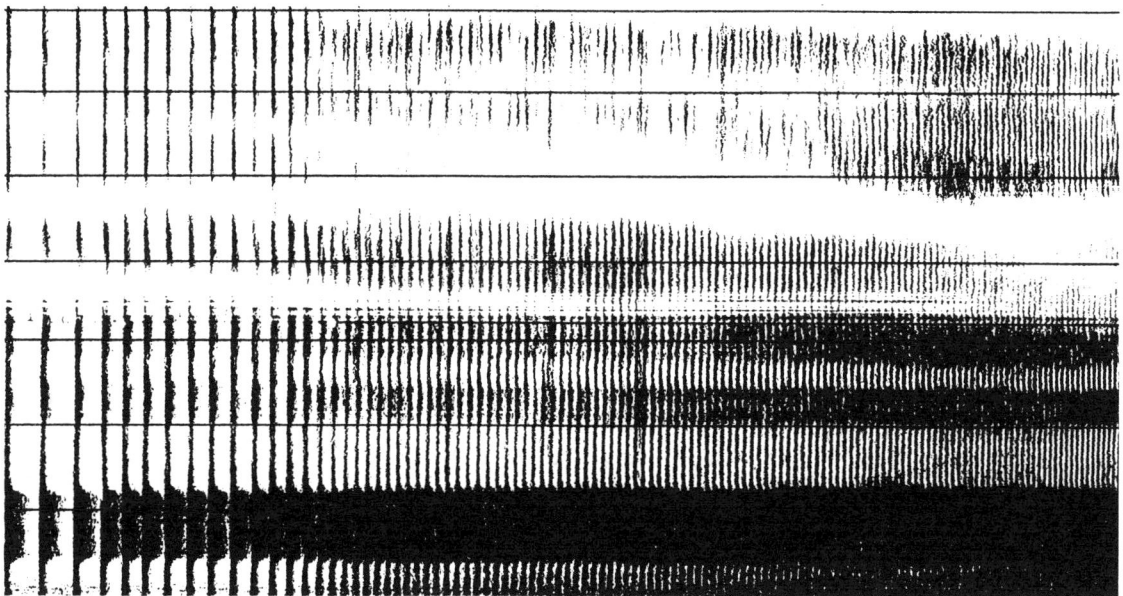

1. Use this spectrogram to answer the following:

   a. Was this spectrogram produced with a relatively narrow- or wide-band analysis filter? How do you know?

   b. Was the vocal frequency constant throughout the phonation? If so, what was the speaker's F_0? If not, how did it change? Explain.

   c. Were the formants consistent throughout the phonation? If not, how did they change?

The spectrogram on the next page was produced using the same instrument and speaker prolonging a different vocalization. In this case, the frequency scale extends from 0 to 8000 Hz (the thin frequency line marks are spaced every 500 Hz).

---

[1] Model 7800 is a hybrid (analog/digital) spectrograph; see Baken (1987, p. 344) for a description of the instrument.

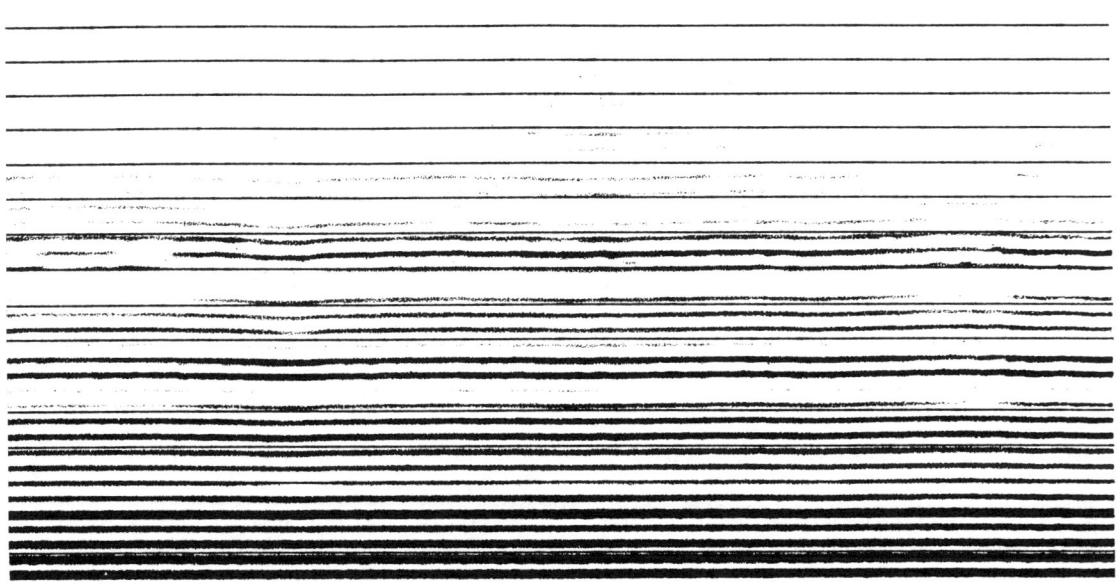

2. Use this spectrogram to answer the following:

   a. Was this spectrogram produced with a relatively narrow- or wide-band analysis filter? How do you know?

   b. Was the vocal frequency constant throughout the phonation? If so, what was this speaker's vocal F_0? If not, how did it change? Explain.

   c. Were the formants consistent throughout the phonation? If not, how did they change?

3. Summarize your conclusions about vocal source and vocal tract filter contributions to a vowel signal by completing the summary table on the hand-in sheet. In each blank space enter "vocal sound source" or "vocal tract filter" as appropriate.

4. For each of the following conditions, indicate on the hand-in sheet whether the problem is most likely to affect the vocal source or the vocal tract filter, and state whether the harmonics and/or the formants are most likely to be affected:

   a. Dysphonia due to vocal nodules;

   b. Dysarthria;

   c. Abnormal vocal mutation;

   d. Delayed speech maturation;

   e. Stuttering; and

   f. Hypernasality.

READ MORE ABOUT IT!

Baken, R. J. (1987). *Clinical measurement of speech and voice* (pp. 326–384). Boston: Little, Brown.

Borden, G. J., & Harris, K. S. (1984). *Speech science primer: Physiology, acoustics, and perception of speech* (2nd ed.) Baltimore: Williams and Wilkins.

Fant, G. (1960). *Acoustic theory of speech production.* The Hague: Mouton.

Farmer, A. (1984). Spectrography. In C. Code & M. Ball (eds.), *Instrumentation in speech-language pathology* (pp. 21–40). San Diego: College-Hill Press.

Gerratt, B. R. (1983). Formant frequency fluctuation as an index of motor steadiness in the vocal tract. *Journal of Speech and Hearing Research, 26,* 297–304.

Imaizumi, S. (1986). Spectrographic evaluation of laryngeal pathology. In C. W. Cummings & J. M. Fredrickson (Eds.), *Otolaryngology — Head and neck surgery* (Vol. 3, pp. 1838–1845). St. Louis: Mosby.

Isshiki, N., Ohkawa, M., & Goto, M. (1985). Stiffness of the vocal cord in dysphonia — Its assessment and treatment. *Acta Otolaryngologica, suppl. 419,* 167–174.

Kent, R. D. (1993). Vocal tract acoustics. *Journal of Voice, 7,* 97–117.

Kent, R. D., & Read, C. (1992). *The acoustic analysis of speech.* San Diego: Singular Publishing Group.

Ladefoged, P. (1982). *A course in phonetics* (2nd ed.). New York: Harcourt Brace Jovanovich.

Lieberman, P. (1977). *Speech physiology and acoustic phonetics.* New York: Macmillan.

Ohde, R. N., & Sharf, D. J. (1992). *Phonetic analysis of normal and abnormal speech.* New York: Merrill.

Pickett, J. M. (1980). *The sounds of speech communication.* Austin, TX: Pro-Ed.

Potter, R. K., & Peterson, G. E. (1948). The representation of vowels and their movements. *Journal of the Acoustical Society of America, 20,* 528–535.

Rothman, H. (1976). An acoustic investigation of consonant-vowel transitions in the speech of deaf adults. *Journal of Phonetics, 4,* 95–102.

Sasaki, Y., Okamura, H., & Yumoto, E. (1991). Quantitative analysis of hoarseness using a digital sound spectrograph. *Journal of Voice, 5,* 36–40.

Shoup, J. E., Lass, N. J., & Kuehn, D. P. (1982). Acoustics of speech. In N. J. Lass, J. L. Northern, & D. E. Yoder (Eds.), *Speech, language, and hearing* (Vol. 1, pp. 193–218). Philadelphia: Saunders.

Simmons, N. N. (1983). Acoustic analysis of ataxic dysarthria: An approach to monitoring treatment. In W. R. Berry (Ed.), *Clinical dysarthria* (pp. 283–294). San Diego: College-Hill Press.

Stevens, K. N., & House, A. S. (1961). An acoustics theory of vowel production and some of its implications. *Journal of Speech and Hearing Research, 4,* 303–320.

Stevens, K. N., & Klatt, D. H. (1972). Current models of sound sources for speech. In B. D. Wyke (Ed.), *Ventilatory and phonatory control systems.* New York: Oxford.

Weismer, G. (1984). Acoustic descriptions of dysarthric speech: Perceptual correlates and physiological inferences. *Seminars in Speech and Language, 5,* 293–314.

Weismer, G., & Liss, J. M. (1991). Acoustic/perceptual taxonomies of speech production deficits in motor speech disorders. In C. A. Moore, K. M. Yorkston, & D. R. Beukelman (Eds.), *Dysarthria and apraxia of speech: Perspectives on management* (pp. 245–270). Baltimore: Paul H. Brookes.

Wood, S. (1986). The role of the pharynx in speech. In C. W. Cummings & J. M. Fredrickson (Eds.), *Otolaryngology — Head and neck surgery* (Vol. 3, pp. 1776–1788). St. Louis: Mosby.

Yanagihara, N. (1967). Significance of harmonic changes and noise components in hoarseness. *Journal of Speech and Hearing Research, 10,* 531–541.

Student _____   Date _____

SOUND SPECTROGRAPHY II — IDENTIFYING "SOURCE" AND "FILTER" CONTRIBUTIONS TO THE SPEECH SIGNAL

I. CHANGING THE FILTER

First spectrogram: /i:u:i:/   Filter bandwidth _____ Hz

Second spectrogram: /i:u:i:/   Filter bandwidth _____ Hz

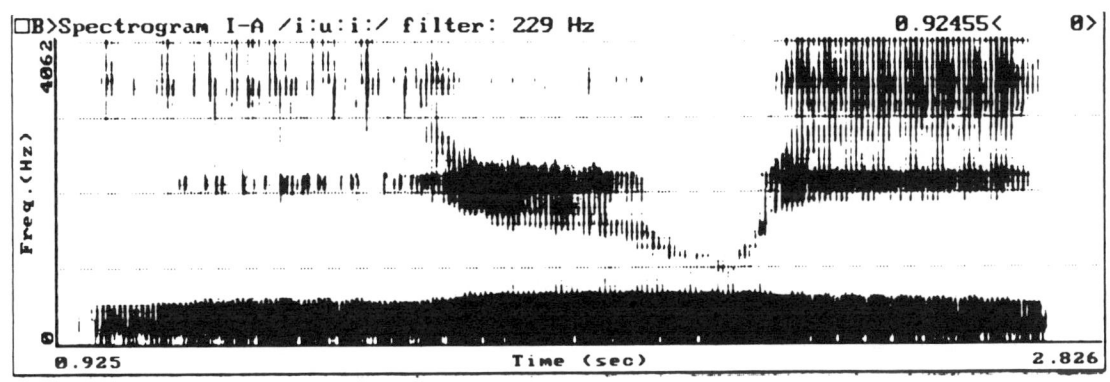

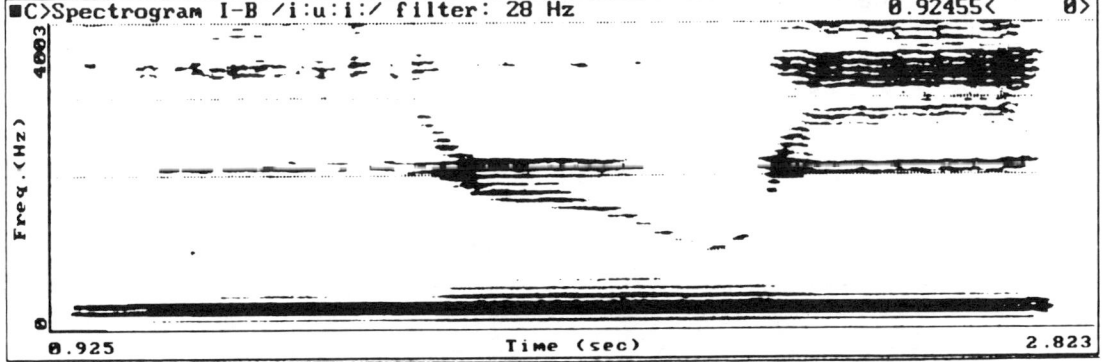

Attach your labeled spectrograms to this page.

Student _____ Date _____

5. Harmonics are shown better in the first or in the second spectrogram?

6. How is the harmonic line spacing related to vocal F_0? _____

7. What is the relationship between harmonic strength and harmonic frequency?

8. Changing the vowel changes the (circle one):

        harmonics   formants

9. How are formant bands formed? By changing the harmonics or by emphasizing different harmonics?

10. Formants are shown more clearly in the first or in the second spectrogram?

Student   Date

11. Complete the following based on your spectrogram:

Vowel	Formant 1	Formant 2	Formant 3
[i]	_____ Hz	_____ Hz	_____ Hz
[u]	_____ Hz	_____ Hz	_____ Hz

12. How do the harmonics change as the formants shift? _____

_____

_____

_____

13. What is the relationship between formant frequency and harmonic frequency?

_____

_____

_____

_____

14. What is the effect of formants on harmonics? _____

_____

_____

_____

_____

Student _____   Date _____

II. CHANGING THE SOURCE

First spectrogram: /i:i:i:/   Filter bandwidth _____ Hz

Second spectrogram: /i:i:i:/   Filter bandwidth _____ Hz

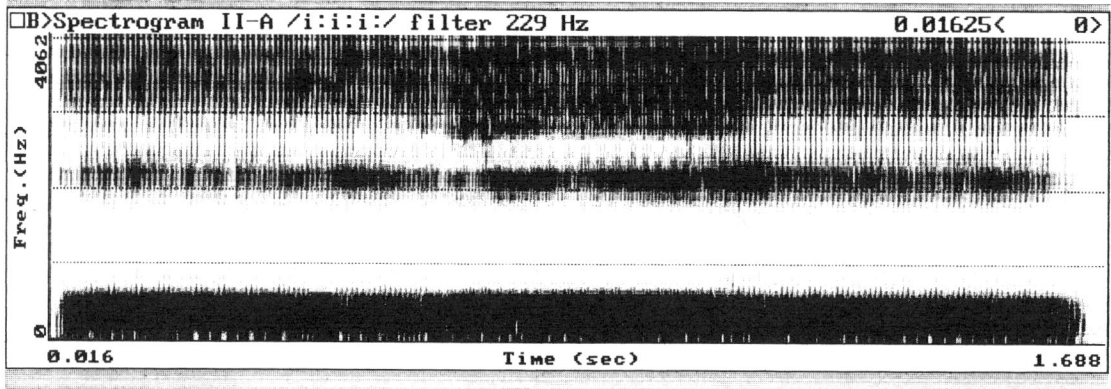

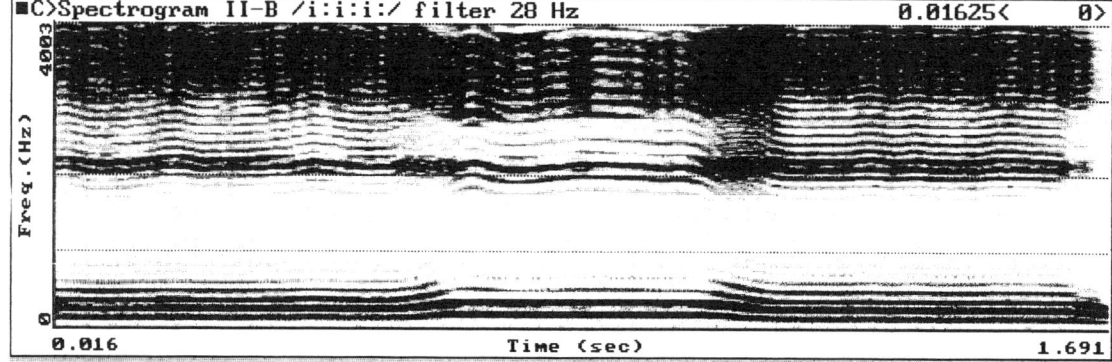

Attach your labeled spectrograms to this page.

Student _____ Date _____

5. What is the relationship between harmonic spacing and vocal F_0? _____
_____
_____
_____

6. Formant change as a function of F_0 change: _____
_____
_____
_____
_____

III. SUMMARY

1. a. Analysis filter used: _____

   Explain: _____
   _____
   _____

   b. Vocal F_0: _____
   _____
   _____
   _____

   c. Vowel formants: _____
   _____
   _____
   _____

Student _____ Date _____

2. a. Analysis filter used: _____

Explain: _____

_____

_____

_____

b. Vocal F_0: _____

_____

_____

_____

_____

_____

c. Vowel formants: _____

_____

_____

_____

Student _____   Date _____

3. Complete the following summary table:

Spectrogram Characteristics	Origin
Harmonic line spacing	
Noise between harmonics	
Decrease of harmonic strength with increasing frequency	
Glottal pulses	
Movement of harmonic lines	
Formant bands	

4. Complete the following table concerning the effects of various communication disorders/symptoms:

Condition	Origin: Source/Filter	Effect on: Harmonics/Formants
a. Dysphonia (vocal nodules)		
b. Dysarthria		
c. Abnormal vocal mutation		
d. Delayed speech maturation		
e. Stuttering		
f. Hypernasality		

UNIT 29

Clinical Application: Spectrography — Vowel Formants

The frequency values of vowel formants depend on the length and shape of the vocal tract. An evaluation of formant frequencies not only reveals the accuracy with which a speaker can produce the vowels of her language, but also provides information about vocal tract length and configuration.

Purpose: These exercises will teach you how to estimate the formant frequencies of vowels and how to plot the results of your measurements in a widely accepted and clinically useful format.

Equipment: A sound spectrograph, microphone and speaker system.

General preparation: Review the basic information about vowel formants. (Good sources include Baken, 1987, pp. 353–365; Borden & Harris, 1984, pp. 105–111; Kent & Read, 1992, pp. 87–100; and Pickett, 1980, pp. 41–78.) Also review the operating manual for your sound spectrograph to be sure that you understand how to generate wide-band sound spectrograms.

I. MEASURING FORMANT FREQUENCIES

1. Prepare a wide-band spectrogram (0–4000 Hz) of the statement "She saw ten tops." Adjust the display parameters so that the formant bands of the vowels are optimally distinct.

2. Examine the spectrogram and identify the four vowels and the formant bands of each.

3. The formants are probably not constant. That is, their frequency is likely to change across the syllable. Consider why this should be. (Hint: formants are determined by the configuration of the vocal tract.)

4. Measure the frequency of the first and second formant (usually abbreviated F1 and F2, respectively) of each vowel. The frequency is determined at the point that is half of the formant band's thickness.[1] If the vowel has a relatively steady portion, measure the formant frequency there. Otherwise, measure the frequency at the midpoint of the vowel. (You will probably find it most convenient to do these measurements using the spectrograph's cursor.) Tabulate the formant frequencies on the hand-in sheet.

5. How do the formant frequencies you have measured compare to published norms? Propose an explanation for any differences.

6. Print the spectrogram. Label it to indicate the filter bandwidth used in the analysis. Label each of the vowels and draw a line through each F1 and F2. Write the formant frequency next to each formant line. Attach the spectrogram to the hand-in sheet.

II. GRAPHIC ANALYSIS OF FORMANT FREQUENCIES

Formant frequencies change in a regular way from vowel to vowel.[2] The most common way of visualizing the relationship of the formant structure of different vowels is to plot the formant frequencies on a special graph that depicts the "F1–F2 plane."

1. You will evaluate 10 English vowels in /hVd/ syllables. The stimuli are:

    /hid/   /hɪd/   /hɛd/   /hæd/   /hɑd/

    /hɔd/   /hʊd/   /hud/   /hʌd/   /hɝd/

2. Prepare wide-band spectrograms of all of these syllables spoken by an adult female, an adult male, and a young child (perhaps 5 or 6 years old). Sample spectrograms are provided on the hand-in sheets.

3. Identify the first two formants of each production and measure their frequency. Enter your data into the table on the hand-in sheet. Print your spectrograms, label the vowels, and clip them to the hand-in sheets.

---

[1] Remember that formants are *peak* frequencies in the vocal tract transfer.

[2] That's to say that the vocal tract must be configured differently to produce different vowels!

4. The graph provided on the hand-in sheet has the frequency for F1 on the horizontal (x) axis, and the frequency of F2 on the vertical (y) axis. The space created is sometimes called the "F1–F2 plane." On it, plot the formant frequencies for the female speaker. Connect points for /i, ɛ, æ, ɑ, ɔ, u/ (beginning with /i/ and continuing around until you reach /i/ once again) using a RED pen. You should have a roughly trapezoidal polygon when finished.

5. Do the same for the formant frequencies of the male speaker, but this time use a BLUE pen to connect the vowel points.

6. Finally, plot the formant data for the child speaker. This time use a GREEN pen when connecting vowel points.

7. What relationship do you see between the polygon for a single speaker and the standard IPA vowel quadrilateral? How can you explain this relationship?

8. Use a standard black pencil to connect the points representing /i/ by the three speakers. Do the same for /æ/. What relationship is there between speaker category (male, female, child) and formant position on the F1–F2 plane? How do you explain this orderly progression of formant locations for the three categories of speaker?

9. If possible, plot the first and second formants of these ten vowels as produced by a speaker with an articulatory disorder. What conclusions can you draw about this patient's articulation?

READ MORE ABOUT IT!

Angelocci, A. A., Kopp, G. A., & Holbrook, A. (1964). The vowel formants of deaf and normal-hearing eleven- to fourteen-year-old boys. *Journal of Speech and Hearing Disorders, 29,* 156–170.

Baken, R. J. (1987). *Clinical measurement of speech and voice.* Boston: Little, Brown.

Borden, G. J., & Harris, K. S. (1984). *Speech science primer: Physiology, acoustics, and perception of speech* (2nd ed.). Baltimore: Williams and Wilkins.

Buhr, R. D. (1980). The emergence of vowels in an infant. *Journal of Speech and Hearing Research, 23,* 73–94.

Eguchi, S., & Hirsh, I. J. (1969). Development of speech sounds in children. *Acta Oto-laryngologica, suppl. 257,* 5–43.

Fairbanks, G., & Grubb, P. (1961). A psychophysical investigation of vowel formants. *Journal of Speech and Hearing Research, 4,* 203–219.

Gilbert, J. H. (1970). Formant concentration positions in the speech of children at two levels of linguistic development. *Journal of the Acoustical Society of America, 48,* 1404–1406.

Holbrook, A., & Fairbanks, G. (1962). Diphthong formants and their movements. *Journal of Speech and Hearing Research, 5,* 38–58.

Howell, P., & Williams, M. (1992). Acoustic analysis and perception of vowels in children's and teenagers' stuttered speech. *Journal of the Acoustical Society of America, 91,* 1697–1706.

Howell, P., & Vause, L. (1986). Acoustic analysis and perception of vowels in stuttered speech. *Journal of the Acoustical Society of America, 79,* 1571–1579.

Kahane, J. C. (1979). Pathophysiological effects of Möbius syndrome on speech and hearing. *Archives of Otolaryngology, 105,* 29–34.

Kent, R. D. (1976). Anatomical and neuromuscular maturation of the speech mechanism: Evidence from acoustic studies. *Journal of Speech and Hearing Research, 18,* 421–447.

Kent, R. D. (1979). Isovowel lines for the evaluation of formant structure in speech disorder. *Journal of Speech and Hearing Disorders, 44,* 513–521.

Kent, R. D., & Forner, L. L. (1979). Developmental study of vowel formant frequencies in an imitation task. *Journal of the Acoustical Society of America, 65,* 208–217.

Kent, R. D., & Murray, A. D. (1982). Acoustic features of vocalic utterances at 3, 6, and 9 months. *Journal of the Acoustical Society of America, 72,* 353–365.

Kent, R. D., Osberger, M. J., Netsell, R., & Hustedde, C. G. (1987). Phonetic development in identical twins differing in auditory function. *Journal of Speech and Hearing Disorders, 52,* 64–75.

Kent, R. D., & Read, C. (1992). *The acoustic analysis of speech.* San Diego: Singular Publishing Group.

Kent, R. D., & Rosenbek, J. C. (1983). Acoustic patterns of apraxia of speech. *Journal of Speech and Hearing Research, 26,* 231–249.

Ladefoged, P. (1982). *A course in phonetics* (2nd ed.). New York: Harcourt Brace Jovanovich.

Lindblom, B. (1963). Spectrographic study of vowel reduction. *Journal of the Acoustical Society of America, 35,* 1773–1781.

Manning, W. H., Moore, J. N., Dunham, M. J., Lu, F. L., & Domico, E. (1992). Vowel production in a prelinguistic child following cochlear implantation. *Journal of the American Academy of Audiology, 3,* 16–21.

Monsen, R. B. (1976). Normal and reduced phonological space: The production of English vowels by deaf adolescents. *Journal of Phonetics, 4,* 189–198.

Peterson, G. E. (1959). Vowel formant measurements. *Journal of Speech and Hearing Research, 2,* 173–183.

Peterson, G. E. (1961). Parameters of vowel quality. *Journal of Speech and Hearing Research, 4,* 10–29.

Peterson, G. E., & Barney, H. L. (1952). Control methods used in a study of the vowels. *Journal of the Acoustical Society of America, 24,* 175–184.

Peterson, G. E., & Coxe, M. S. (1953). The vowels [e] and [o] in American speech. *Quarterly Journal of Speech, 39,* 33–41.

Pickett, J. M. (1980). *The sounds of speech communication.* Austin, TX: Pro-Ed.

Potter, R. K., Kopp, G. A., & Green, H. G. (1966). *Visible speech.* New York: Dover.

Potter, R. K., & Peterson, G. E. (1948). The representation of vowels and their movements. *Journal of the Acoustical Society of America, 20,* 528–535.

Shoup, J. E., Lass, N. J., & Kuehn, D. P. (1982). Acoustics of speech. In N. J. Lass, J. L. Northern, & D. E. Yoder (Eds.), *Speech, language and hearing* (Vol. 1, pp. 193–218). Philadelphia: Saunders.

Stevens, K. N., & House, A. S. (1961). An acoustical theory of vowel production and some of its implications. *Journal of Speech and Hearing Research, 4,* 303–320.

Wood, S. (1986). The role of the pharynx in speech. In C. W. Cummings & J. M. Fredrickson (Eds.), *Otolaryngology–Head and neck surgery* (Vol. 3, pp. 1776–1788). St. Louis: Mosby.

Student   Date

SOUND SPECTROGRAPHY: VOWEL FORMANTS

I. MEASURING FORMANT FREQUENCIES

Spectrogram: "She saw ten tops"   Filter bandwidth _____ Hz

Speaker: _____

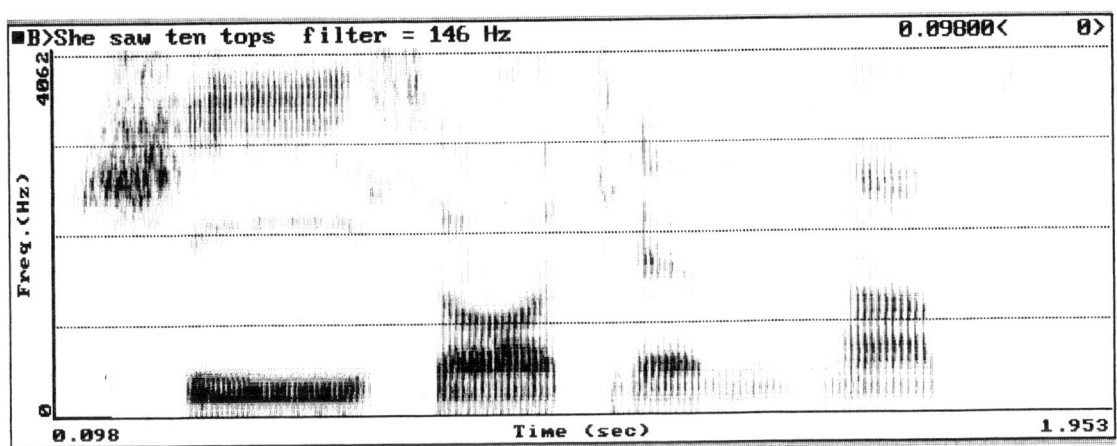

Attach your labeled spectrogram to this page.

Student _____   Date _____

3. Why are the formant bands not constant over the duration of the vowel?

_____
_____
_____
_____
_____

4. Formant frequencies of the vowels in "She saw ten tops":

Vowel	Formant 1	Formant 2
[i]	_____ Hz	_____ Hz
[ɔ]	_____ Hz	_____ Hz
[ɛ]	_____ Hz	_____ Hz
[ɑ]	_____ Hz	_____ Hz

5. Comparison of formant frequencies to norms and explanation of differences:

_____
_____
_____
_____
_____
_____
_____

Student   Date

II. GRAPHIC ANALYSIS OF FORMANT FREQUENCIES

Attach your labeled spectrograms to these pages.

Sample wide-band spectrograms of an adult male speaker:

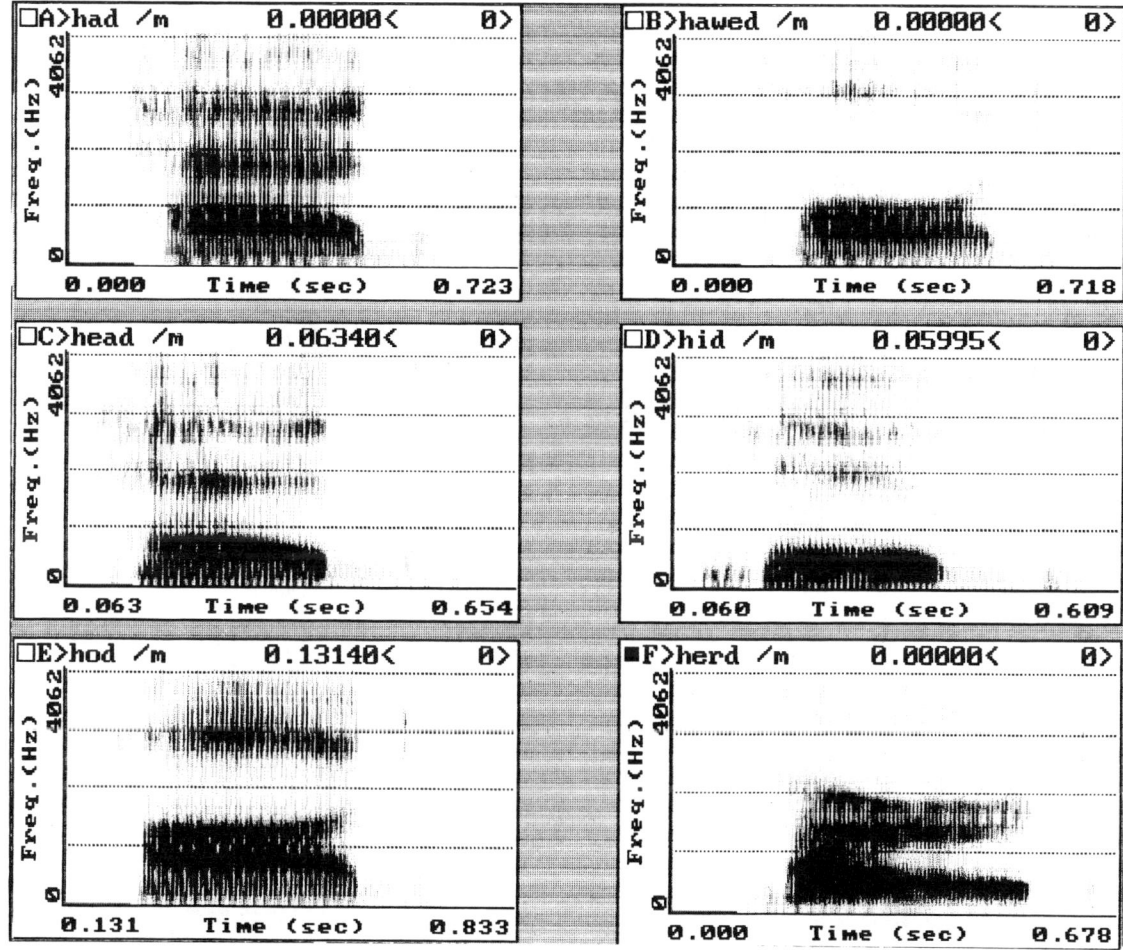

Student   Date

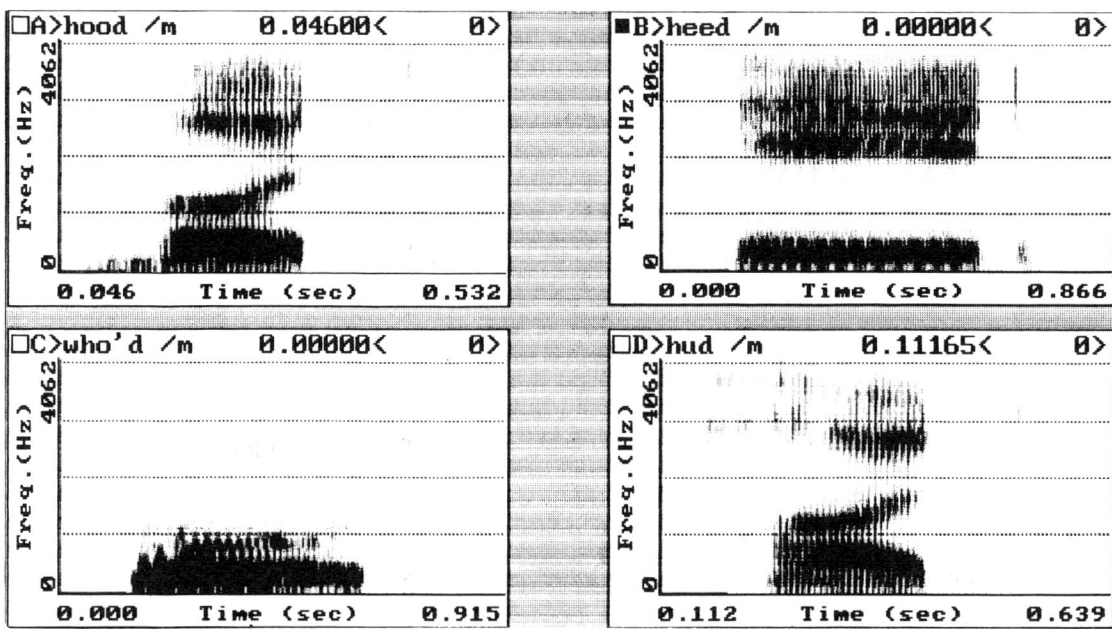

Student   Date

Sample wide-band spectrograms of an adult female speaker:

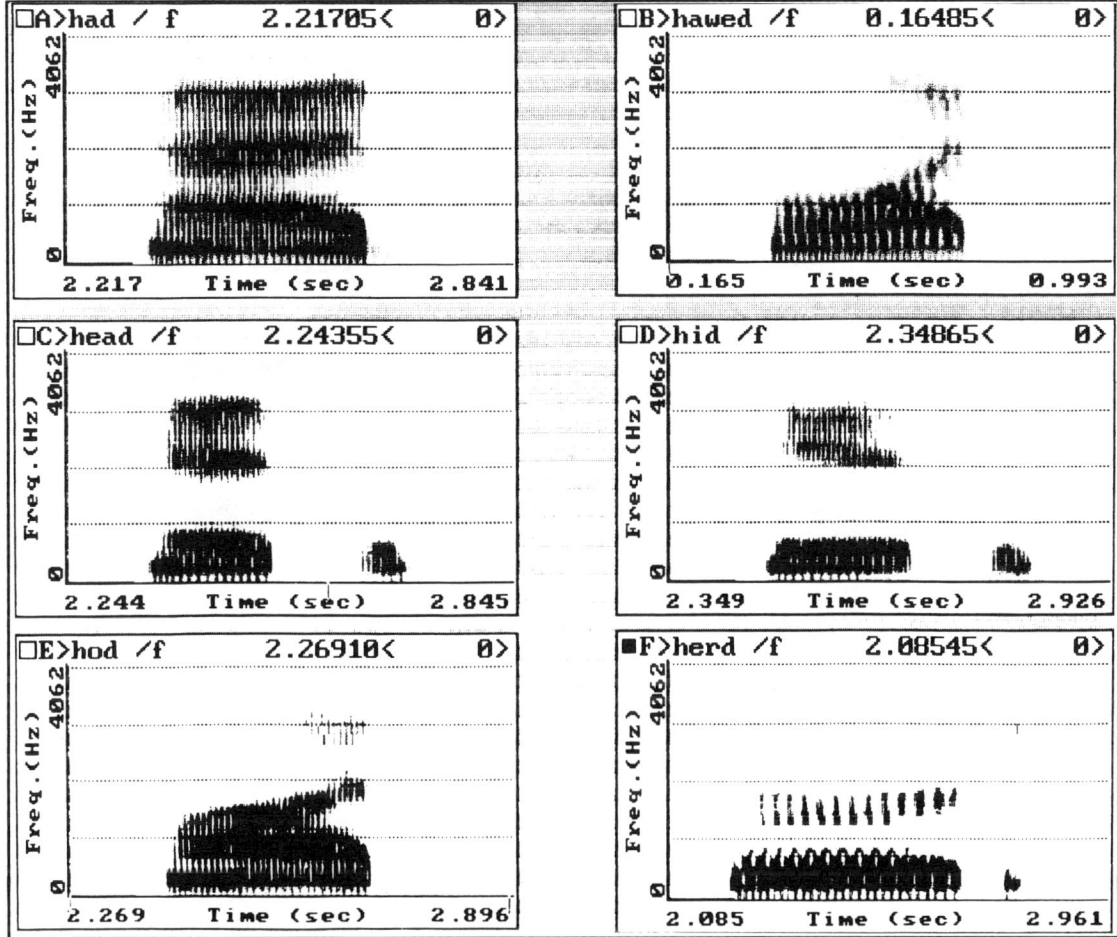

Student _____   Date _____

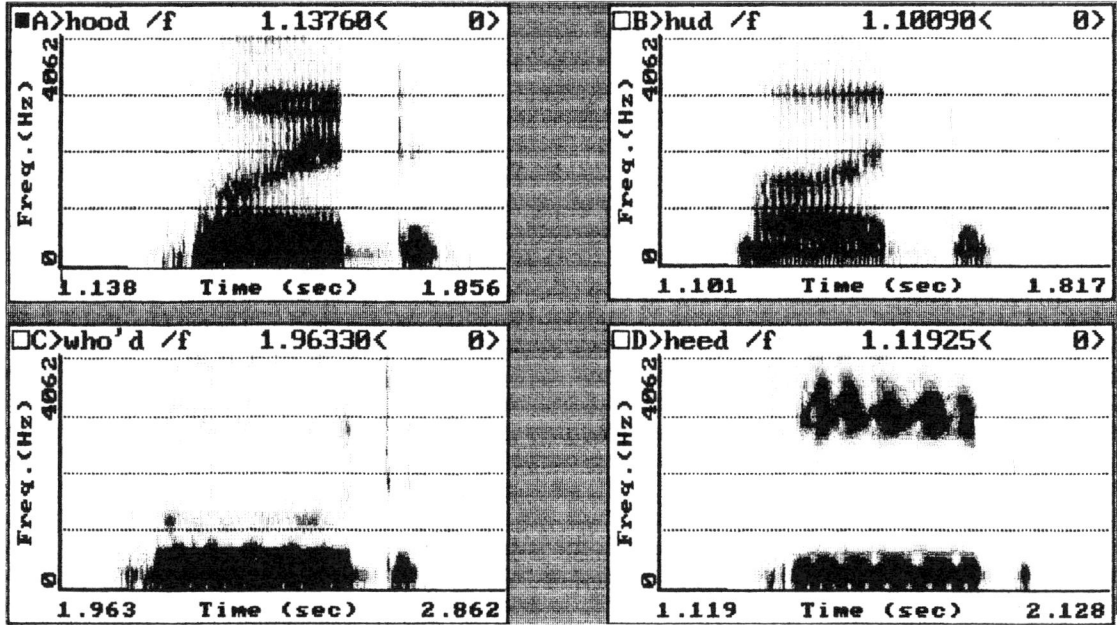

Student   Date

Sample wide-band spectrograms of a 5-year-old girl:

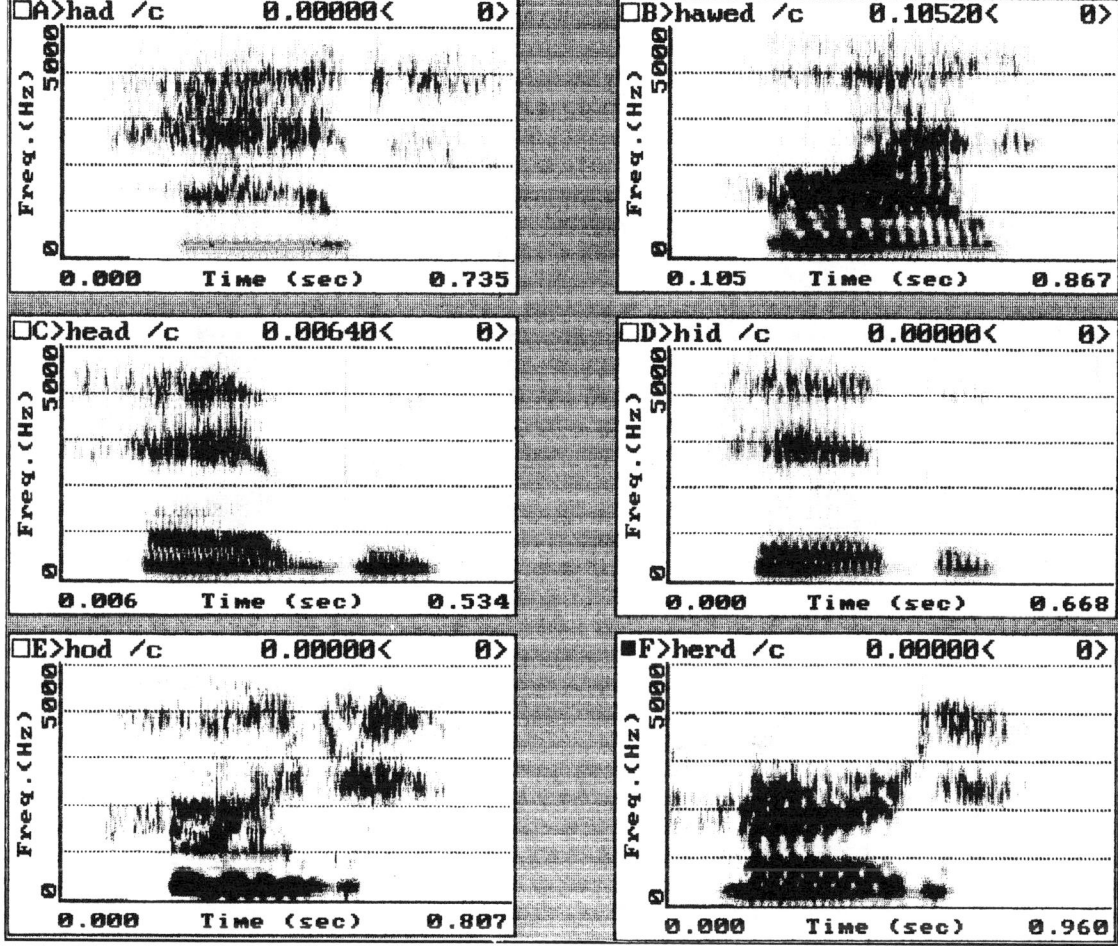

Student   Date

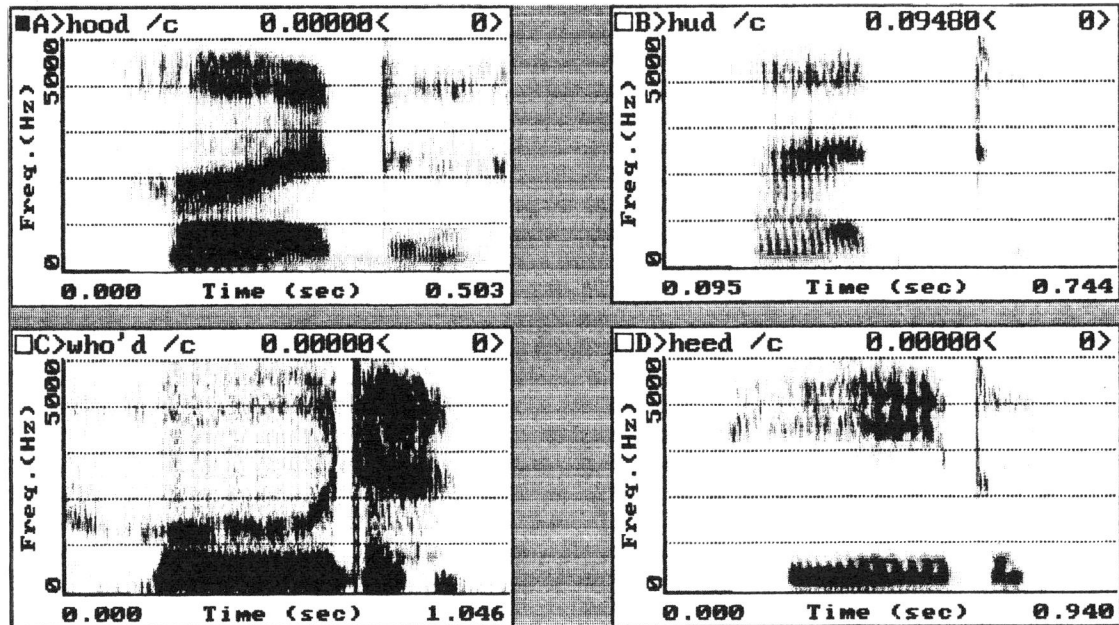

Student _____   Date _____

1. Complete the following table based on your formant data:

		Formant Frequencies (in Hz)					
		Male		Female		Child	
	Vowel	F1	F2	F1	F2	F1	F2
[i]	heed	_____	_____	_____	_____	_____	_____
[ɪ]	hid	_____	_____	_____	_____	_____	_____
[ɛ]	head	_____	_____	_____	_____	_____	_____
[æ]	had	_____	_____	_____	_____	_____	_____
[ɑ]	hod	_____	_____	_____	_____	_____	_____
[ɔ]	hawed	_____	_____	_____	_____	_____	_____
[ʊ]	hood	_____	_____	_____	_____	_____	_____
[u]	who'd	_____	_____	_____	_____	_____	_____
[ʌ]	hud	_____	_____	_____	_____	_____	_____
[ɝ]	herd	_____	_____	_____	_____	_____	_____

Student _____ Date _____

4–6. Use the following graph to plot the F1–F2 planes of each of your speakers.

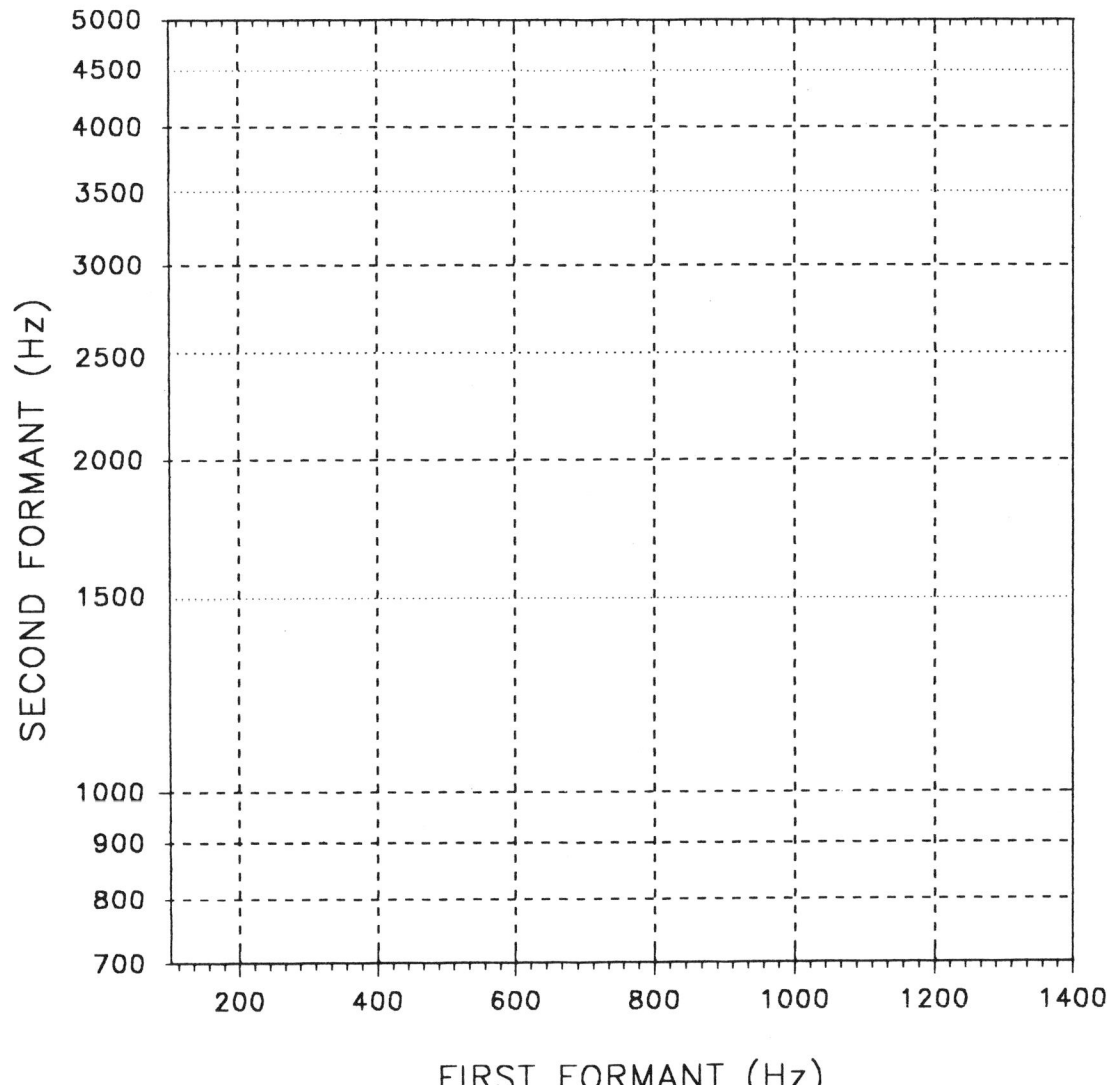

Student _____ Date _____

7. Relationship of formant locations in the F1–F2 plane and the vowel quadrilateral:

_____
_____
_____
_____
_____
_____
_____
_____
_____

8. Change in location of formants as a function of speaker category: _____

_____
_____
_____
_____
_____
_____
_____
_____
_____

Student   Date

9. Patient description: _____

_____

_____

_____

Attach your patient's spectrograms to this page. The following samples are from a 4½-year-old female speaker with delayed articulatory maturation.

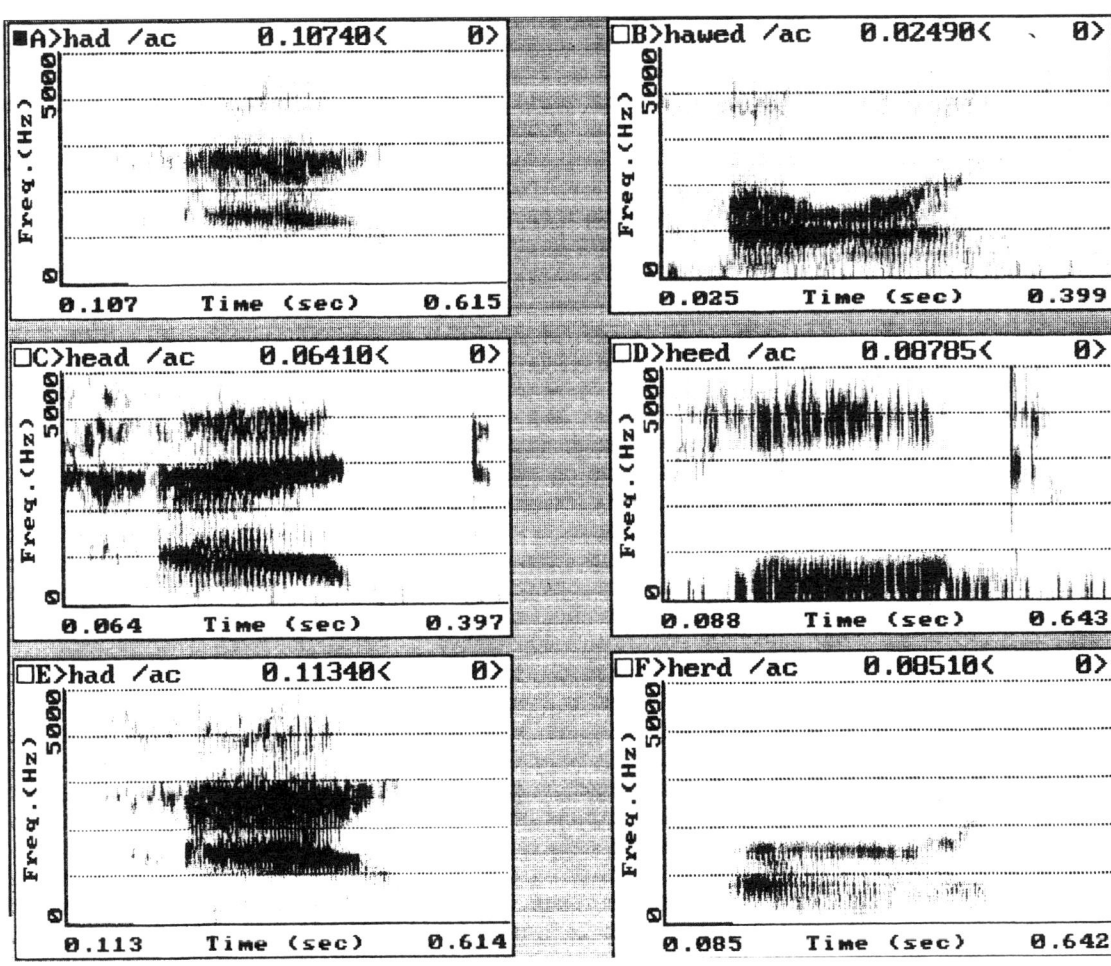

Student   Date

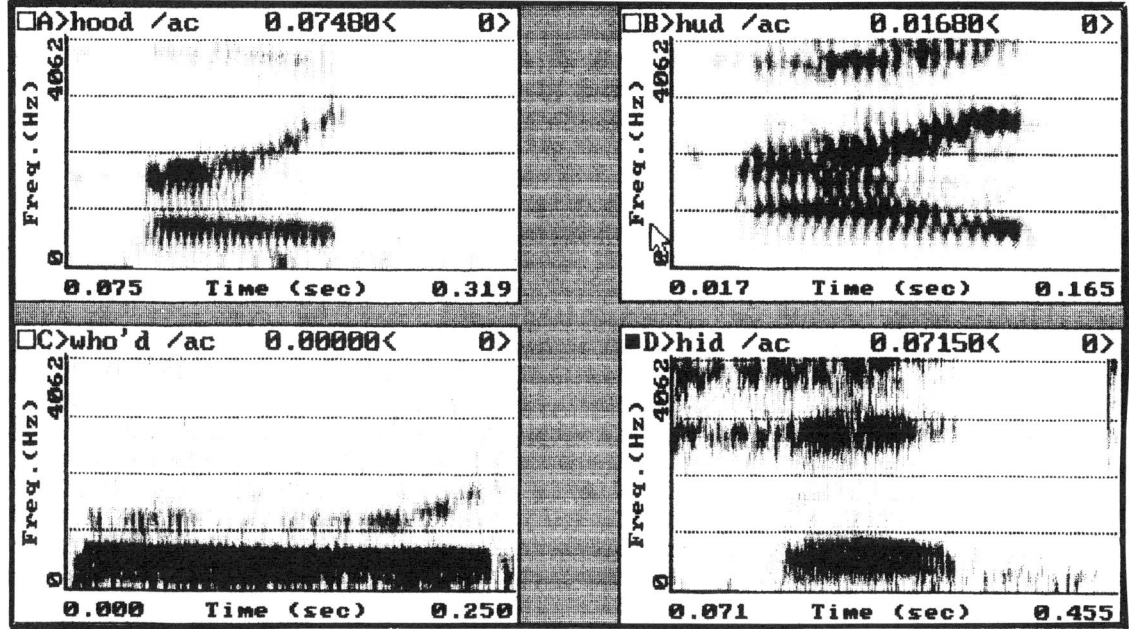

Complete the following table using your patient's formant data:

Vowel		Formant Frequencies (in Hz)	
		F1	F2
[i]	heed	_____	_____
[ɪ]	hid	_____	_____
[ə]	head	_____	_____
[æ]	had	_____	_____
[ɑ]	hod	_____	_____
[ɔ]	hawed	_____	_____
[ʊ]	hood	_____	_____
[u]	who'd	_____	_____
[ʌ]	hud	_____	_____
[ɝ]	herd	_____	_____

Student _____   Date _____

Use the following graph to plot the F1–F2 plane of your patient.

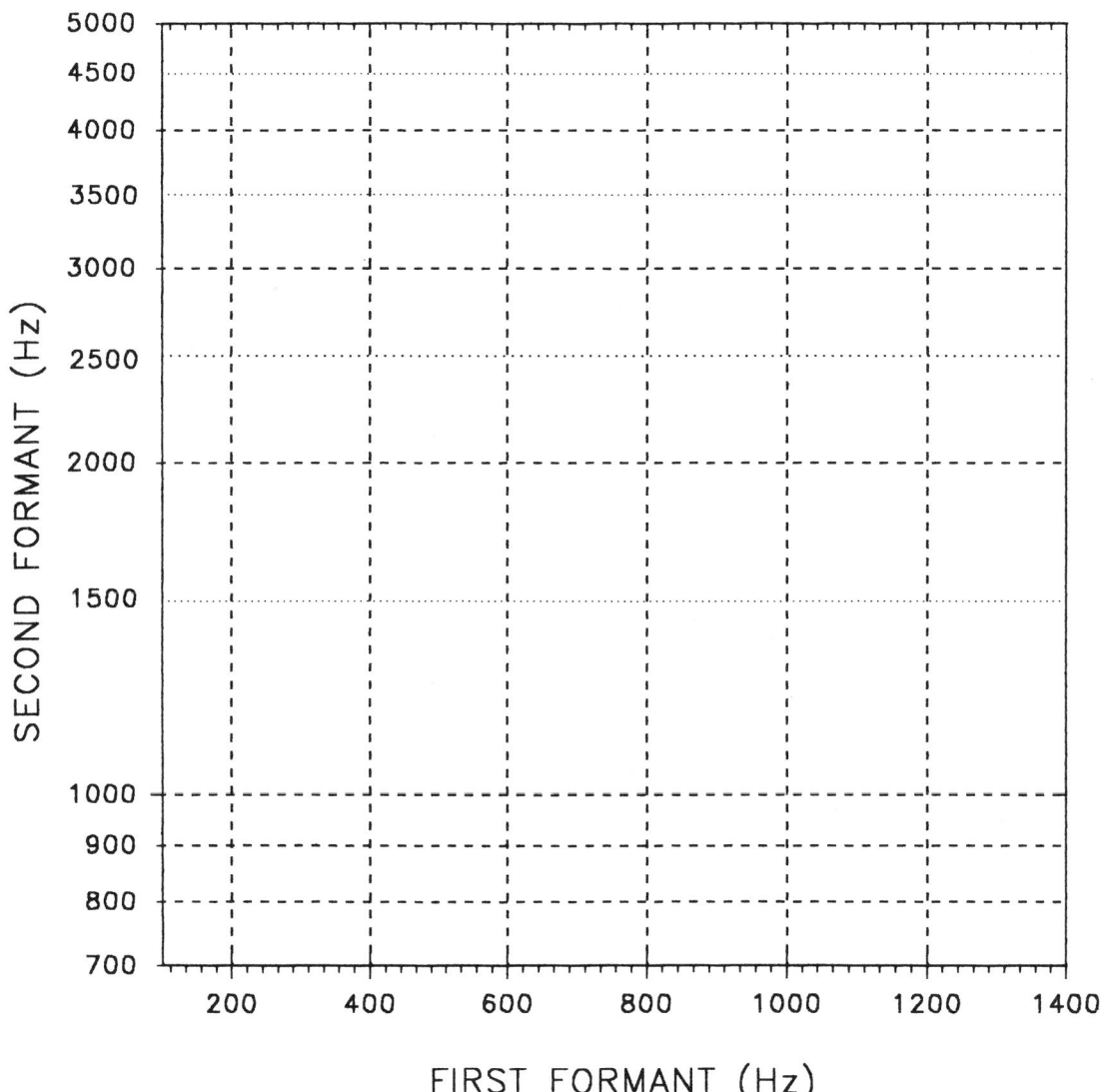

UNIT 30

Clinical Application: Spectrography — Sonorants

A *sonorant* is a consonant that depends on a manipulation of vocal tract resonance for its production. Therefore, formant targets — largely of F2 and F3 — and transitions are their most salient characteristic. Sonorants include *nasal* (/m/, /n/, and /ŋ/) and *approximant* consonants. The approximants may be further subdivided into *liquids* (/r/ and /l/) and *glides* (/w/ and /j/), also known as *semivowels*.

In general, the production of an approximant involves a greater constriction than is used in the production of pure vowels and a quicker, more extreme movement of the vocal tract than is used for diphthongs. However, these movements and the resulting formant transitions are considerably slower than those of all other consonants. This, and the general reduction in acoustic energy caused by the increased vocal tract constriction, make them rather distinctive on the spectrogram.

Nasal consonants are characterized by a great deal of low frequency energy (in the vicinity of the fundamental frequency), called a *nasal murmur*. There is often a clear distinction between an adjacent vowel and a nasal consonant that reflects the relatively quick onset of oral closure. The place of nasal consonant articulation is largely tied to the second formant transition as well as to the location of acoustic zeros (or *antiresonances*) in the spectra (see Pickett, 1980, pp. 73–77 and 121–128).

Because the production of sonorants requires a carefully timed and coordinated vocal tract adjustment, they are among those consonants most commonly misarticulated by patients with dysarthria or with disrupted or delayed speech learning.

Purpose: In these exercises you will become familiar with the spectral characteristics of nasal and approximant consonants. You will also perform some rudimentary spectral analyses of misarticulated sonorants.

Equipment: A microphone and/or tape recorder and sound spectrograph (analog or digital).

General preparation: Read about the formant structure of nasal and approximant consonants (Ohde & Sharf, 1992; Pickett, 1980). Review what is known about the influence of speech rate, sound position, and coarticulatory effects on them.

I. NASAL CONSONANTS

1. Using either a tape recorder or a direct microphone input to a spectrograph,[1] have a normal speaker say "mow" and "no" at a moderate rate.

2. Obtain a wide-band spectrogram of these utterances (with the audio waveform, if possible with your system).

3. Locate and label each phone on each of the spectrographic records. (Sample records from a normal male speaker are available on the hand-in sheet.)

   a. Draw a vertical line separating the initial consonant from the adjacent vowel. Do this for "mow" and "no."

   b. Looking only to the left of each line (that is, during nasal consonant production), locate and label the nasal murmur, the first and second formants, and any apparent antiresonances. What spectral differences do you note?

   c. Looking to the right of each line (that is, during the following vowel), locate and identify the second formant transition. Compare and contrast the two spectrograms.

4. Obtain a wide-band spectrogram of another normal speaker saying the words "some" and "sun" at a moderate rate. Again, print these spectrograms with a simultaneous acoustic trace at the top. Be sure to label this record as you did before.

5. Compare and contrast these spectrograms with those you obtained earlier for "mow" and "no."

II. APPROXIMANTS

1. Obtain a wide-band spectrogram of a normal speaker's production of the phrases "a ray," "a lay," "a way," and "a yea" with their respective acoustic waveforms. (Again, sample records from a normal male speaker are available on the hand-in sheet.)

---

[1] Extraneous room noise will degrade the recording and potentially confound the analysis. Therefore, it is best to place your patient in a quiet or sound-attenuating room (IAC booth).

2. Locate and label each phone on the spectrographic record.

3. Compare [r] and [l]. Determine the relative frequency of F1, F2, and F3. Also determine whether the acoustic energy present at the higher frequencies is relatively high or low. (See the table on the hand-in sheet.)

4. Based on this information, speculate on the salient acoustic characteristics that distinguish these consonants.

5. Compare [w] and [j] as you did [r] and [l] to complete the table on the hand-in sheet.

6. Based on this information, speculate on the salient acoustic characteristics that distinguish these two consonants.

7. Obtain spectrograms of the same phrases spoken by a patient with an articulatory disorder. After carefully labeling the spectrograms and oscillograms, compare the displays with those you had gotten earlier from the normal speaker. In particular, assess this patient's spectrograms with respect to: (a) duration; (b) acoustic energy; (c) formant transition/trajectory; (d) continuity; (e) voicing and voice quality; and (f) extraneous noise.

An example (of the phrase "a yea" /ə jeɪ/) obtained from a 58-year-old dysarthric man is provided below.

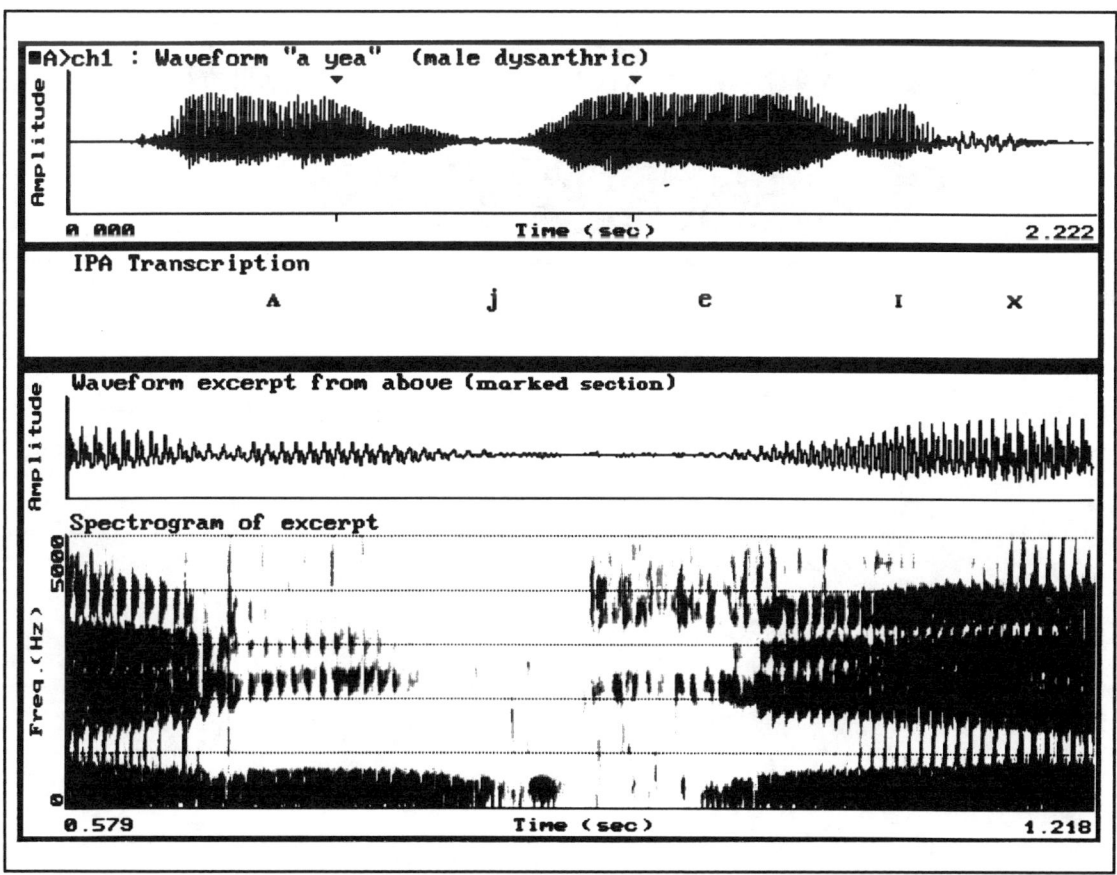

8. Tape record the same or another patient reading the Rainbow Passage (Appendix D) at a comfortable rate. From this sample extract a word or short phrase containing one or more sonorants for spectrographic analysis. Label the phones in the spectrogram and evaluate it as you did above.

Examples (of the word "colors") are shown below as spoken by the same dysarthric patient and on the next page as spoken by a normal adult woman.

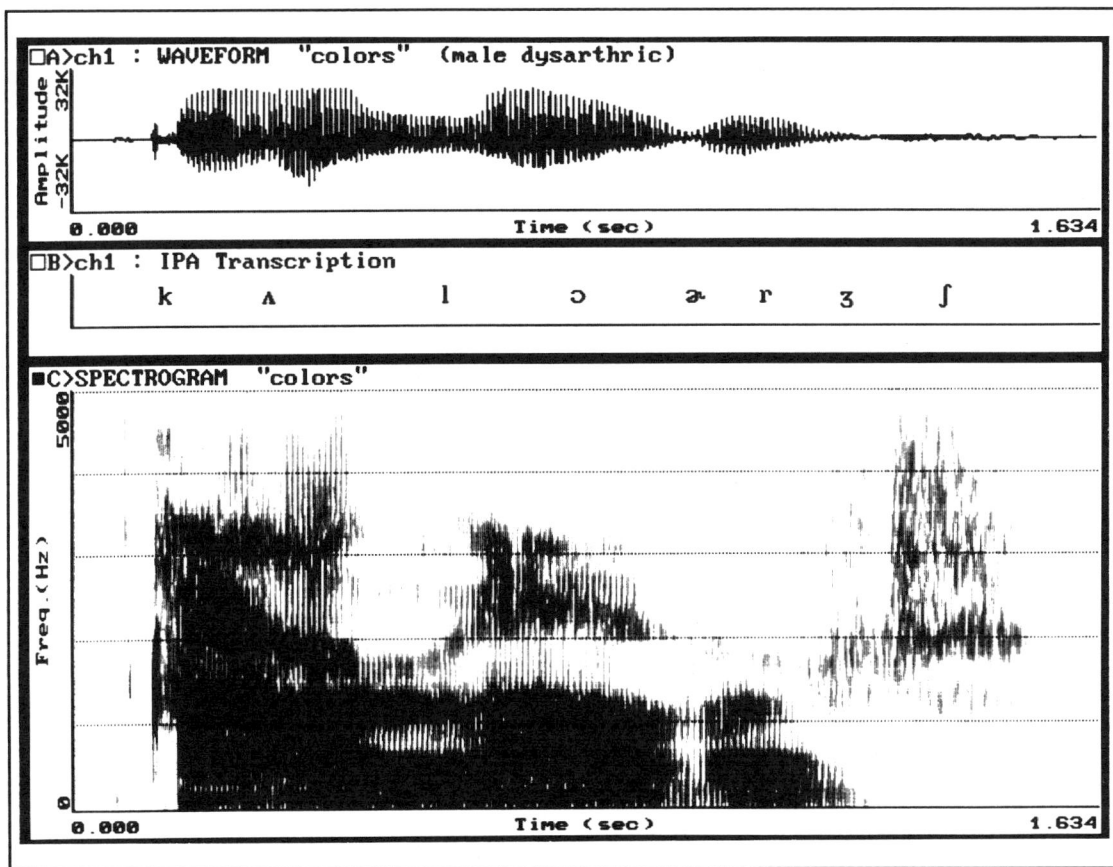

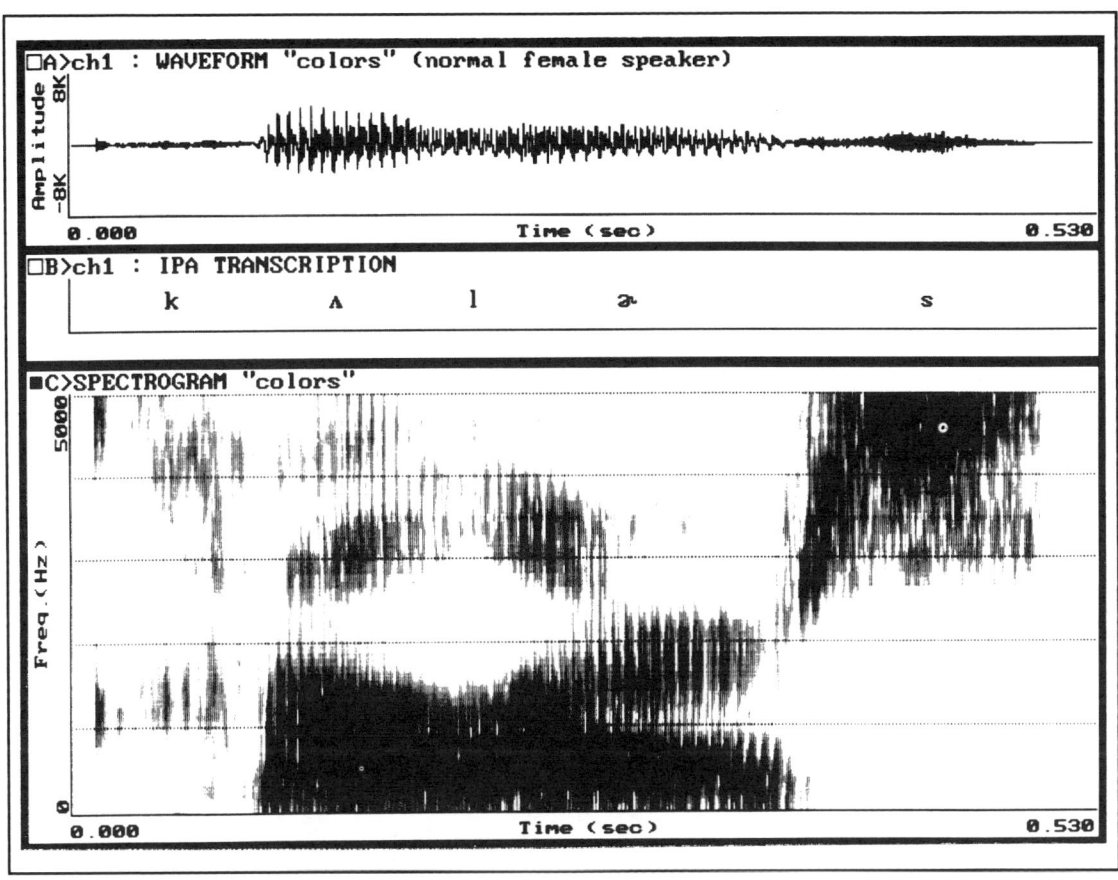

READ MORE ABOUT IT!

Baken, R. J. (1987). *Clinical measurement of speech and voice* (pp. 365–375). Boston: Little, Brown.

Curtis, J. F., & Hardy, J. C. (1959). A phonetic study of misarticulation of /r/. *Journal of Speech and Hearing Research, 2,* 244–257.

Dalston, R. M. (1975). Acoustic characteristics of English /w, r, l/ spoken correctly by young children and adults. *Journal of the Acoustical Society of America, 57,* 462–469.

Fujimura, O. (1962). Analysis of nasal consonants. *Journal of the Acoustical Society of America, 34,* 1865–1875.

Hoffman, P. R., Schuckers, G. H., & Daniloff, R. G. (1989). *Children's phonetic disorders: Theory and treatment.* Boston: Little, Brown.

Hoffman, P. R., Schuckers, G. H., & Ratusnik, D. L. (1977). Contextual-coarticulatory inconsistency of /r/ misarticulation. *Journal of Speech and Hearing Research, 20,* 631–643.

Klein, R. P. (1971). Acoustic analysis of the acquisition of acceptable r in American English. *Child Development, 42,* 543–550.

Kurowski, K., & Blumstein, S. E. (1984). Perceptual integration of the murmur and formant transitions for place of articulation in nasal consonants. *Journal of the Acoustical Society of America, 76,* 383–390.

Kurowski, K., & Blumstein, S. E. (1987). Acoustic properties for place of articulation in nasal consonants. *Journal of the Acoustical Society of America, 81,* 1917–1927.

Lehiste, I., & Peterson, G. E. (1961). Transitions, glides, and diphthongs. *Journal of the Acoustical Society of America, 33,* 268–277.

Lisker, L. (1957). Minimal cues for separating /w, j, r, l/ in intervocalic position. *Word, 13,* 256–267.

O'Connor, J. D., Gerstman, L. J., Liberman, A. M., Delattre, P. G., & Cooper, F. S. (1957). Acoustic cues for the perception of initial /w, j, r, l/ in English. *Word, 13,* 24–43.

Ohde, R. N., & Sharf, D. J. (1992). *Phonetic analysis of normal and abnormal speech* (pp. 55–93). New York: Merrill.

Pickett, J. M. (1965). Some acoustic cues for synthesis of the /n-d/ distinction. *Journal of the Acoustical Society of America, 38,* 474–477.

Pickett, J. M. (1980). *The sounds of speech communication.* Austin, TX: Pro-Ed.

Repp, B. H. (1986). Perception of the [m]-[n] distinction in CV syllables. *Journal of the Acoustical Society of America, 79,* 1987–1999.

Sharf, D. J., & Benson, P. J. (1982). Identification of synthesized /r-w/ continua for adult and child speakers. *Journal of the Acoustical Society of America, 71,* 1008–1015.

Sharf, D. J., & Ohde, R. N. (1983). Perception of distorted "r" sounds in the synthesized speech of children and adults. *Journal of Speech and Hearing Research, 26,* 516–524.

Student   Date

SPECTROGRAPHY: SONORANTS

I. NASAL CONSONANTS

Below is the acoustic waveform and respective wide-band spectrograms of the words "mow" and "no" spoken by a normal man. The "tags" or "wedges" above the oscillogram correspond to the beginning and end of each spectrographic display. This record was obtained using the Kay Elemetrics Computerized Speech Lab (CSL™) system.

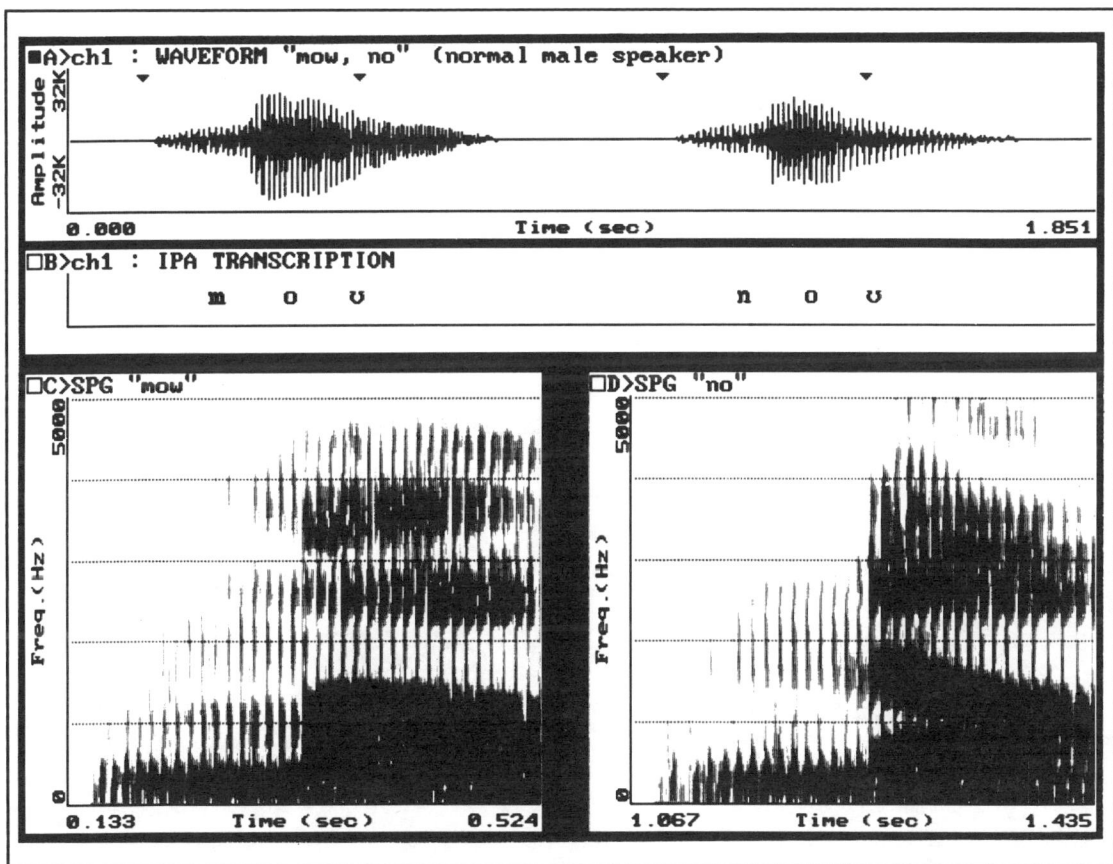

Attach your labeled spectrograms to this page.

Student _____   Date _____

3. b. Spectral differences, [m] vs. [n]: _____

_____
_____
_____
_____
_____
_____

c. Compare and contrast (vowel portion): _____

_____
_____
_____
_____
_____
_____

5. Compare and contrast ("some" and "sun" vs. "mow" and "no"):

_____
_____
_____
_____
_____
_____
_____

Student   Date

II. APPROXIMANTS

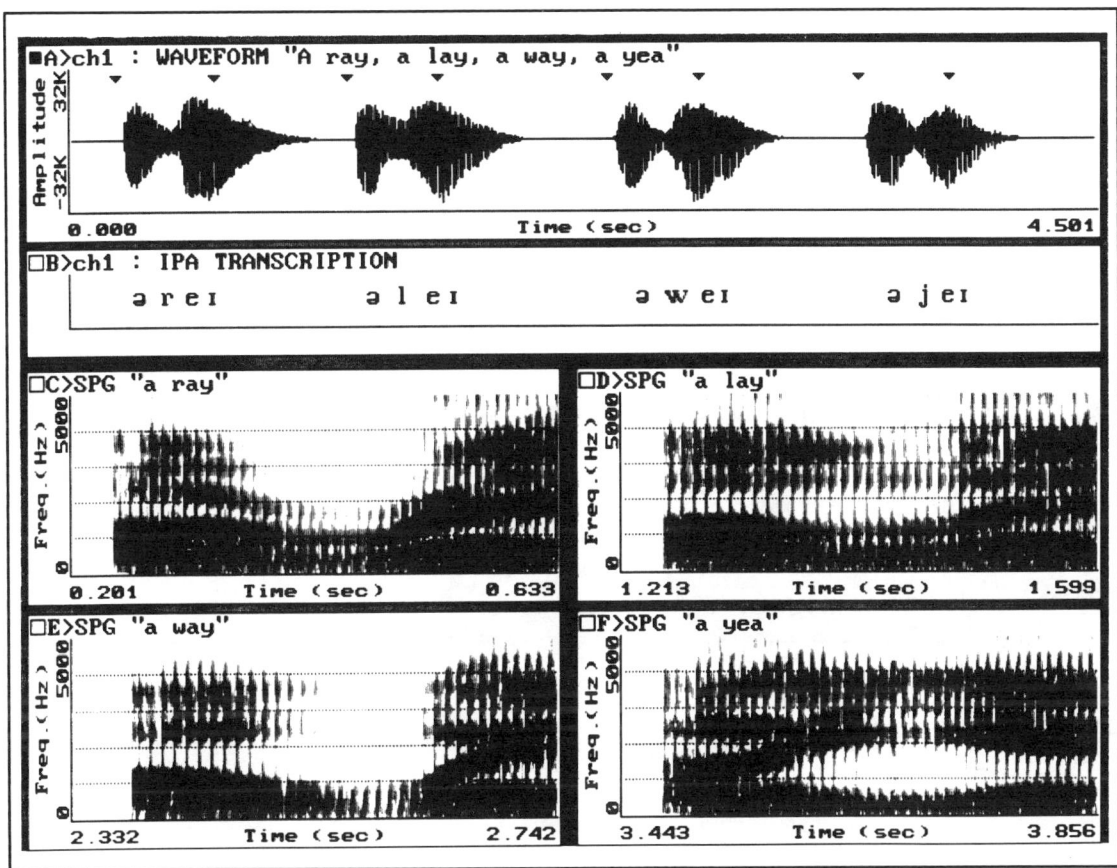

Student _____ Date _____

3. Comparison of [r] and [l]. Circle your answer:

Consonant	Formant Characteristics		
[r]	F1 frequency is relatively:	low	high
	F2 frequency is relatively:	low	high
	F3 frequency is relatively:	low	high
	Energy at higher formants is relatively:	low	high
[l]	F1 frequency is relatively:	low	high
	F2 frequency is relatively:	low	high
	F3 frequency is relatively:	low	high
	Energy at higher formants is relatively:	low	high

4. Salient acoustic characteristics: _____

_____

_____

_____

_____

_____

_____

Student _____ Date _____

3. Comparison of [w] and [j]. Circle your answer.

Consonant	Formant Characteristics		
[w]	F1 frequency is relatively:	low	high
	F2 frequency is relatively:	low	high
	F3 frequency is relatively:	low	high
	Energy at higher formants is relatively:	low	high
[j]	F1 frequency is relatively:	low	high
	F2 frequency is relatively:	low	high
	F3 frequency is relatively:	low	high
	Energy at higher formants is relatively:	low	high

6. Salient acoustic characteristics: _____

_____

_____

_____

_____

_____

_____

Student _____   Date _____

7. Patient: _____

   Utterances: _____

   _____

   Assessment/comparison: _____

   _____

   _____

   _____

   _____

   _____

   _____

   _____

   _____

   _____

8. Patient: _____

   Extracted word(s): _____

   Spectrographic analysis: _____

   _____

   _____

   _____

   _____

   _____

   _____

   _____

   _____

   _____

UNIT 31

Clinical Application: Spectrography — Fricatives

Fricatives are consonants whose production depends on the placement of a narrow constriction that results in a turbulent airflow at some point in the vocal tract. The turbulence noise, distributed over various frequency ranges (depending on the place of articulation), is called *frication*. Fricative consonants are further classified as either *sibilant* or *nonsibilant*. The sibilant consonants include /s/, /z/, /ʃ/ and /ʒ/. They are characterized by greater turbulence noise, especially at the higher frequencies. This results in a more "strident" quality than the nonsibilant sounds (/h/, /f/, /v/, /θ/, and /ð/). "Lisping" occurs when a fricative such as /s/ and /z/ loses its sibilant quality; that is, frication energy shifts from the higher to the lower frequencies in the spectrum (Daniloff, Wilcox, & Stephens, 1980). Other pathologies, such as cleft palate and the motor speech disorders, often result in inappropriately placed vocal tract occlusions that produce frication noise falling outside normal allophonic variation. Thus bilabial (/ɸ/, /β/), velar (/x/, /ɣ/), uvular (/χ/, /ʁ/), and pharyngeal (/ħ/, /ʕ/) fricatives (Ladefoged, 1982) are commonly produced by such patients as a distortion of the intended consonant.

Purpose: In these exercises you will practice identifying the spectral characteristics associated with normally and abnormally produced fricative consonants.

Equipment: A microphone and/or tape recorder and sound spectrograph (analog or digital).

General preparation: Read about the spectral properties of sibilant and nonsibilant consonants (Ohde & Sharf, 1992; Pickett, 1980). Review what is known about the influence of speech rate, sound position, and coarticulatory effects on these sounds.

I. SIBILANTS

1. Using either a tape recorder or a direct microphone input to a spectrograph, have a normal speaker say "sigh" and "shy" at a moderate rate.

2. Obtain a wide-band spectrogram of these utterances (with the audio waveform, if possible). Be sure that the frequency range of your spectrogram extends up to at least 8000 Hz.

3. Locate and label each phone on each of the spectrographic records. (Sample records from a normal female speaker are available on the hand-in sheet.)

4. What spectral features distinguish these fricatives from the vowel and from each other?

5. Obtain a wide-band spectrogram of another normal speaker saying the words "sue" and "zoo" at a moderate rate. Again, print these spectrograms with a simultaneous oscillogram. (See the hand-in sheet for sample spectrograms of these words.) Be sure to label this record as you did before.

6. What acoustic characteristics distinguish these cognates?

7. Obtain spectrograms of isolated words or short phrases spoken by a patient with an articulatory disorder likely to affect sibilant production. After carefully labeling the spectrograms, compare the displays with those you had gotten earlier from the normal speaker. In particular, assess your patient's spectrograms with respect to (a) duration; (b) acoustic energy; (c) distribution of acoustic energy; (d) voicing; and (e) continuity.

   Examples (of the word "soup" /sup/) obtained from a 28-year-old woman with a lateral lisp are shown on the next page, both pre- and post-therapy.

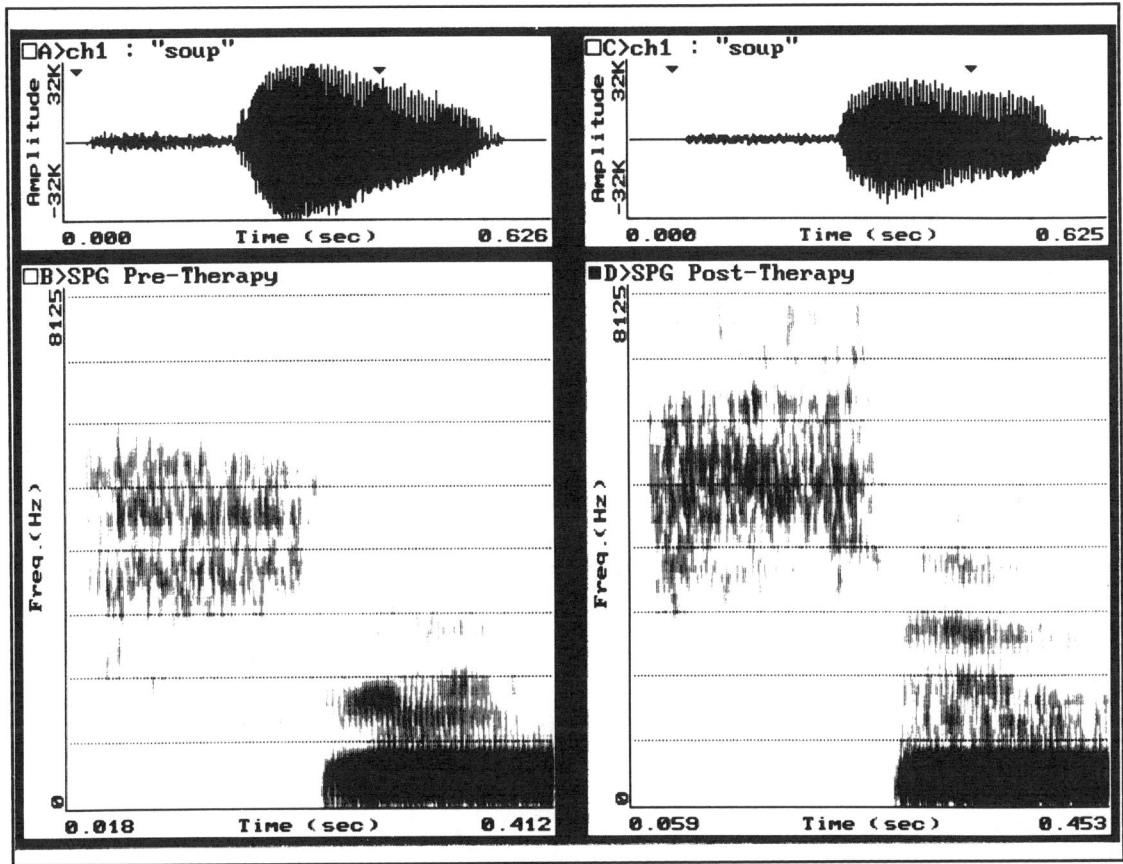

II. NONSIBILANTS

1. Obtain a wide-band spectrogram of a normal speaker's production of the words "high," "fie," and "thigh" with their respective acoustic waveforms.

2. Locate and label each phone on the spectrographic record. (A sample is provided on the hand-in sheet.) What spectral features distinguish these fricatives from each other?

3. How do these sounds differ from the sibilants you analyzed earlier?

4. Obtain a wide-band spectrogram of a normal speaker saying the words "ether" (/i θ ɚ)/) and "either" (/i ð ɚ/) at a moderate rate. Again, print these spectrograms with the audio waveforms. Be sure to label this record as you did before.

5. What characteristic(s) distinguish these voiced/voiceless cognates? Compare these spectrograms to those you obtained earlier of "sue" and "zoo."

6. Tape record a patient reading a standard passage at a comfortable rate. From this sample extract a word or short phrase containing one or more fricatives for spectrographic analysis. Label each of the phones and provide a detailed analysis.

Examples (of the phrase "path high above") are shown below as spoken by a 43-year-old dysarthric male and on the next page as spoken by a normal adult male.

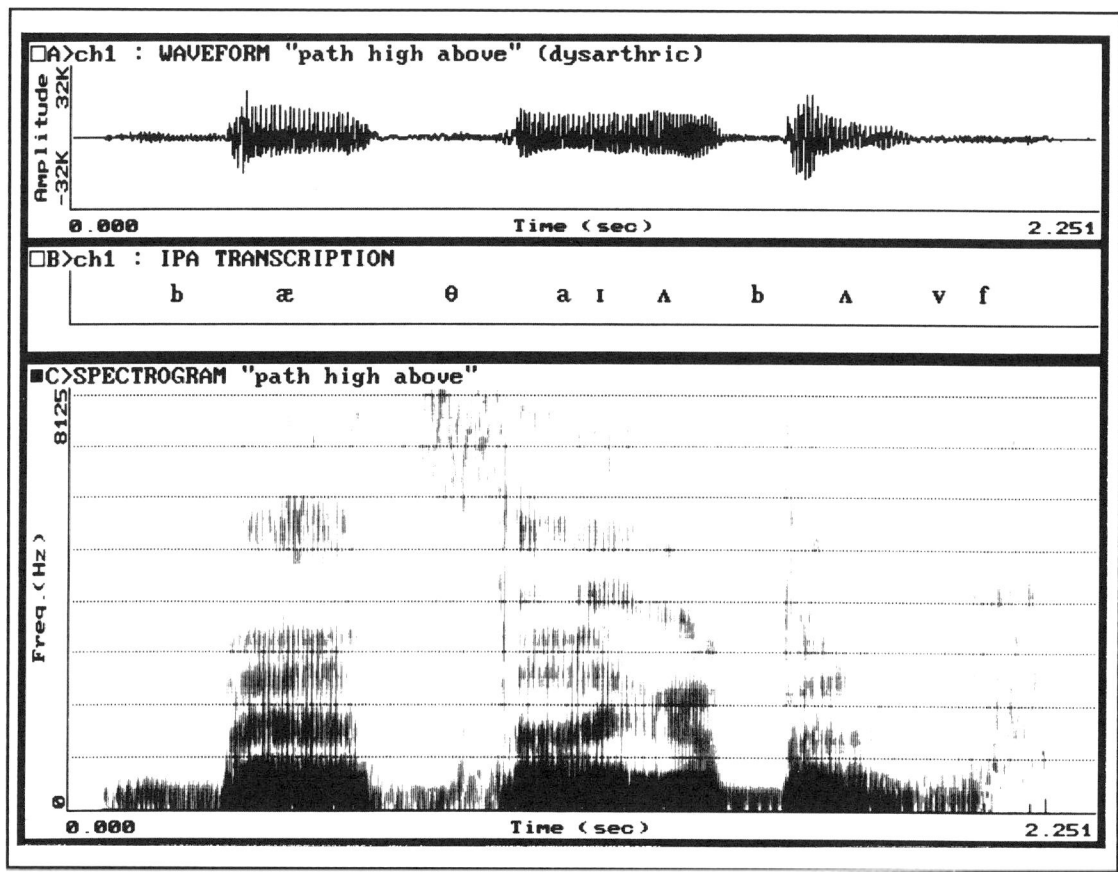

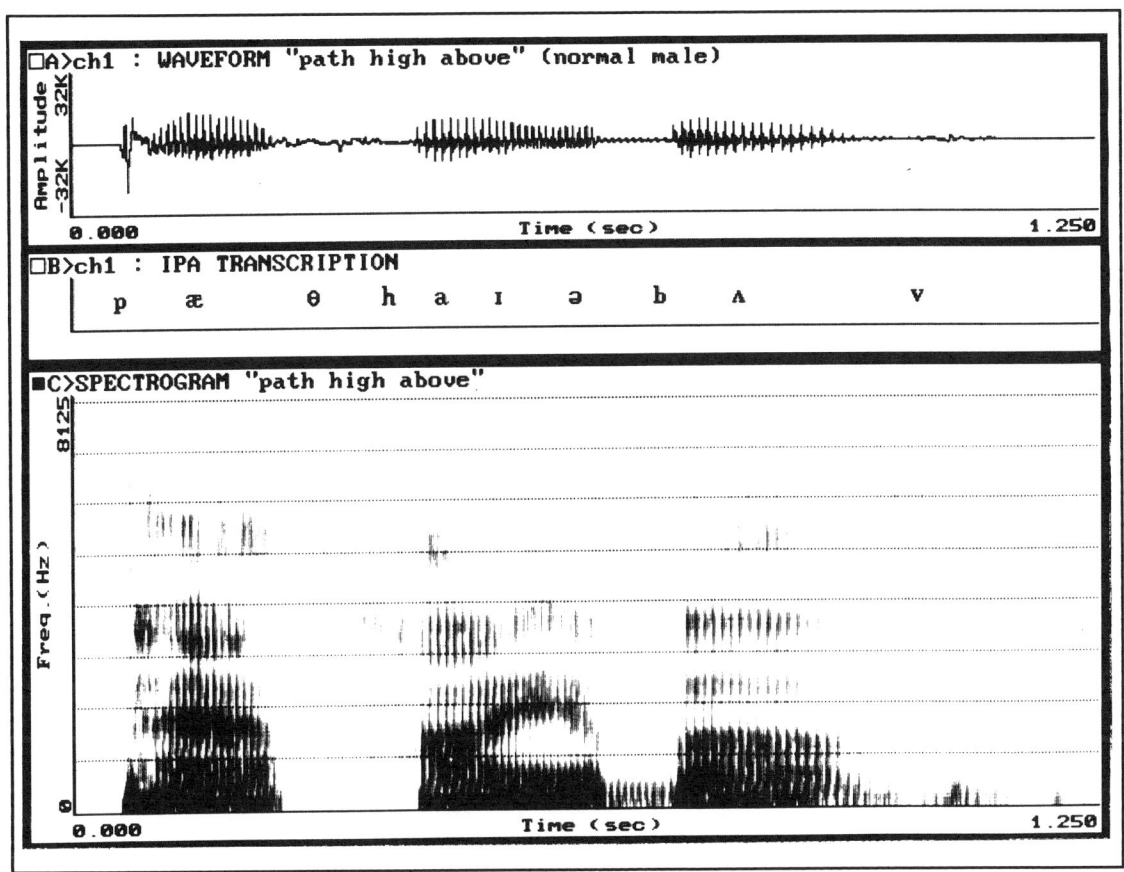

READ MORE ABOUT IT!

Baken, R. J. (1987). *Clinical measurement of speech and voice* (pp. 366–369). Boston: Little, Brown.

Bauer, H. R., & Kent, R. D. (1987). Acoustic analyses of infant fricative and trill vocalizations. *Journal of the Acoustical Society of America, 81,* 505–511.

Behrens, S. J., & Blumstein, S. E. (1988). Acoustic characteristics of English voiceless fricatives: A descriptive analysis. *Journal of Phonetics, 16,* 295–298.

Daniloff, R. G., Wilcox, K., & Stephens, M. I. (1980). An acoustic-articulatory description of children's defective /s/ productions. *Journal of Communication Disorders, 13,* 347–363.

Harris, K. S. (1958). Cues for the discrimination of American English fricatives in spoken syllables. *Language and Speech, 1,* 1–7.

Heinz, J. M., & Stevens, K. N. (1961). On the properties of voiceless fricative consonants. *Journal of the Acoustical Society of America, 33,* 589–596.

Hughes, G. W., & Halle, M. (1956). Spectral properties of fricative consonants. *Journal of the Acoustical Society of America, 28,* 303–310.

Kawano, M., Isshiki, N., Harita, Y., & Tanokuchi, F. (1985). Laryngeal fricative in cleft palate speech. *Acta Otolaryngologica, Suppl. 419,* 180–188.

Ladefoged, P. (1982). *A course in phonetics* (2nd ed., pp. 143–153). New York: Harcourt Brace Jovanovich.

Mazza, P. L., Schuckers, G. H., & Daniloff, R. G. (1979). Contextual-coarticulatory inconsistency of /s/ misarticulation. *Journal of Phonetics, 7,* 57–69.

Nittrouer, S., Studdert-Kennedy, M., & McGowan, R. S. (1989). The emergence of phonetic segments: Evidence from the spectral structure of fricative-vowel syllbles spoken by children and adults. *Journal of Speech and Hearing Research, 32,* 120–132.

Ohde, R. N., & Sharf, D. J. (1992). *Phonetic*

analysis of normal and abnormal speech (pp. 190–207). New York: Merrill.

Pentz, A., Gilbert, H. R., & Zawadzki, P. (1979). Spectral properties of fricative consonants in children. *Journal of the Acoustical Society of America, 66,* 1891–1893.

Pickett, J. M. (1980). *The sounds of speech communication* (pp. 128–131). Austin, TX: PRO ED.

Schwartz, M. F. (1967). Transitions in American English /s/ as cues to the identification of adjacent stop consonants. *Journal of the Acoustical Society of America, 42,* 898–899.

Soli, S. D. (1981). Second formants in fricatives: Acoustic consequences of fricative-vowel coarticulation. *Journal of the Acoustical Society of America, 70,* 976–984.

Stevens, K. N. (1971). Airflow and turbulence noise for fricative and stop consonants: Static considerations. *Journal of the Acoustical Society of America, 50,* 1180–1192.

Strevens, P. (1960). Spectra of fricative noise in human speech. *Language and Speech, 3,* 32–49.

Uldall, E. (1964). Transitions in fricative noise. *Language and Speech, 7,* 13–14.

Weismer, G., & Elbert, M. (1982). Temporal characteristics of "functionally" misarticulated /s/ in 4- to 6-year-old children. *Journal of Speech and Hearing Research, 25,* 275–287.

Student   Date

SPECTROGRAPHY: FRICATIVES

I. SIBILANTS

Below is the acoustic waveform and corresponding wide-band spectrogram of the words "sigh" and "shy" spoken by a normal woman. This record was obtained using the Kay Elemetrics Computerized Speech Lab (CSL™) system.

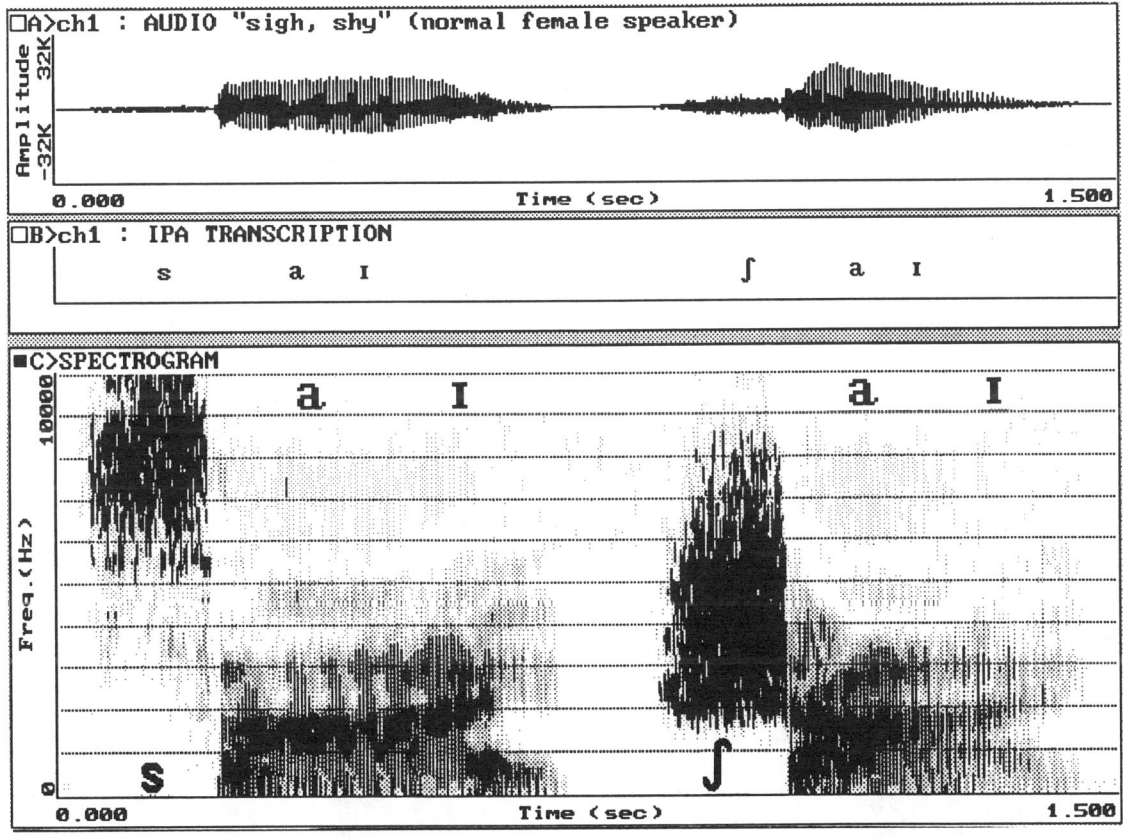

Attach your labeled spectrograms to this page.

Student _____ Date _____

4. Spectral differences: _____

_____

_____

_____

_____

_____

_____

_____

A similar waveform/spectrographic display obtained from the same normal female speaker is shown below:

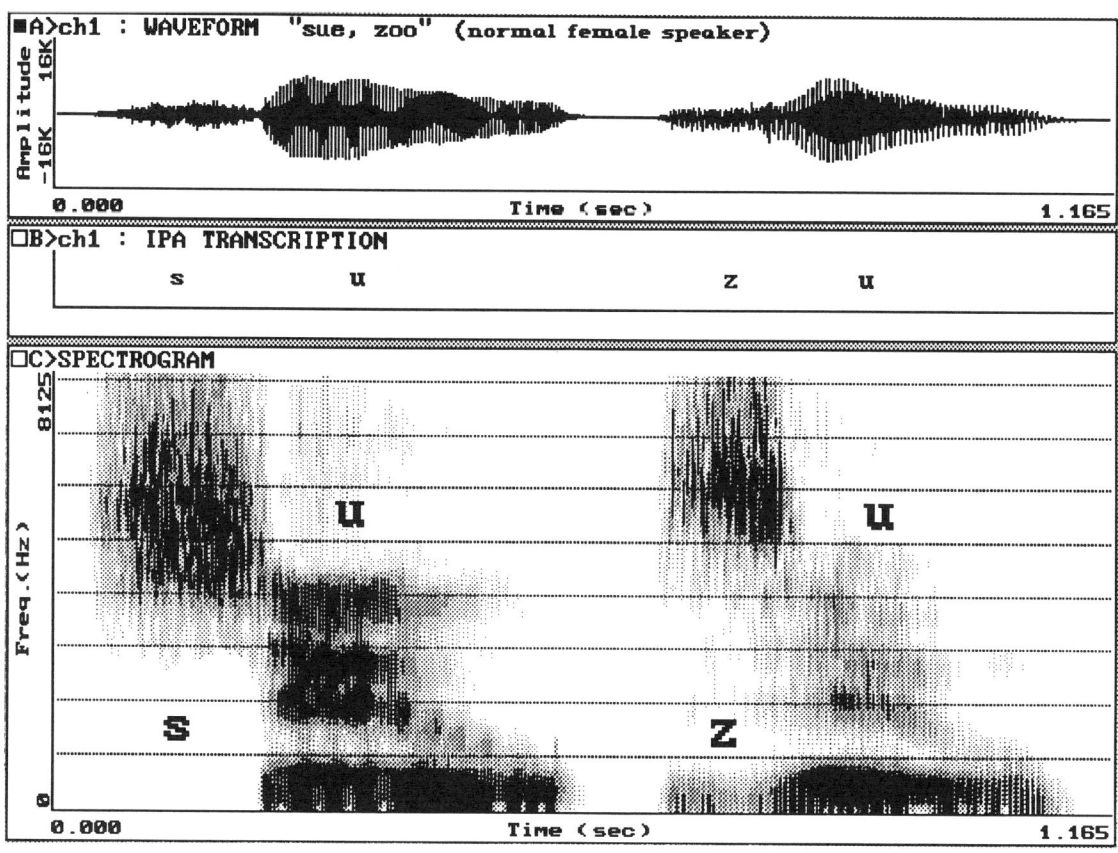

Student _____   Date _____

6. Spectral differences: _____

_____

_____

_____

_____

_____

_____

_____

7. Patient: _____

Utterance(s): _____

_____

Assessment/comparison: _____

_____

_____

_____

_____

_____

_____

_____

_____

Student _____ Date _____

II. NONSIBILANTS

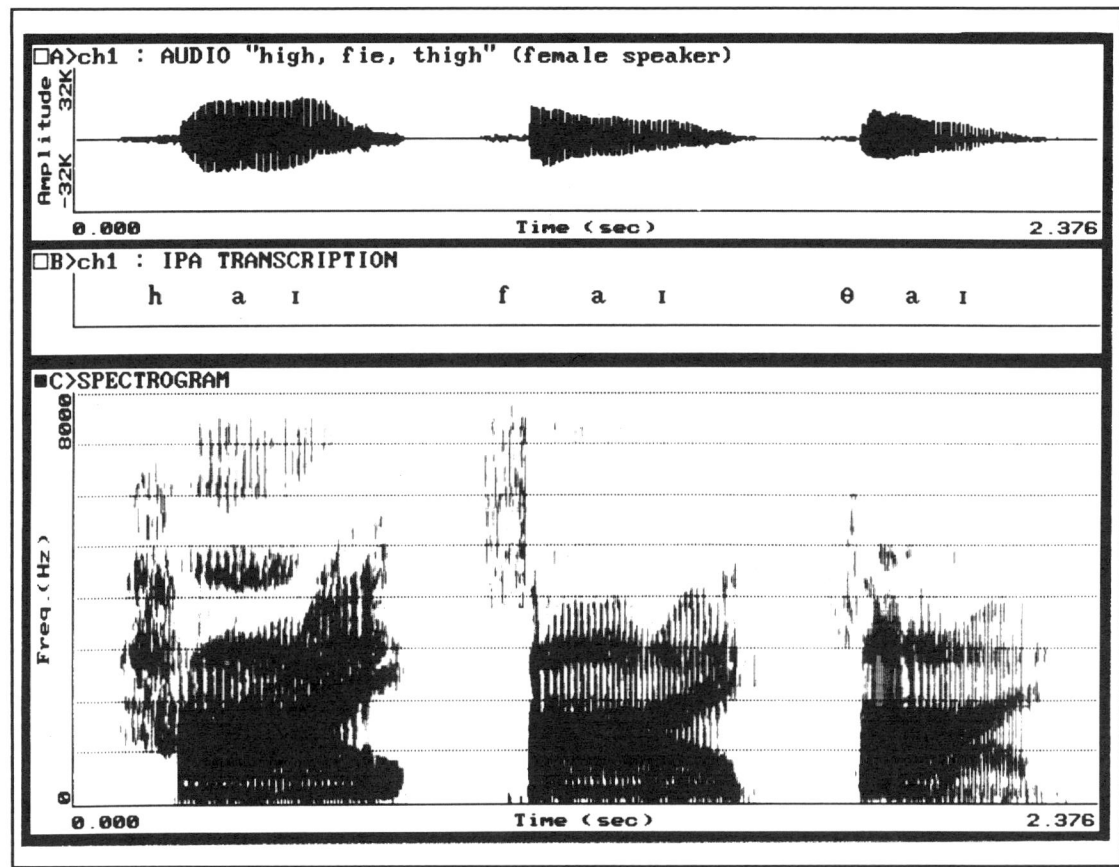

2. Spectral differences: _____

_____

_____

_____

_____

_____

_____

_____

Student _____   Date _____

3. Nonsibilants vs. sibilants: _____

_____

_____

_____

_____

_____

_____

_____

_____

5. [θ] vs. [ð]: _____

_____

_____

_____

_____

_____

_____

_____

_____

_____

_____

_____

Student _____   Date _____

6. Patient: _____

Extracted word(s): _____

Spectrographic analysis: _____

_____

_____

_____

_____

_____

_____

_____

_____

_____

_____

_____

UNIT 32

Clinical Application: Spectrography — Plosives and Affricates

Plosives (also known as stops[1] or stop-plosives) and affricates are consonants produced by completely occluding the vocal tract, temporarily arresting acoustic energy, and then suddenly releasing the tract constriction, resulting in an acoustic burst, or plosion. The presence of minor turbulence noise following the burst is called *aspiration*, and, in English at least, is to be expected in some phonetic contexts. The English plosives include /p/, /b/, /t/, /d/, /k/, and /g/. There is also a glottal plosive, /ʔ/, as produced in [ʔʌʔoʊ] ("uh-oh"); While it is an allophone of /t/ in many dialects — as in [kʌʔn] ("cotton") and [bʌʔn] ("button") — it is commonly used by cleft palate speakers to substitute for other plosives. Both structural and neurological damage may prevent a speaker from generating intraoral pressure (P_{io}) sufficient for plosion. This may be due to a ventilatory impairment and/or an inability to completely occlude the vocal tract. Of course, precision and timing are also of great importance. An incomplete or poorly coordinated closure may result in frication rather than plosion. A fricative-like distortion of the plosive consonant is called *spirantization* (Weismer, 1984a, 1984b).

Affricates are produced when a plosive is released, not into a vocalic segment, but into frication (see Unit 31 "Spectrography — Fricatives"). Thus affricates are associated with a silent period during which stop closure is maintained, a plosive burst, and then frication. When an affricate precedes a vowel, the frication, in some phonetic contexts, may be followed by brief aspiration before voicing begins. In English, the affricates include /tʃ/, and its voiced cognate /dʒ/. Common among dysarthrics is the tendency toward *deaffrication*. This occurs when the speaker is un-

---

[1] Because they are produced with an occluded oral cavity, nasals are sometimes included among those consonants referred to as stops; The term "stop-nasal" may be encountered as well.

able to appropriately and completely close the vocal tract, resulting in a fricative-like distortion of the intended affricate.

Purpose: In these exercises you will practice identifying the spectral characteristics associated with normally and abnormally produced plosives and affricates.

Equipment: A microphone and/or tape recorder and sound spectrograph (analog or digital).

General preparation: Read about the spectral properties of plosive and affricate consonants, especially as they relate to manner, place and voicing (Baken, 1987; Kent & Read, 1992; Ohde & Sharf, 1992; Pickett, 1980). Review what is known about the influence of speech rate, sound position, and coarticulatory effects on these sounds.

I. PLOSIVES

While there are many cues to the voicing of plosives, the *voice onset time* (VOT) is the most robust. The VOT is defined as the time between stop release (the burst) and the onset of glottal pulsing. For voiced English plosives, the VOT is relatively short, in general less than 25 ms. Voicing may even precede the burst (prevoicing), resulting in a negative VOT, and is, in fact, very common when a voiced plosive occurs between vocalic segments. Voiceless English plosives tend to have VOTs greater than 45 ms or so. Abnormal VOTs have been identified in the fluent speech of stutterers, as well as in the speech of dysarthrics, apraxics, and phonologically disordered children — even in cases in which the categorically perceived voiced/voiceless distinction is maintained. It is important to remember that the "appropriate" VOT is specified by the phonological rules of a given a language. Language aside, the VOT used by normal speakers does not vary significantly from one repetition of the stimulus to another. Thus high VOT variability, as well as excessive prevoicing or an extended voicing lag, reflect poor coordination between laryngeal function and articulatory movement.

On the next page are the acoustic signals of the words (a) "pig" and (b) "big" spoken in isolation by a normal adult male speaker of American English. From each waveform the release burst and several cycles of glottal pulses have been extracted and a wide-band spectrogram of the excerpt was obtained. To facilitate VOT measurement, vertical lines have been drawn at the burst and at the start of glottal pulsing. The onset of glottal pulsing is usually identified by looking for evidence of the first "glottal striation" in the vicinity of the second formant frequency.[2]

In the case of "pig," the VOT interval extends over 8.9 divisions. Because the time scale is 0.01 seconds/division, the VOT for [p] is 0.089 seconds (or 89 milli-

---

[2] A notable exception to this is when there is evidence of prevoicing. In these cases the first glottal striation identified in the vicinity of the fundamental frequency marks the onset of glottal pulsing.

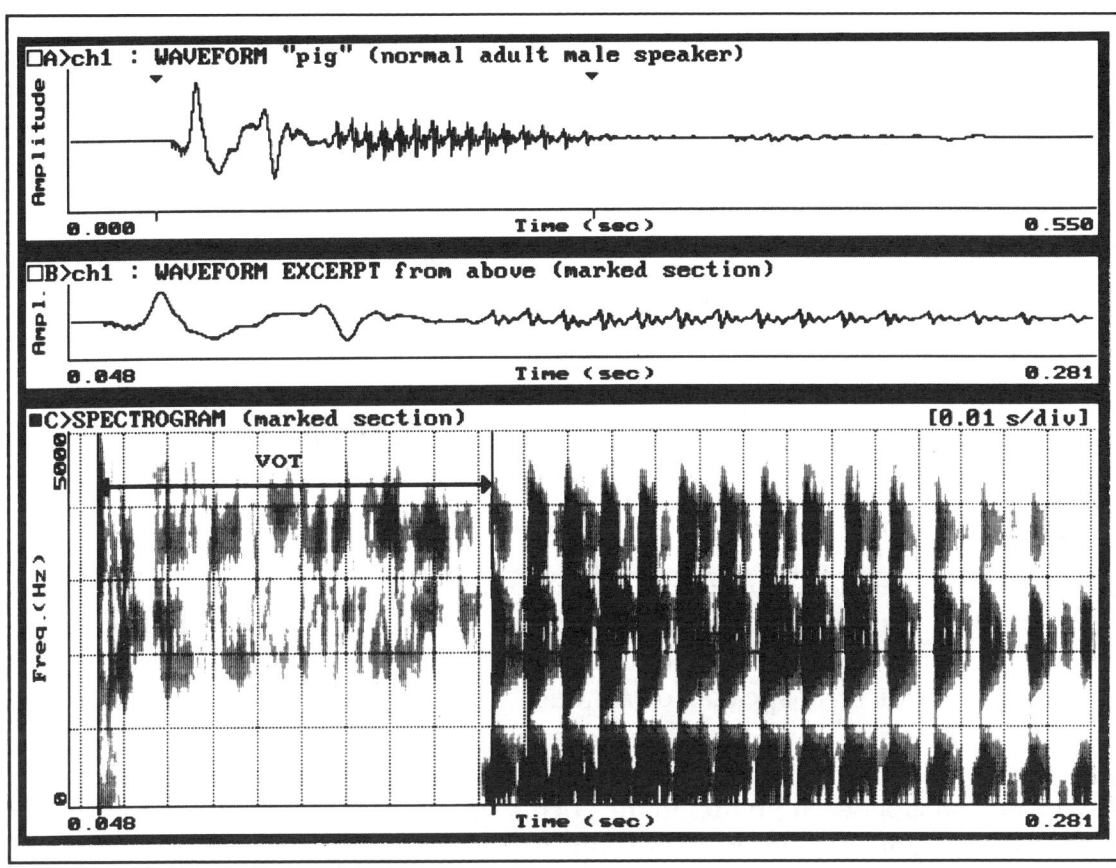
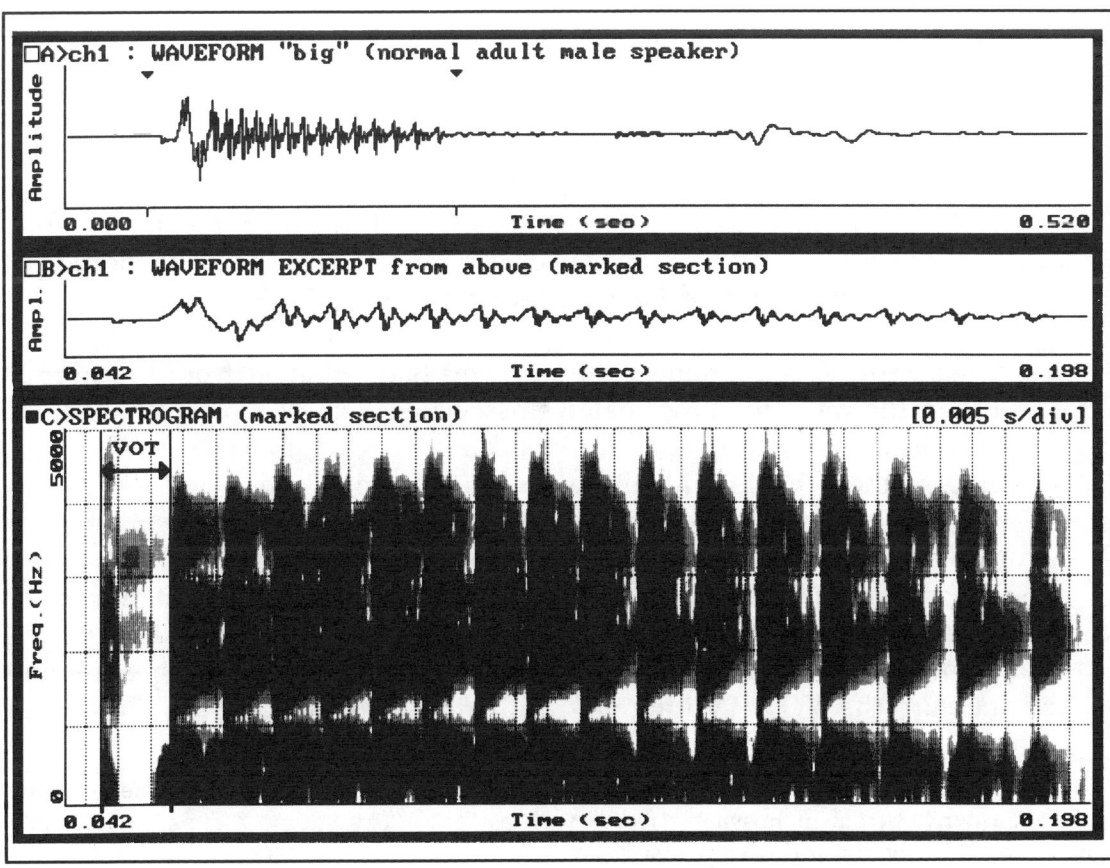

seconds). As for "big," the VOT covers 2.1 divisions. At 0.005 s/div, the VOT for [b] is therefore 0.0105 s (or 10.5 ms).

Using the data displays on the next page, determine the VOTs for the same words spoken by a normal 2-year-old female speaker of American English. Be sure to mark the burst and start of glottal pulsing. How did you select these points? Compare these VOTs with those from the adult speaker.

EXERCISES

1. Using either a tape recorder or a direct microphone input to a spectrograph, have a normal speaker repeat the phrases "It's a peat" and "It's a beat" at a comfortable rate.[3]

2. From each utterance, isolate the last words and obtain wide-band spectrograms of them along with simultaneous audio waveforms. If possible, print the spectrograms with a time scale or timing marks. (Sample spectrograms from a normal 5-year-old male speaker of American English are provided on the hand-in sheet.)

3. Locate and label each phone on the spectrographic record. Mark the location of each burst and the onset of voicing. Indicate any aspiration.

4. **a.** Determine the VOTs for the plosive consonants.

   b. Are they normal for your speaker's age, sex, and native language? According to whom?

5. Obtain similar spectrograms from a patient saying the same phrases. As before, locate and label each phone on the spectrographic record. Mark the location of each burst and the onset of voicing. Indicate any aspiration, if present.

6. **a.** Compare this spectrogram to the one you had obtained from the normal speaker. Indicate any abnormalities associated with the plosive burst.

   b. Compare these VOTs with those you measured above.

7. Record a patient with a known articulatory disorder as he reads the Rainbow Passage (Appendix D). Obtain a wide-band spectrogram of an isolated word or short phrase containing one or more plosives, and be sure to label it. Mark the location of the release burst and the onset of glottal pulsing on the spectrogram and measure the VOT. Indicate any aspiration, if present.

---

[3] To minimize contextual variability while eliciting a more "natural" utterance, VOT measures are most often derived from monosyllabic words such as "pay"/"bay," "time"/"dime," and "coat"/"goat" embedded within a carrier phrase such as "It's a _____" or "Say _____ again."

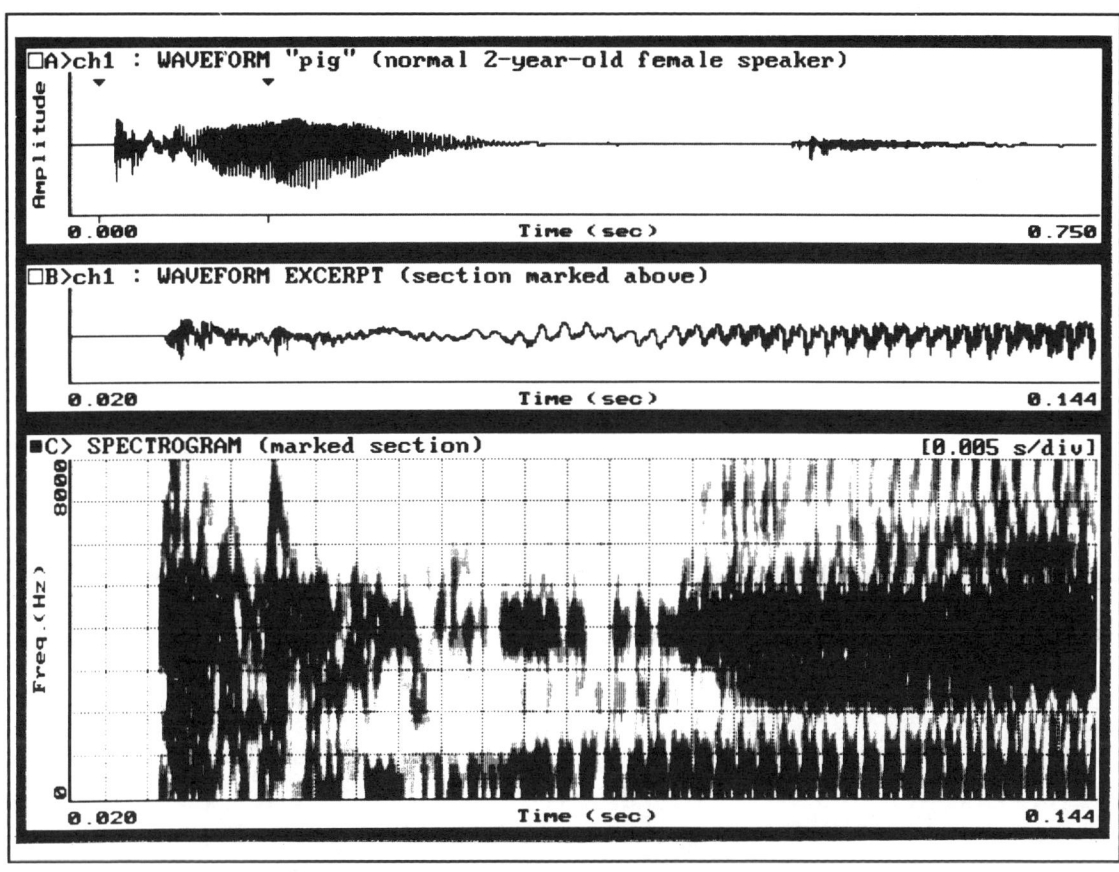
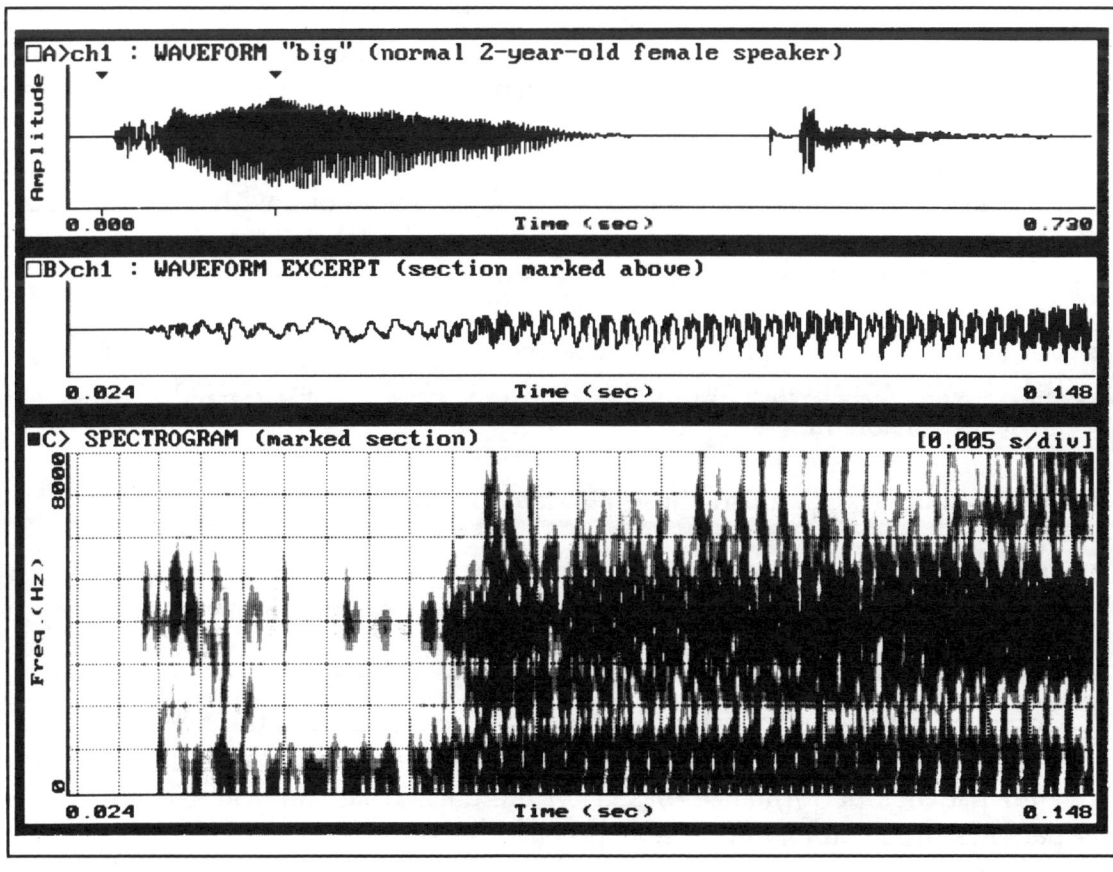

8. Repeat #7 using a normal speaker of similar age and sex. Extract the same recorded segment, and label your spectrogram as you did for your patient.

9. Compare VOTs and describe any other remarkable differences between the two spectrographic displays. (Sample spectrograms from a dysarthric and from a normal speaker are provided on the hand-in sheet.)

II. AFFRICATES

1. Obtain wide-band spectrograms of a normal speaker's production of the words "cheer" (/tʃiɚ/) and "tear" (/tiɚ/) spoken at a comfortable rate. Print these spectrograms along with their respective acoustic waveforms. (Sample spectrograms from a normal adult speaker are provided on the hand-in sheet.)

2. Label your spectrograms and identify each release burst and the onset of glottal pulsing. How do the initial consonants differ? Explain.

3. Compare these spectrograms with those of the words "jeer" (/dʒiɚ/) and "dear" (/diɚ/) as produced by the same normal speaker at approximately the same moderate rate.

4. The spectrogram on the facing page was obtained from a 62-year-old hyperkinetic dysarthric speaker. How does this patient's performance compare with the normal speaker you examined? What are the most salient abnormalities?

5. Obtain a wide-band spectrogram of a normal speaker's production of the phrases "a cheap" (/ə tʃip/) and "a jeep" (/ə dʒip/) along with their respective acoustic waveforms. (Sample spectrograms obtained from a normal adult speaker are available on the hand-in sheet.)

6. Locate and label each phone on the spectrographic record. Mark the location of the burst, frication, and the onset of voicing associated with each affricate consonant.

7. What features distinguish these affricates from each other?

8. Obtain similar spectrograms from a patient with an articulatory disorder attempting the same phrases. As before, locate and label each phone on the spectrographic record.

9. Compare the spectrograms to the ones you obtained from the normal speaker. Indicate any abnormalities associated with the release burst or frication. Assess your patient's performance. Based on the data, what can you say about your patient's articulatory timing and precision?

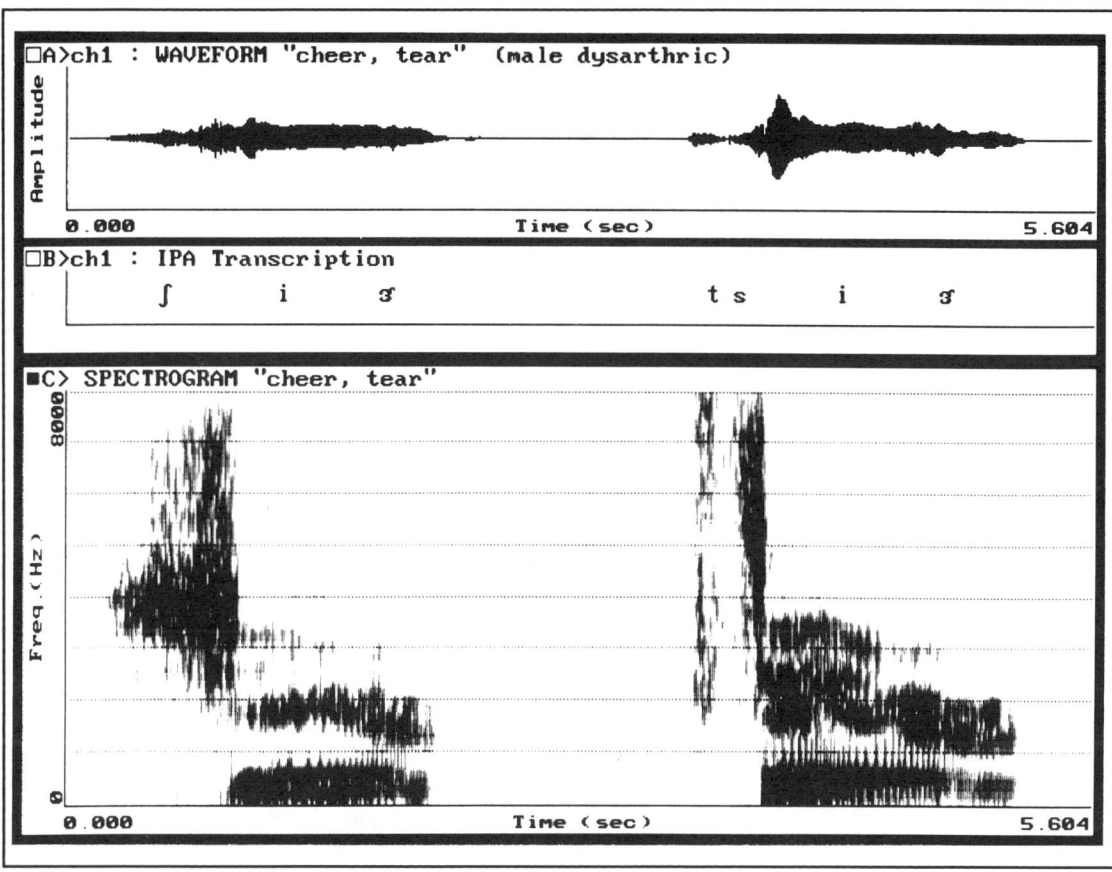

READ MORE ABOUT IT!

Agnello, J. G. (1975). Measurements and analysis of visible speech. In S. Singh (Ed.), *Measurement procedures in speech, hearing, and language* (pp. 379–397). Baltimore: University Park Press.

Allen, G. D., & Norwood, J. A. (1988). Cues for intervocalic /t/ and /d/ in children and adults. *Journal of the Acoustical Society of America, 84*, 868–875.

Baken, R. J. (1987). *Clinical measurement of speech and voice* (pp. 369–379). Boston: Little, Brown.

Baran, J. A., Laufer, M. Z., & Daniloff, R. (1977). Phonological contrastivity in conversation: A comparative study of voice onset time. *Journal of Phonetics, 5*, 339–350.

Bond, Z. S., & Wilson, H. F. (1980). Acquisition of the voicing contrast by language-delayed and normal-speaking children. *Journal of Speech and Hearing Research, 23*, 152–161.

Borden, G. J., & Harris, K. S. (1984). *Speech science primer* (2nd ed.) Baltimore: Williams & Wilkins.

Borden, G. J., Kim, D. H., & Spiegler, K. (1987). Acoustics of stop consonant-vowel relationships. *Journal of Fluency Disorders, 12*, 175–184.

Eguchi, S., & Hirsh, I. J. (1969). Development of speech sounds in children. *Acta Otolaryngologica, Suppl. 257*, 5–43.

Freeman, F. J., Sands, E. S., & Harris, K. S. (1978). Temporal coordination of phonation and articulation in a case of verbal apraxia: A voice onset time study. *Brain and Language, 6*, 106–111.

Gilbert, J. H. V. (1977). A voice onset time analysis of apical stop production in three-year-olds. *Journal of Child Language, 4*, 103–110.

Kawano, M. Honjo, I., Kojima, H., Kurata, K., Tanokuchi, F., & Kido, N. (1991). Laryngeal constriction on glottal stops in cleft palate speech. *Studia Phonologica, 25*, 7–13.

Kent, R. D. (1976). Anatomical and neuromuscular maturation of the speech mechanism: Evidence from acoustic studies. *Journal of Speech and Hearing Research, 18*, 421–447.

Kent, R. D., & Read, C. (1992). *The acoustic analysis of speech* (pp. 105–121). San Diego: Singular Publishing Group.

Klatt, D. H. (1975). Voice onset time, frication, and aspiration in word-initial consonant clusters. *Journal of Speech and Hearing Research, 18*, 686–706.

Lieberman, A. M., Harris, K. S., Hoffman, H. S., & Griffith, B. C. (1957). The discrimination of speech sound within and across phoneme boundaries. *Journal of Experimental Psychology, 54*, 358–368.

Lisker, L., & Abramson, A. S. (1964). A cross-language study of voicing in initial stops: Acoustical measurements. *Word, 20*, 384–422.

Lisker, L., & Abramson, A. S. (1967). Some effects of context on voice onset time in English. *Language and Speech, 10*, 1–28.

Macken, M. A., & Barton, D. (1980). The acquisition of the voicing contrast in English: A study of voice onset time in word-initial stop consonants. *Journal of Child Language, 7*, 41–74.

Menyuk, P., & Klatt, M. (1975). Voice onset time in consonant cluster production by children and adults. *Journal of Child Language, 2*, 223–231.

Monsen, R. B. (1976). Second formant transitions of selected consonant-vowel combinations in the speech of deaf and normal-hearing children. *Journal of Speech and Hearing Research, 19*, 279–289.

Morris, R. J. (1989). VOT and dysarthria: A descriptive study. *Journal of Communication Disorders, 22*, 23–33.

Ohde, R. N., & Sharf, D. J. (1992). *Phonetic analysis of normal and abnormal speech*. New York: Merrill.

Pickett, J. M. (1965). Some acoustic cues for synthesis of the /n-d/ distinction. *Journal of the Acoustical Society of America, 38*, 474–477.

Pickett, J. M. (1980). *The sounds of speech communication*. Austin, TX: PRO-ED.

Port, R. F., & Rotunno, R. (1979). Relation between voice-onset time and vowel duration. *Journal of the Acoustical Society of America, 66*, 654–662.

Shewan, C. M., Leeper, H. A., Jr., & Booth, J. C. (1984). An analysis of voice onset time (VOT) in aphasic and normal subjects. In J. C. Rosenbek, M. R. McNeil, & A. E. Aronson (Eds.), *Apraxia of speech: Physiology, acoustics, linguistics, management* (pp. 197–220). San Diego: Singular Publishing Group.

Sweeting, P. M., & Baken, R. J. (1982). Voice onset time in a normal-aged population. *Journal of Speech and Hearing Research, 25*, 129–134.

Weismer, G. (1979). Sensitivity of VOT measures to certain segmental features in speech production. *Journal of Phonetics, 7*, 197–204.

Weismer, G. (1984a). Acoustic descriptions of dysarthric speech: Perceptual correlates and physiological inferences. *Seminars in Speech and Language, 5*, 293–313.

Weismer, G. (1984b). Articulatory characteristics of Parkinsonian dysarthria: Segmental and phrase-level timing, spirantization, and glottal-supraglottal coordination. In M. R. McNeil, J. C. Rosenbek, & A. E. Aronson (Eds.), *The dysarthrias: Physiology, acoustics, perception, management* (pp. 101–130). San Diego: Singular Publishing Group.

Zlatin, M. A. (1974). Voicing contrast: Perceptual and productive voice onset time characteristics of adults. *Journal of the Acoustical Society of America, 56*, 981–994.

Zlatin, M. A., & Koenigsknecht, R. A. (1976). Development of the voicing contrast: A comparison of voice onset time in stop perception and production. *Journal of Speech and Hearing Research, 19*, 93–111.

Student _____   Date _____

SPECTROGRAPHY: PLOSIVES AND AFFRICATES

Attach all of your labeled spectrograms to this page.

I. PLOSIVES

Two-year-old female speaker

a. VOT for [p] in "pig": _____

b. VOT for [b] in "big": _____

Selection of burst and onset of glottal pulsing: _____

_____

_____

_____

_____

Comparison with adult speaker: _____

_____

_____

_____

_____

Student _____   Date _____

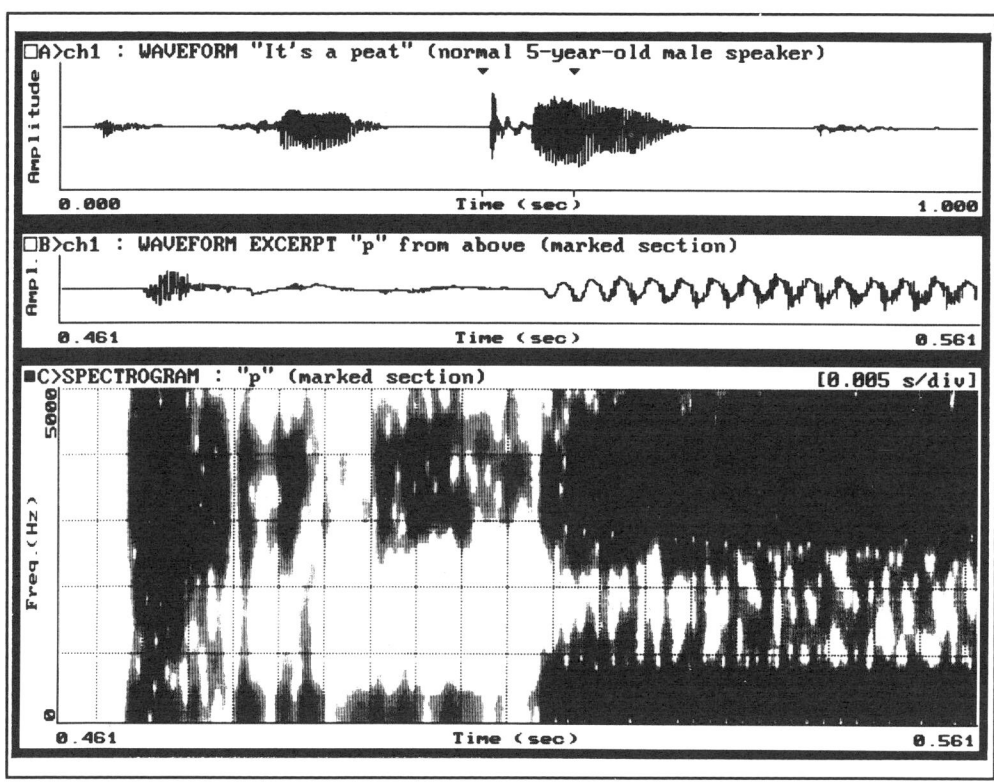

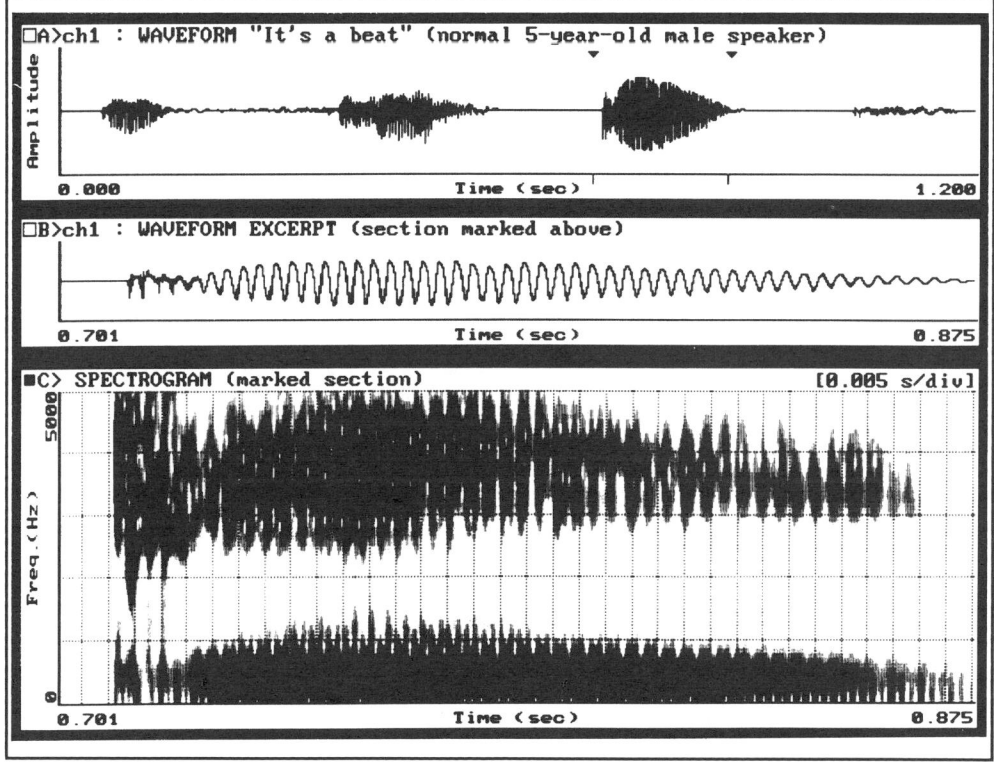

Student _____ Date _____

3. Speaker: _____

Speaker characteristics: _____

4. a. VOT for [p] in "peat": _____

VOT for [b] in "beat": _____

b. Normal? _____

_____

_____

_____

_____

_____

Source(s): _____

_____

5. Patient: _____

Patient characteristics: _____

_____

6. a. VOT for [p] in "peat": _____

VOT for [b] in "beat": _____

b. Comparison/analysis: _____

_____

_____

_____

_____

Student   Date

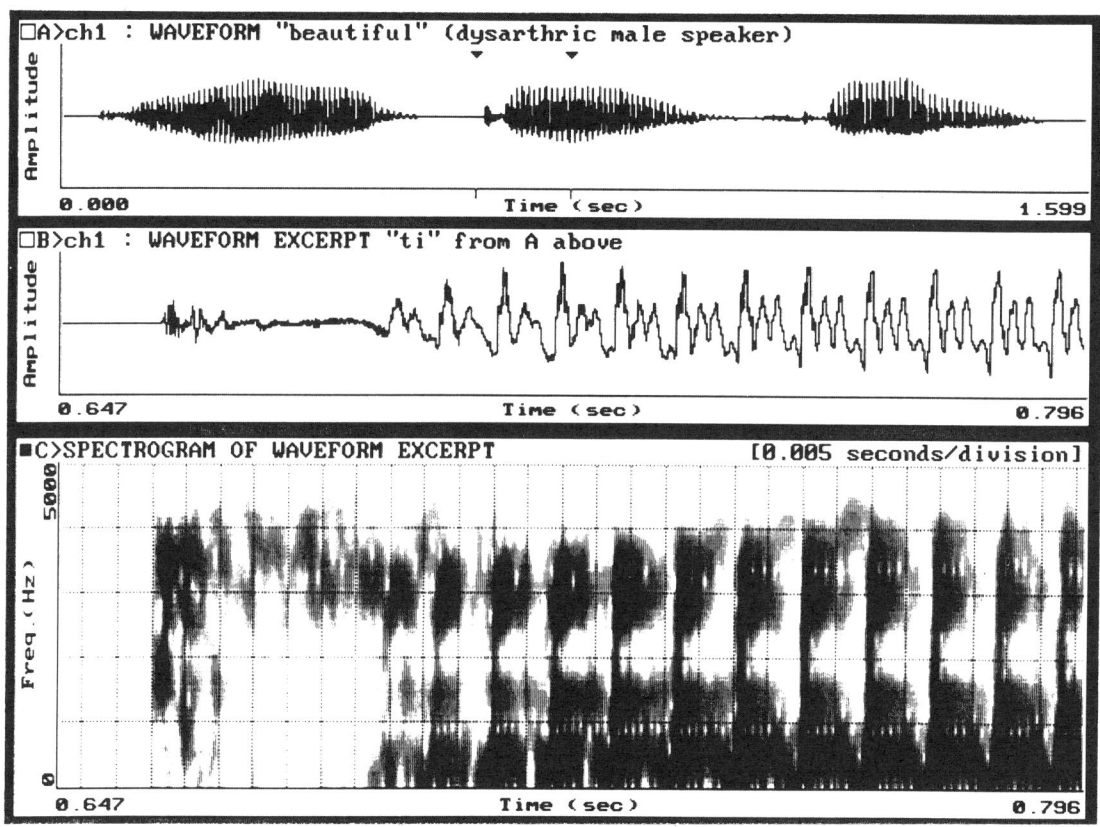

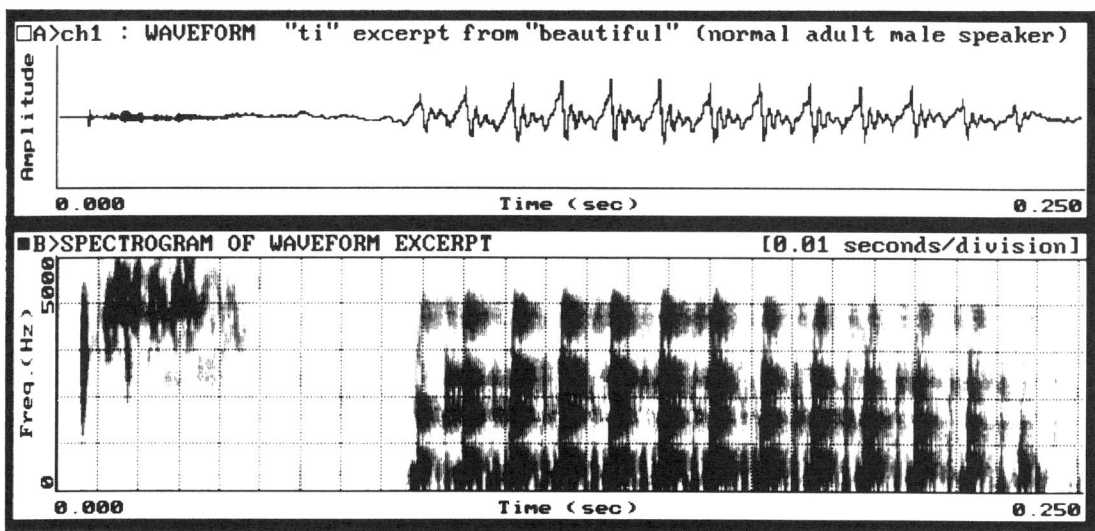

Student _____ Date _____

7. Patient: _____

   Patient characteristics: _____

   _____

   VOT for [ ] in "_____": _____

8. Normal speaker: _____

   Speaker characteristics: _____

   _____

   VOT for [ ] in "_____": _____

9. Comparison of patient with normal speaker: _____

   _____

   _____

   _____

   _____

   _____

   _____

   _____

   _____

   _____

   _____

   _____

Student   Date

II. AFFRICATES

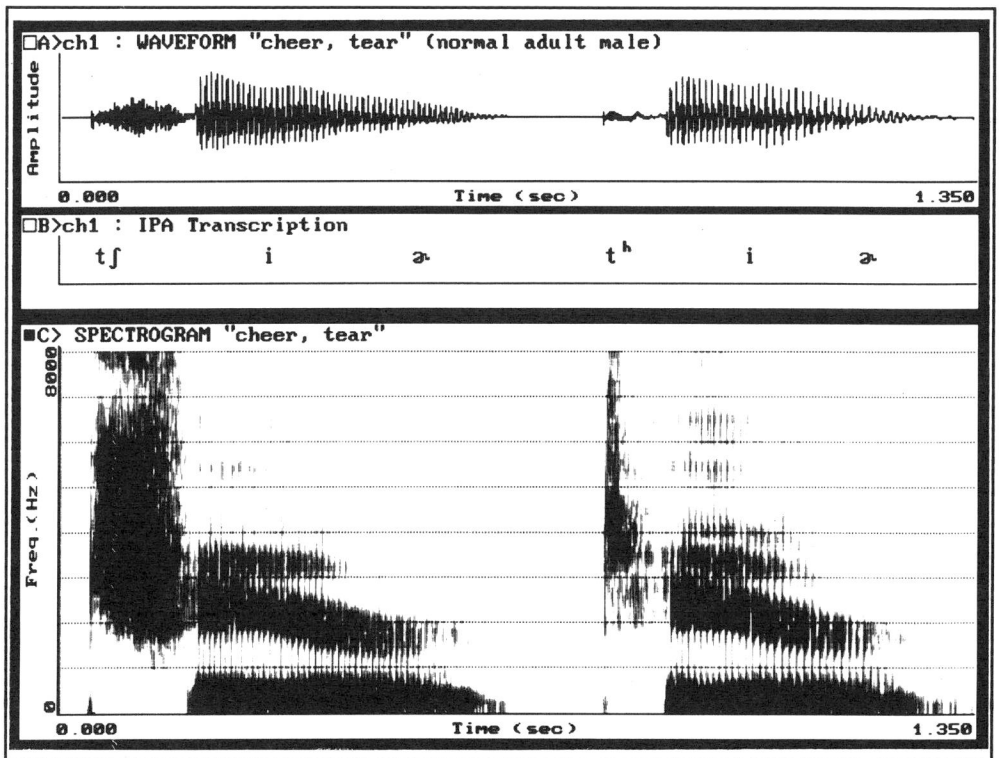

Student _____ Date _____

2. Normal speaker: _____

   Speaker characteristics: _____
   _____

   Comparison of [tʃ] and [t] in "cheer" and "tear": _____
   _____
   _____
   _____
   _____
   _____
   _____
   _____
   _____

3. Comparison of [dʒ] and [d] in "jeer" and "dear": _____
   _____
   _____
   _____
   _____
   _____
   _____
   _____
   _____
   _____

Student   Date

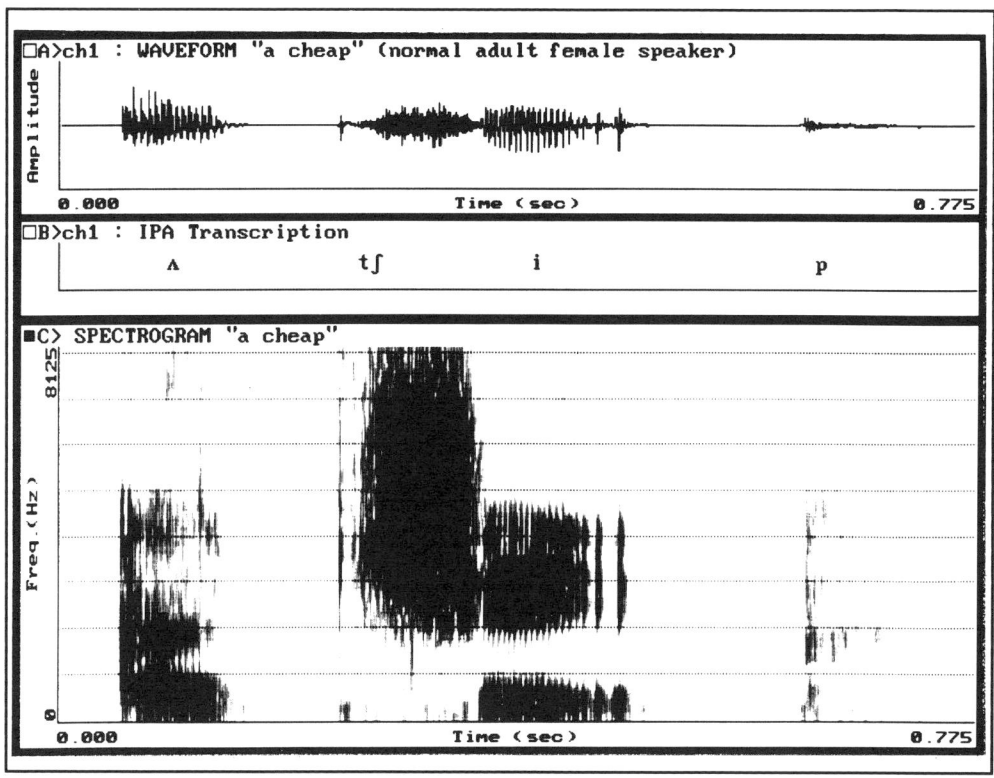

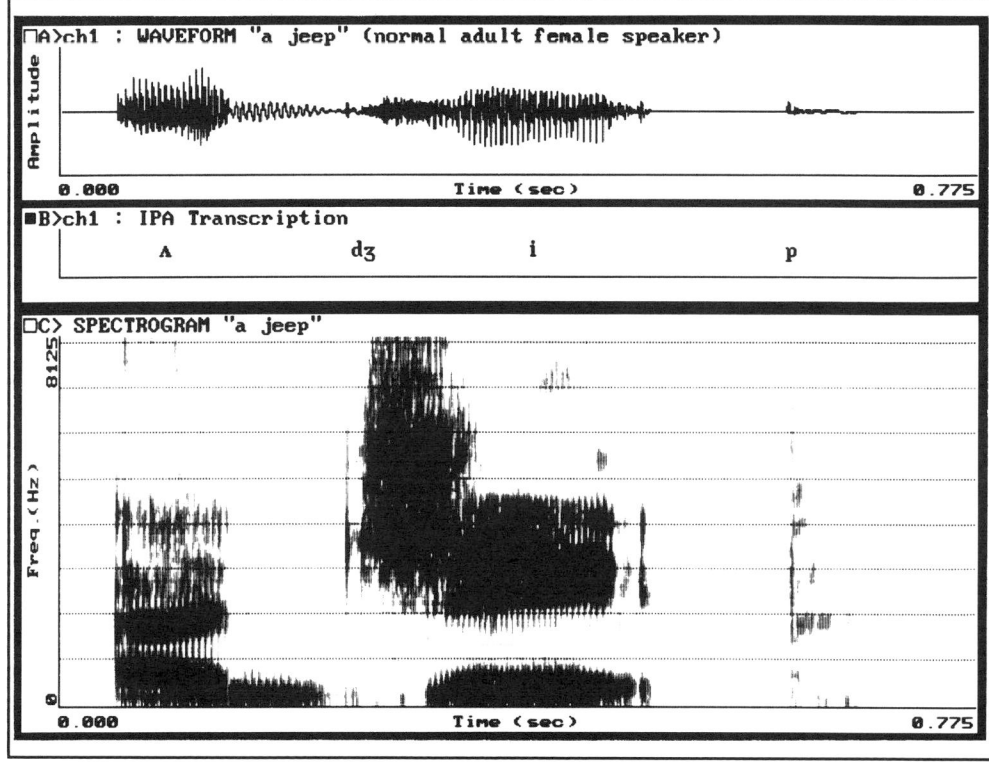

Student   Date

4. Patient: _62-year-old hyperkinetic dysarthric male_

   Patient characteristics: _Native American English speaker, congenital cerebral palsy (athetosis)_

   Comparison/Assessment: _____

   _____

   _____

   _____

   _____

   _____

   _____

   _____

   _____

5. Normal speaker: _____

   Patient characteristics: _____

   _____

7. Comparison of [tʃ] and [dʒ]: _____

   _____

   _____

   _____

   _____

   _____

   _____

Student _____ Date _____

9. Patient: _____

Patient characteristics: _____

_____

Comparison/analysis: _____

_____
_____
_____
_____
_____
_____
_____
_____
_____
_____
_____
_____
_____

APPENDIXES

APPENDIX A

Sample Vocal Tract Examination Form

Sample Examination Form

Patient _____   Date of Birth _____

Presenting Complaint _____   Date of Exam _____

_____   Examiner _____

STRUCTURE   DESCRIPTION
_____

FACE _____

_____

LIPS _____

_____

TONGUE _____

_____

HARD PALATE _____

_____

VELUM _____

_____

MANDIBLE _____

_____

OCCLUSION _____

_____

DENTITION _____

_____

OROPHARYNX _____

_____

LARYNGOPHARYNX _____

_____

NASOPHARYNX/NASAL CAVITY _____

_____

CRANIAL NERVES V and VII	Sensory function _____ _____ _____ Motor function _____ _____ _____
CRANIAL NERVES IX and X	Ingestive function _____ _____ _____ Volitional nonspeech function _____ _____ _____ Speech function _____ _____ _____
CRANIAL NERVE XI	Motor function _____ _____ _____
CRANIAL NERVE XII	Ingestive function _____ _____ _____ Volitional nonspeech function _____ _____ _____ Speech function _____ _____ _____

APPENDIX B

The Angle Classification System of Malocclusions

At the turn of the 20th century, an American dentist named Edward H. Angle (1855–1930) proposed a system that divided abnormal occlusion (or *malocclusion*) into three major classes. This classification system continues to be used in its original or in modified form. It is important to remember that the "Angle Class" system is meant to relate the orientation of the upper and lower jaws (the maxilla and mandible) and is not generally intended to describe the relationship of the upper and lower teeth. However, the position of the maxillary and mandibular first permanent molars with the jaws closed is used as a guide to the occlusal relationship.

CLASS I

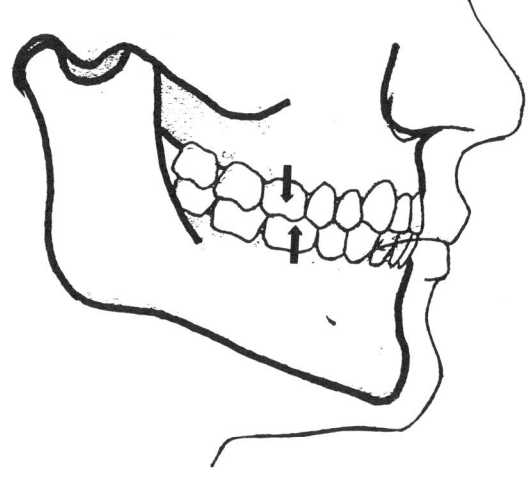

Neutrocclusion: A normal anteroposterior relationship of the upper and lower jaws. Cusps of the maxillary first molars are slightly behind those of the mandibular first molars. A class I *malocclusion* means that, although the jaw relationship is normal, the position of the anterior teeth is not.

CLASS II

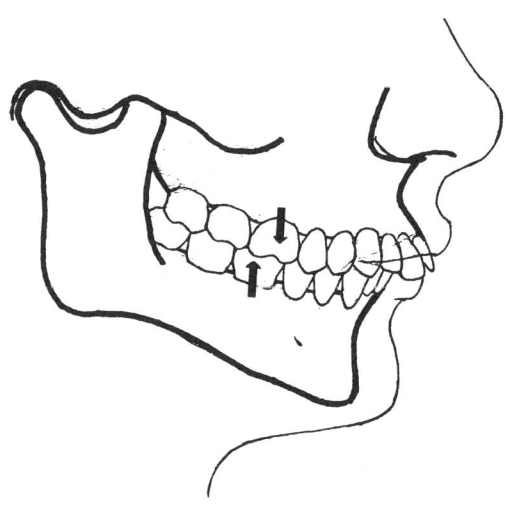

Distocclusion: A retruded (or recessed) mandible, also known as *retrognathism*. Cusps of the maxillary first molars are in front of the opposing first molars.
Division 1: Distocclusion with extreme protrusion, that is, labioversion, of the upper incisors (as shown).
Division 2: Distocclusion with extreme retrusion, that is, linguoversion, of the upper incisors.

CLASS III

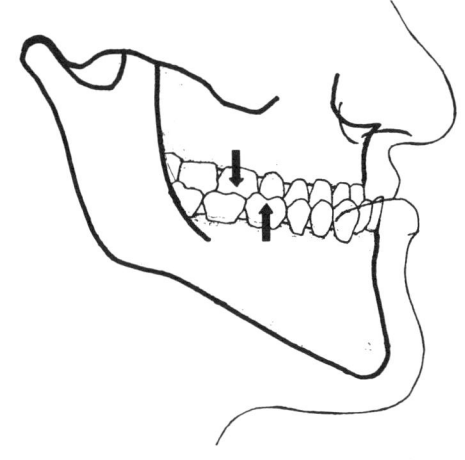

Mesiocclusion: A protruding mandible, also known as *prognathism*. Cusps of the maxillary and first molars are substantially posterior to those of the opposing mandibular first molars.

SOURCES OF INFORMATION

Angle, E. H. (1907). *Malocclusion of the teeth* (7th ed.). Philadelphia: S. S. White Dental Manufacturing Co.

Barrett, R. H., & Hanson, M. L. (1974). *Oral myofunctional disorders* (pp. 31–55). St. Louis: Mosby.

Bloomer, H. H. (1971). Speech defects associated with dental malocclusions and related abnormalities. In L. E. Travis (Ed.), *Handbook of speech pathology and audiology* (pp. 715–766). New York: Appleton-Century-Crofts.

Harvold, E. P. (1970). Speech articulation and oral morphology. *ASHA Reports, 5,* 69–75.

Hixon, E. H. (1970). Development of the facial complex. *ASHA Reports, 5,* 33–48.

Langley, L. L., & Cheraskin, E. (1956). *The physiology of dental practice.* St. Louis: Mosby.

Lischer, B. E. (1912). *Principles and methods of orthodontics.* Philadelphia: Lea and Febiger.

Saltzman, J. A. (1957). *Orthodontics: Principles and prevention.* Philadelphia: Lippincott.

Zemlin, W. R. (1988). *Speech and hearing science: Anatomy and physiology* (3rd ed., pp. 235–247). Englewood Cliffs, NJ: Prentice-Hall.

APPENDIX C

Common Logarithm Table

	.00	.01	.02	.03	.04	.05	.06	.07	.08	.09
0.0		-2.000	-1.699	-1.523	-1.398	-1.301	-1.222	-1.155	-1.097	-1.046
0.1	-1.000	-0.959	-0.921	-0.886	-0.854	-0.824	-0.796	-0.770	-0.745	-0.721
0.2	-0.699	-0.678	-0.658	-0.638	-0.620	-0.602	-0.585	-0.569	-0.553	-0.538
0.3	-0.523	-0.509	-0.495	-0.481	-0.469	-0.456	-0.444	-0.432	-0.420	-0.409
0.4	-0.398	-0.387	-0.377	-0.367	-0.357	-0.347	-0.337	-0.328	-0.319	-0.310
0.5	-0.301	-0.292	-0.284	-0.276	-0.268	-0.260	-0.252	-0.244	-0.237	-0.229
0.6	-0.222	-0.215	-0.208	-0.201	-0.194	-0.187	-0.180	-0.174	-0.167	-0.161
0.7	-0.155	-0.149	-0.143	-0.137	-0.131	-0.125	-0.119	-0.114	-0.108	-0.102
0.8	-0.097	-0.092	-0.086	-0.081	-0.076	-0.071	-0.066	-0.060	-0.056	-0.051
0.9	-0.046	-0.041	-0.036	-0.032	-0.027	-0.022	-0.018	-0.013	-0.009	-0.004
1.0	0.000	0.004	0.009	0.013	0.017	0.021	0.025	0.029	0.033	0.037
1.1	0.041	0.045	0.049	0.053	0.057	0.061	0.064	0.068	0.072	0.076
1.2	0.079	0.083	0.086	0.090	0.093	0.097	0.100	0.104	0.107	0.111
1.3	0.114	0.117	0.121	0.124	0.127	0.130	0.134	0.137	0.140	0.143
1.4	0.146	0.149	0.152	0.155	0.158	0.161	0.164	0.167	0.170	0.173
1.5	0.176	0.179	0.182	0.185	0.188	0.190	0.193	0.196	0.199	0.201
1.6	0.204	0.207	0.210	0.212	0.215	0.217	0.220	0.223	0.225	0.228
1.7	0.230	0.233	0.236	0.238	0.241	0.243	0.246	0.248	0.250	0.253
1.8	0.255	0.258	0.260	0.262	0.265	0.267	0.270	0.272	0.274	0.276
1.9	0.279	0.281	0.283	0.286	0.288	0.290	0.292	0.294	0.297	0.299
2.0	0.301	0.303	0.305	0.307	0.310	0.312	0.314	0.316	0.318	0.320
2.1	0.322	0.324	0.326	0.328	0.330	0.332	0.334	0.336	0.338	0.340
2.2	0.342	0.344	0.346	0.348	0.350	0.352	0.354	0.356	0.358	0.360
2.3	0.362	0.364	0.365	0.367	0.369	0.371	0.373	0.375	0.377	0.378
2.4	0.380	0.382	0.384	0.386	0.387	0.389	0.391	0.393	0.394	0.396
2.5	0.398	0.400	0.401	0.403	0.405	0.407	0.408	0.410	0.412	0.413
2.6	0.415	0.417	0.418	0.420	0.422	0.423	0.425	0.427	0.428	0.430
2.7	0.431	0.433	0.435	0.436	0.438	0.439	0.441	0.442	0.444	0.446
2.8	0.447	0.449	0.450	0.452	0.453	0.455	0.456	0.458	0.459	0.461
2.9	0.462	0.464	0.465	0.467	0.468	0.470	0.471	0.473	0.474	0.476
3.0	0.477	0.479	0.480	0.481	0.483	0.484	0.486	0.487	0.489	0.490
3.1	0.491	0.493	0.494	0.496	0.497	0.498	0.500	0.501	0.502	0.504
3.2	0.505	0.507	0.508	0.509	0.511	0.512	0.513	0.515	0.516	0.517
3.3	0.519	0.520	0.521	0.522	0.524	0.525	0.526	0.528	0.529	0.530
3.4	0.531	0.533	0.534	0.535	0.537	0.538	0.539	0.540	0.542	0.543
3.5	0.544	0.545	0.547	0.548	0.549	0.550	0.551	0.553	0.554	0.555
3.6	0.556	0.558	0.559	0.560	0.561	0.562	0.563	0.565	0.566	0.567
3.7	0.568	0.569	0.571	0.572	0.573	0.574	0.575	0.576	0.577	0.579
3.8	0.580	0.581	0.582	0.583	0.584	0.585	0.587	0.588	0.589	0.590
3.9	0.591	0.592	0.593	0.594	0.595	0.597	0.598	0.599	0.600	0.601
4.0	0.602	0.603	0.604	0.605	0.606	0.607	0.609	0.610	0.611	0.612
4.1	0.613	0.614	0.615	0.616	0.617	0.618	0.619	0.620	0.621	0.622
4.2	0.623	0.624	0.625	0.626	0.627	0.628	0.629	0.630	0.631	0.632
4.3	0.633	0.634	0.635	0.636	0.637	0.638	0.639	0.640	0.641	0.642
4.4	0.643	0.644	0.645	0.646	0.647	0.648	0.649	0.650	0.651	0.652
4.5	0.653	0.654	0.655	0.656	0.657	0.658	0.659	0.660	0.661	0.662
4.6	0.663	0.664	0.665	0.666	0.667	0.667	0.668	0.669	0.670	0.671
4.7	0.672	0.673	0.674	0.675	0.676	0.677	0.678	0.679	0.679	0.680
4.8	0.681	0.682	0.683	0.684	0.685	0.686	0.687	0.688	0.688	0.689
4.9	0.690	0.691	0.692	0.693	0.694	0.695	0.695	0.696	0.697	0.698

	0	1	2	3	4	5	6	7	8	9
5.0	0.699	0.700	0.701	0.702	0.702	0.703	0.704	0.705	0.706	0.707
5.1	0.708	0.708	0.709	0.710	0.711	0.712	0.713	0.713	0.714	0.715
5.2	0.716	0.717	0.718	0.719	0.719	0.720	0.721	0.722	0.723	0.723
5.3	0.724	0.725	0.726	0.727	0.728	0.728	0.729	0.730	0.731	0.732
5.4	0.732	0.733	0.734	0.735	0.736	0.736	0.737	0.738	0.739	0.740
5.5	0.740	0.741	0.742	0.743	0.744	0.744	0.745	0.746	0.747	0.747
5.6	0.748	0.749	0.750	0.751	0.751	0.752	0.753	0.754	0.754	0.755
5.7	0.756	0.757	0.757	0.758	0.759	0.760	0.760	0.761	0.762	0.763
5.8	0.763	0.764	0.765	0.766	0.766	0.767	0.768	0.769	0.769	0.760
5.9	0.771	0.772	0.772	0.773	0.774	0.775	0.775	0.776	0.777	0.777
6.0	0.778	0.779	0.780	0.780	0.781	0.782	0.782	0.783	0.784	0.785
6.1	0.785	0.786	0.787	0.787	0.788	0.789	0.790	0.790	0.791	0.792
6.2	0.792	0.793	0.794	0.794	0.795	0.796	0.797	0.797	0.798	0.799
6.3	0.799	0.800	0.801	0.801	0.802	0.803	0.803	0.804	0.805	0.806
6.4	0.806	0.807	0.808	0.808	0.809	0.810	0.810	0.811	0.812	0.812
6.5	0.813	0.814	0.814	0.815	0.816	0.816	0.817	0.818	0.818	0.819
6.6	0.820	0.820	0.821	0.822	0.822	0.823	0.823	0.824	0.825	0.825
6.7	0.826	0.827	0.827	0.828	0.829	0.829	0.830	0.831	0.831	0.832
6.8	0.833	0.833	0.834	0.834	0.835	0.836	0.836	0.837	0.838	0.838
6.9	0.839	0.839	0.840	0.841	0.841	0.842	0.843	0.843	0.844	0.844
7.0	0.845	0.846	0.846	0.847	0.848	0.848	0.849	0.849	0.850	0.851
7.1	0.851	0.852	0.852	0.853	0.854	0.854	0.855	0.856	0.856	0.857
7.2	0.857	0.858	0.859	0.859	0.860	0.860	0.861	0.862	0.862	0.863
7.3	0.863	0.864	0.865	0.865	0.866	0.866	0.867	0.867	0.868	0.869
7.4	0.869	0.870	0.870	0.871	0.872	0.872	0.873	0.873	0.874	0.874
7.5	0.875	0.876	0.876	0.877	0.877	0.878	0.879	0.879	0.880	0.880
7.6	0.881	0.881	0.882	0.883	0.883	0.884	0.884	0.885	0.885	0.886
7.7	0.886	0.887	0.888	0.888	0.889	0.889	0.890	0.890	0.891	0.892
7.8	0.892	0.893	0.893	0.894	0.894	0.895	0.895	0.896	0.897	0.897
7.9	0.898	0.898	0.899	0.899	0.900	0.900	0.901	0.901	0.902	0.903
8.0	0.903	0.904	0.904	0.905	0.905	0.906	0.906	0.907	0.907	0.908
8.1	0.908	0.909	0.910	0.910	0.911	0.911	0.912	0.912	0.913	0.913
8.2	0.914	0.914	0.915	0.915	0.916	0.916	0.917	0.918	0.918	0.919
8.3	0.919	0.920	0.920	0.921	0.921	0.922	0.922	0.923	0.923	0.924
8.4	0.924	0.925	0.925	0.926	0.926	0.927	0.927	0.928	0.928	0.929
8.5	0.929	0.930	0.930	0.931	0.931	0.932	0.932	0.933	0.933	0.934
8.6	0.934	0.935	0.936	0.936	0.937	0.937	0.938	0.938	0.939	0.939
8.7	0.940	0.940	0.941	0.941	0.942	0.942	0.943	0.943	0.943	0.944
8.8	0.944	0.945	0.945	0.946	0.946	0.947	0.947	0.948	0.948	0.949
8.9	0.949	0.950	0.950	0.951	0.951	0.952	0.952	0.953	0.953	0.954
9.0	0.954	0.955	0.955	0.956	0.956	0.957	0.957	0.958	0.958	0.959
9.1	0.959	0.960	0.960	0.960	0.961	0.961	0.962	0.962	0.963	0.963
9.2	0.964	0.964	0.965	0.965	0.966	0.966	0.967	0.967	0.968	0.968
9.3	0.968	0.969	0.969	0.970	0.970	0.971	0.971	0.972	0.972	0.973
9.4	0.973	0.974	0.974	0.975	0.975	0.975	0.976	0.976	0.977	0.977
9.5	0.978	0.978	0.979	0.979	0.980	0.980	0.980	0.981	0.981	0.982
9.6	0.982	0.983	0.983	0.984	0.984	0.985	0.985	0.985	0.986	0.986
9.7	0.987	0.987	0.988	0.988	0.989	0.989	0.989	0.990	0.990	0.991
9.8	0.991	0.992	0.992	0.993	0.993	0.993	0.994	0.994	0.995	0.995
9.9	0.996	0.996	0.997	0.997	0.997	0.998	0.998	0.999	0.999	1.000

APPENDIX D

Standard Reading Passage: The Rainbow

THE RAINBOW PASSAGE*

	Cumulative Word Count
When the sunlight strikes the raindrops in the air, they act	10
like a prism and form a rainbow. The rainbow is	20
a division of white light into many beautiful colors. These	30
take the shape of a long round arch, with its	40
path high above, and its two ends apparently beyond the	50
horizon. There is, according to legend, a boiling pot of	60
gold at one end. People look, but no one ever	70
finds it. When a man looks for something beyond his	80
reach, his friends say he is looking for the pot	90
of gold at the end of the rainbow.	98
Throughout the centuries men have explained the rainbow in various	108
ways. Some have accepted it as a miracle without physical	118
explanation. To the Hebrews it was a token that there	128
would be no more universal floods. The Greeks used to	138
imagine that it was a sign from the gods to	148
foretell war or heavy rain. The Norsemen considered the rainbow	158
as a bridge over which the gods passed from earth	168
to their home in the sky. Other men have tried	178
to explain the phenomenon physically. Aristotle thought that the rainbow	188
was caused by the reflection of the sun's rays by the	198
rain. Since then physicists have found that it is not	208
reflection, but refraction by the raindrops which causes the rainbow.	218
Many complicated ideas about the rainbow have been formed. The	228
difference in the rainbow depends considerably upon the size of	238
the water drops, and the width of the colored band	248
increases as the size of the drops increases. The actual	258
primary rainbow observed is said to be the effect of	268
superposition of a number of bows. If the red of	278
the second bow falls upon the green of the first,	288
the result is to give a bow with an abnormally	298
wide yellow band, since red and green lights when mixed	308
form yellow. This is a very common type of bow,	318
one showing mainly red and yellow, with little or no	328
green or blue.	331

* Source: Fairbanks, G. (1960). *Voice and articulation drillbook* (2nd ed.). New York: Harper and Bros., p. 127. [Used with permission.]

APPENDIX

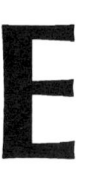

Mathematical Definitions of Vocal Jitter Measures

Calculation of mean absolute jitter*:

$$J_{abs} = \frac{1}{n-1}\left[\sum_{i=1}^{n-1}|t_i - t_{i+1}|\right]$$

Calculation of mean percent jitter*:

$$J(\%) = \frac{\frac{1}{n-1}\left[\sum_{i=1}^{n-1}|t_i - t_{i+1}|\right]}{\frac{1}{n}\sum_{i=1}^{n}t_i} \times 100$$

Calculation of jitter factor**:

$$JF = \frac{\frac{1}{n-1}\left[\sum_{i=1}^{n-1}|F_{0_i} - F_{0_{i+1}}|\right]}{\frac{1}{n}\sum_{i=1}^{n}F_{0_i}} \times 100$$

---

* Where t_i equals the period of the ith cycle and n equals the number of periods (cycles) in the sample.

** Where F_{0_i} equals the fundamental frequency of the ith cycle and n equals the number of cycles in the sample.

Calculation of relative average perturbation*:

$$\text{RAP}(\%) = \frac{\dfrac{1}{n-2}\left[\displaystyle\sum_{i=2}^{n-1}\left|\dfrac{t_{i-1} + t_i + t_{i+1}}{3} - t_i\right|\right]}{\dfrac{1}{n}\displaystyle\sum_{i=1}^{n} t_i} \times 100$$

Calculation of frequency perturbation quotient (5-point)*:

$$\text{FPQ}(\%) = \frac{\dfrac{1}{n-4}\left[\displaystyle\sum_{i=3}^{n-1}\left|\dfrac{t_{i-2} + t_{i-1} + t_i + t_{i+1} + t_{i+2}}{5} - t_i\right|\right]}{\dfrac{1}{n}\displaystyle\sum_{i=1}^{n} t_i} \times 100$$

NOTE: This measure is sometimes called the pitch perturbation quotient (PPQ). Greater than 5-point averaging is also possible.

---

*Where t_i equals the period of the ith cycle and n equals the number of periods (cycles) in the sample.

APPENDIX

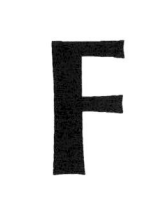

Mathematical Definitions of Vocal Shimmer Measures

Calculation of mean percent shimmer*:

$$\text{Shimmer (\%)} = \frac{\frac{1}{n-1}\left[\sum_{i=1}^{n-1} |A_i - A_{i+1}|\right]}{\frac{1}{n}\sum_{i=1}^{n} A_i} \times 100$$

Calculation of mean shimmer in decibels*:

$$\text{Shimmer (dB)} = \frac{\sum_{i=1}^{n-1} |20 \times \log(A_i/A_{i+1})|}{n-1}$$

Calculation of amplitude perturbation quotient (APQ)*:

$$\text{APQ (\%)} = \frac{\frac{1}{n-10}\left[\sum_{i=6}^{n-5}\left|\frac{A_{i-5} + A_{i-4} + \ldots + A_i + \ldots + A_{i+4} + A_{i+5}}{11} - A_i\right|\right]}{\frac{1}{n}\sum_{i=1}^{n} A_i} \times 100$$

---

*Where A_i equals the amplitude of the ith cycle and n equals the number of amplitude data (cycles) in the sample.

APPENDIX G

Predicted Normal Forced Vital Capacity (FVC)

[Note: Age in years, height in centimeters]

WOMEN

FVC in mL = [21.78 − (0.101 × Age)] × Height

MEN

FVC in mL = [27.63 − (0.112 × Age)] × Height

CHILDREN

	HEIGHT RANGE	FORMULA
Girls	98–113	FVC = (27.8 × Height) − 1900
	118–138	FVC = (32.2 × Height) − 2400
	143–163	FVC = (43.2 × Height) − 3970
	168–173	FVC = (26.5 × Height) − 1200
Boys	98–118	FVC = (27.4 × Height) − 1770
	123–148	FVC = (40.0 × Height) − 3330
	153–173	FVC = (63.0 × Height) − 6730
	178–188	FVC = (30.0 × Height) − 1050

APPENDIX H

Low-Flow Reading Passage

MARVIN WILLIAMS

Marvin Williams is only nine. Marvin lives with his mother on Monroe Avenue in Vernon Valley. Marvin loves all movies, even eerie ones with evil villains in them. Whenever a new movie is in the area, Marvin is usually an early arrival. Nearly every evening Marvin is in row one along the aisle.

APPENDIX

High-Flow Reading Passage

HARRISON COOK

Just fifteen minutes ago, I had a fairly respected person visit my toy store on Cherry Blossom Street. Called Harrison Cook, he is a highly influential official in this town. His daughter Christine is a student at the local university. My son says that she is perhaps the prettiest teenager in the whole country. Why such a successful fellow would come to my humble shop is still a mystery.